Metabolic Complications of Acute Arterial Occlusions and Related Conditions (Myonephropathic-Metabolic Syndrome)

by
Henry Haimovici, M.D., F.A.C.S.

Clinical Professor Emeritus of Surgery
Albert Einstein College of Medicine
Bronx, New York

Chief Emeritus Vascular Surgery
Montefiore Medical Center
Bronx, New York

Foreign Corresponding Member
French National Academy of Medicine
Paris, France

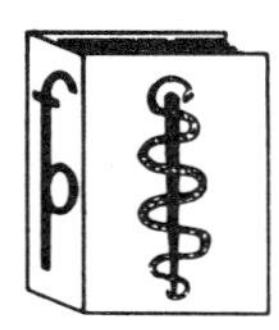

Futura Publishing Company, Inc.
Mount Kisco, New York
1988

Library of Congress Cataloging-in-Publication Data

Haimovici, Henry, 1907–
Metabolic complications of acute arterial occlusions and related conditions: myonephropathic-metabolic syndrome / by Henry Haimovici.
p. cm.
Dedicated to Walter Bradford Cannon.
Bibliography: p.
Includes index.
ISBN 0-87993-324-0
1. Rhabdomyolysis. 2. Arterial occlusions—Complications and sequelae. I. Cannon, Walter B. (Walter Bradford), 1871–1945. II. Title.
[DNLM: 1. Acute Disease. 2. Arterial Occlusive Diseases—complications. 3. Embolism—complications. 4. Leg—blood supply. 5. Rhabdomyolysis—etiology. WG 510 H151m]
RC935.R45H35 1988
616.1′35—dc19
DNLM/DLC 87-36477
for Library of Congress CIP

Published by
Futura Publishing Company, Inc.
295 Main Street, P.O. Box 330
Mount Kisco, New York 10549

L.C. no.: 87-36477
ISBN no.: 087993-324-0

Printed in the United States of America.

Dedicated with Admiration and Reverence
to
Walter Bradford Cannon

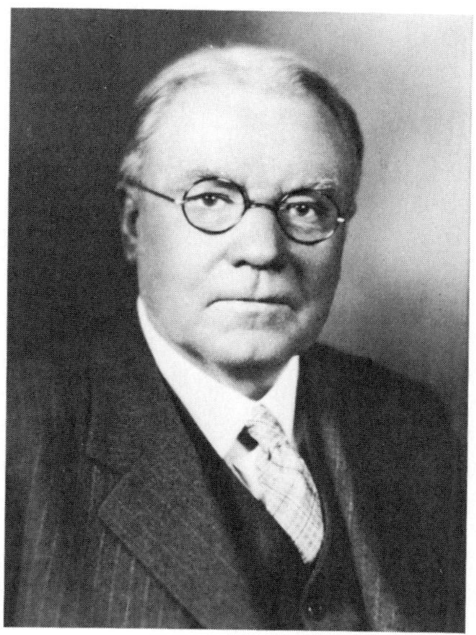

This dedication is most fitting as the central topic of this monograph deals with the effects of acute ischemia of skeletal muscle, a subject for which Cannon pioneered during World War I by elucidating many biologic facets of skeletal muscle-induced ischemic injury.

But Cannon's fame, which is worldwide, is reflected by an uninterrupted flow of enduring and pioneering contributions during his life-long activities starting with the first application of X-rays (1896) in physiology when still a medical student and ending his scientific achievements with the "Law of Denervation," related to the supersensitivity of denervated structures.

Of the many pioneering contributions, the discovery of sympathin E and I had a lasting impact which led to the origin of alpha- and beta-adrenergic blockers, drugs of invaluable clinical applications today.

This succinct dedication would be incomplete without one word about his gentleness as a human being which was only matched by his greatness as an incomparable man of science, whose legacy represents landmarks in the history of physiology.

This monograph is dedicated
with love to my wife
Nelicia

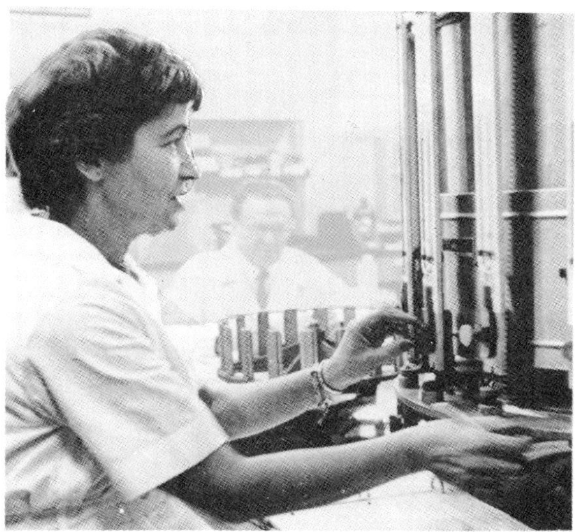

Dr. Maier* Checking Enzyme Action

whose perseverance in urging me to write this book led to its completion. This achievement is largely due to her. As a biochemist herself, who in 1954 initiated the pioneering investigations of the role of enzymes in the metabolism of the arterial wall in atherogenesis, she also took a keen interest and encouraged me in the present studies of the metabolism of the ischemic skeletal muscle in acute arterial occlusions, the subject of this monograph.

---

*Her professional name.

Preamble

Nature is nowhere wont to reveal her innermost secrets more openly than where she shows faint traces of herself away from the beaten track. Nor is there any surer route to the proper practice of medicine than if someone gives his mind over to discerning the customary law of Nature through the careful investigation of diseases that are of rare occurrence.

(William Harvey, 24 April 1657).*

My interest in this problem dates back to 1959 when I first came across unusual clinical and metabolic complications associated with an acute embolic occlusion of the lower extremity. The extreme severity of the clinicopathologic features of this first case had a particular impact on the then prevailing overall more simplistic concept of an acute ischemia. Indeed, up to that point, largely due to unawareness of such complications, the important role of the ischemic skeletal muscle received only scant attention, if any, in the literature. By uncovering critical biochemical elements mostly released from the ischemic muscular fibers, a new understanding of the cause and nature of the metabolic complications became evident. These clinicopathologic and metabolic facets, formerly unsuspected, thus added *a new dimension to the problem of any acute arterial occlusion that may affect striated muscles.*

To impart to the readers the new vision of this problem, both fascinating and potentially catastrophic, I thought that it might be useful to share with them my first experience, typical of what was to unfold later in ever increasing numbers. By so doing, this approach may also serve at the same time as a graphic introduction to this subject.

*From a letter written by Harvey 7 weeks before his death to a little-known correspondent, included in *The Life of William Harvey* by Geoffrey Keynes, Oxford University Press, 1968, p. 369.

Accordingly, the following is an abbreviated version of the first case which happened to include all the clinical, pathological and metabolic highlights characteristic of this syndrome.

> A 64-year-old white man, *one hour* after a "pull-through" resection of the rectum performed for an adenocarcinoma, complained of severe pain in the right lower extremity. Shortly thereafter,physical examination revealed: (a) coldness of the entire extremity; (b) pronounced waxy pallor of the foot and leg and cyanotic mottling of the thigh; (c) anesthesia to pinprick up to the groin; (d) complete absence of motion of the toes, ankle, and knee; (e) marked stiffness of all these joints; (f) absence of all pulses, including that of the external iliac; (g) presence of all pulses in the left lower and both upper extremities; and (h) blood pressure of 120/80 mmHg. The diagnosis of acute occlusion, possibly embolic, of the right common iliac artery was apparent.
>
> At operation, the right common iliac artery appeared to be slightly dilated and pulseless. A whitish red, firm thrombus was easily extruded, together with some atheromatous material, from this artery. The common, superficial, and deep femoral arteries were also occluded, necessitating distal thrombectomy. At the completion of the procedure, the temperature and color of the limb improved. It is noteworthy that the stiffness of the toes, ankle, and knee persisted despite the anesthesia. During this procedure, the patient received four units of whole blood.
>
> The next day the entire right lower extremity became massively swollen, the edema being extremely hard and nonpitting. As a result, the diagnosis of superimposed venous occlusion was entertained. The foot was cold and mottled although the femoral pulse could easily be felt through the dressing.
>
> In the first 12 hours following operation, the patient's urinary output consisted of 240 cc of cherry red urine, and shortly thereafter ranged from 30 to 60 cc per 24 hours. Electrophoresis demonstrated the urinary pigment to be metmyoglobin.
>
> A few days later, using starch gel electrophoresis, the urinary pigment was identified again as myoglobin. There was a benzidine-positive band with characteristic mobility of myoglobin in the urine, and serum haptoglobin bands were those of type 2-1 or 2-2 and were not saturated by 120 mg/100 cc of hemoglobin. This was considered to indicate that significant hemolysis had not occurred in the recent past.

On the third postoperative day, early gangrene of the right foot and entire leg became apparent, with the femoral pulse still being palpable. Edema of the right thigh had subsided considerably.

The renal shutdown was complete and the blood urea nitrogen (BUN) level kept rising steadily. Sodium exchange resins were administered and over the next four days the potassium level was brought down from 7.3 to 4.5 mEq per liter.

On the tenth postoperative day, with a BUN level of 280 mg/100 cc, the general condition was deteriorating; blood pressure started to fall and reached the level of 60/40 mmHg. Extracorporeal dialysis was attempted as a last resort without any beneficial effect, and the patient died shortly afterward.

In postmortem, the heart failed to display evidence of myocardial infarction or intracardiac thrombosis. The aorta displayed several areas of atheromatous plaques, some of which were ulcerated and had a superimposed thrombus which may have been the source of the embolus. The right iliac, common, and superficial femoral arteries down to Hunter's canal were patent. Dissection of the inferior vena cava, the iliac, femoral, and tibial veins failed to reveal any thrombotic occlusion. The gastrocnemius appeared soft and necrotic while the quadriceps femoris had a normal appearance. Histologic examination of the kidney revealed typical tubular necrosis. Microscopic study of the quadriceps femoris and the gastrocnemius showed foci loss of striation and of sarcolemmal nuclei of muscular fibers. There was no evidence of regeneration. Several muscular vessels exhibited fresh thrombi within their lumina.

The first exposure to a most severe case of acute arterial occlusion was associated with a complex picture of myopathy, renal shutdown, and metabolic events. The most striking features were: (1) *extreme suddenness* of the clinical onset; (2) *excruciating pain* of the entire extremity requiring parenteral morphine administration around the clock; (3) *rigidity* of the entire limb, involving contracture of the calf muscles and frozen joints, preventing any motion of any part of the involved musculoskeletal complex; (4) *myoglobinuria* associated with rapidly progressive anuria leading to complete renal shutdown; (5) *metabolic acidosis,* hyperkalemia, hyperazotemia among the major disturbances; (6) *acute renal tubular necrosis;* (7) *rhabdomyolysis;* and (8) *fatal outcome* in a short time.

From the subsequent publications appearing worldwide in increasing numbers of similar instances, it became evident that we were undoubtedly dealing with a potentially serious aspect of acute arterial occlusions which were up to then unrecognized. Furthermore, as time went on and as a result of expanding experience, it became obvious that the metabolic repercussions were essentially related to skeletal muscle ischemia. The latter then assumed a central role in the development of the metabolic syndrome and finally dominated the outcome of the acute arterial occlusions.*

*Haimovici H: Arterial embolism with acute massive ischemic myopathy and myoglobinuria: Evaluation of a hitherto unreported syndrome with report of two cases. *Surgery* 47:739, 1960.

Preface

The biologic responses of skeletal muscle to acute ischemia have been receiving only recently some detailed biochemical evaluation. Their significance, especially in acute arterial occlusions, has assumed greater importance in the context of the overall metabolic syndrome.

As stated in the Preamble, the present study was conceived to correlate the multiple aspects of muscular, renal, and biochemical repercussions associated with sudden arterial interruptions. Although the initial scope of this monograph was to focus on the responses of the latter involving the extremities, subsequent research into this problem proved to be much more extensive and complex than originally anticipated.

Indeed, as the research of the wider spectrum of vascular lesions expanded, it appeared to involve many other areas from which three important facts emerged: (1) the existence of a great variety of acute vascular entities, other than thromboembolic, that are displaying similar complications related essentially to the skeletal muscles; (2) the nature of most complications remained often unrecognized and consequently attributed to other cardiovascular-renal causes; and (3) numerous nonsurgical and medical conditions, exclusive of trauma or arterial occlusions, exhibited similar clinical features, albeit with some significant differences.

One of the often-stressed factors in this wide spectrum of entities, myoglobin, appeared to represent their common denominator. This biochemical marker, however, failed often to provide uniformity in all cases. Indeed, the myoglobin leakage from the muscle appeared to vary in intensity, duration, degree of damage, and ultimate prognosis of the clinical entity.

Regardless of whether myoglobinemia and myoglobinuria were implicated almost exclusively in all the above entities as a cause for the observed complications, their origin—the skeletal muscle ischemia—received little or inadequately deserved attention as the main source of the biochemical findings. Thus, in most publications myoglobin remains the central, if not the unique, pathogenic factor. Two classic monographs testify to the importance attributed to myoglobin: the first was by Biörk (1949) and the second by Kagen (1973). While myoglobin's significance received its due emphasis, the real culprit, however, is above all the skeletal muscle ischemia or rhabdomyolysis.

This study is, therefore, being designed to stress, besides myoglobin, the central role of ischemic skeletal muscle in terms of the clinical, biochemical, pathological, and therapeutic aspects across the entire spectrum of the various entities. To this end, some basic scientific information was reviewed in relation to the skeletal muscles. This appeared necessary for a better comprehension of our present knowledge of the clinical and therapeutic aspects of the acute rhabdomyolysis of the extremities, its metabolic complications, and their treatment.

This monograph deals with, besides the basic data concerning the normal and pathological morphology and biochemistry of the muscular tissue, the clinical entities of the peripheral arterial occlusive problems and a host of conditions ranging from temporary ischemia secondary to aortic clamping to hyperthermic myoglobinuria, thus covering a total of 28 chapters.

This preface, in brief, wishes to emphasize the significance of a subject whose awareness has received inadequate attention in the medical literature. The facts presented in this monograph hope to fill a gap. Indeed, these data have shown that skeletal muscles play a fundamental role in the above conditions and represent a source of disastrous complications in ischemic situations. Although the muscles constitute 40% of the entire body weight, it is significant to point out that 76% of the lower extremity includes striated muscles which, as emphasized, are highly vulnerable to acute ischemic factors. Metabolic complications emerging from the latter level, caused by the arterial pathology or other allied factors, may indeed contribute the largest percentage of noxious biochemical elements responsible for both limb- and life-threatening situations.

Recently, to the foregoing initial ischemic rhabdomyolysis, a new aspect of metabolic response of skeletal muscle to ischemia has been demonstrated as a result of superoxide free radicals.

Superimposed ischemia during the reperfusion of ischemic rhabdomyolytic muscle may paradoxically further aggravate the local prognosis. To counteract this new ischemic phase, newer agents, free-radical scavengers, given just prior to reperfusion are proving helpful in preventing such complications in myocardial lesions. These new agents may also provide a new dimension in the therapy of necrosis-inducing biochemicals of skeletal muscle. This study is still at its threshold and must await further results.

Finally, it should be pointed out that the incidence of acute rhabdomyolysis and its often deadly metabolic syndrome can be reduced or prevented by awareness of its potential occurrence. Alertness will help in its detection and timely management.

Acknowledgments

A monograph of this nature dealing with basic knowledge of morphology and biochemistry of the skeletal muscle as a basis for the understanding of the clinicopathologic entities, the subject of this monograph, necessitated fundamental information of the complex nature of the skeletal muscle. To this end, I consulted a number of books and articles related to the subject. Of these, I wish to mention specifically *Skeletal Muscle,* edited by Lee D. Peachey, Richard H. Adrian, and Stephen R. Geiger, published by the American Physiological Society, and two volumes published by the New York Academy of Sciences, one on *Muscular Dystrophy and Other Inherited Diseases of Skeletal Muscle in Animals,* published in 1979, and the other on *Transport ATPases,* published in 1982. To the authors of these books I wish to express my indebtedness for the information I gleaned from their articles, indicated in the bibliography.

For the gracious cooperation provided me by Mr. Korn and M. Strauss, of Futura Publishing Company, I wish to express my grateful appreciation. Special thanks go to Ms. Linda Shaw, the Production Editor, for sharing with me my constant concern for achieving high standards of printing and editing.

My appreciation goes also to Ms. Elizabeth Caputo, my secretary, for her skill in typing the manuscript.

Henry Haimovici, M.D.

Contents

I

Basic Considerations

1

Morphology of Skeletal Muscle

Introduction

The skeletal muscle is a tissue that incorporates a multitude of biochemical substances in its structural complex.[215] Being highly vulnerable to anoxia, the muscle may respond by releasing into the circulation some or most of these biochemicals which may be highly harmful or even fatal to the patient. These biochemicals are precisely responsible for the metabolic repercussions of the acute ischemic muscle entities.[113]

Before undertaking the study of the clinicopathological aspects of this complex syndrome, for which I coined the term *myonephropathic-metabolic syndrome*, knowledge of a clear understanding of the *normal* morphology and *normal* biochemistry of the skeletal muscle fiber is indispensable.

Accordingly, a brief section of the basic information concerning (1) the morphologic elements of the muscle fiber (Chapter 1), and (2) its biochemical components (Chapter 2) will be described as they may relate more specifically to this syndrome.

They should serve as a biologic opening window on the clinico-pathological aspects dealt with in this monograph.

Morphological Components

Fibers

The fibers are the smallest independent cellular units of the muslce. They are cylindrical, multinucleate, cellular structures that vary greatly in length. A common average length for a fiber in man is 3 cm, but lengths of 4 cm or more are not uncommon, and the shortest fibers in small muscles are less than 1 mm in length. The diameters of fibers vary from 10 to 100 micromillimeters, so that, in many cases, the fibers are visible to the naked eye.

Usually 10 to 20 fibers are grouped into bundles called fascicles (Figure 1-1). Each fascicle is surrounded by the perimysium, which is a thick connective tissue. Each individual muscle fiber included in the fascicle is surrounded by an endomysium which is a delicate connective tissue originating from the perimysium. In each endomysium, blood vessels and nerves are present, although they are not always easy to identify except under scanning electron microscopy (SEM).

Seen under SEM, the endomysium shows that the surface of a muscle fiber is composed of three parts: the endomysial fibrous network, the basal lamina, and the plasmalemma or sarcolemma. These components form a complex that is not easily separated mechanically.

The thinner filaments appear to intermingle with collagen fibrils. The basal lamina, or basement membrane, represents the outer aspect of the covering of the muscle fiber.

Sarcolemma

The sarcolemma first was observed as a separate structural entity in early light microscopic studies of muscle. The sarcolemma of a muscle fiber is especially apparent in the light microscope when the fibers are damaged so that a retraction of the contractile and other internal structures of the fiber occurs, leaving an empty sarcolemmal tube.

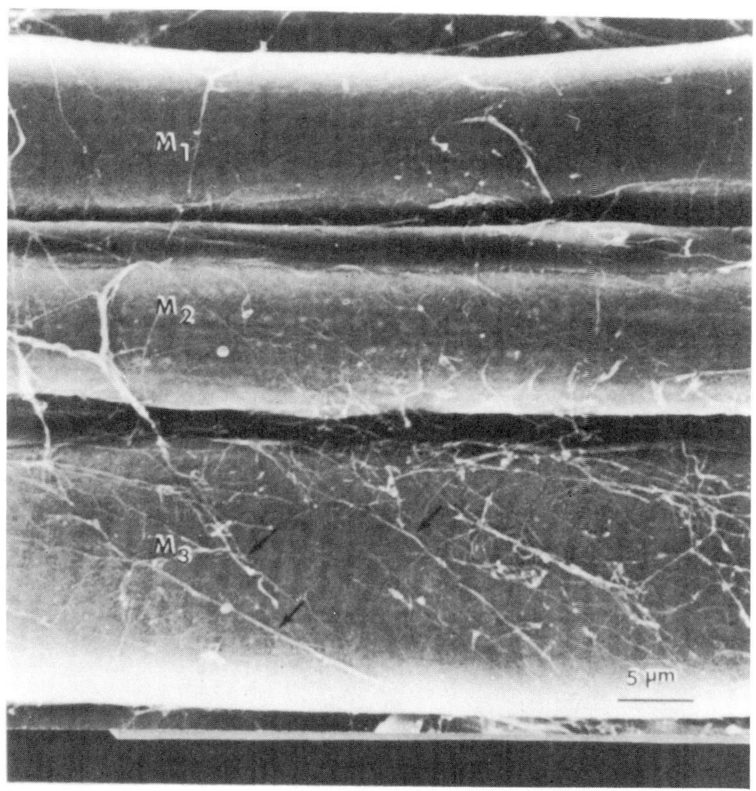

FIGURE 1–1: Skeletal muscle fibers appear as cylindrical units aligned in parallel bundles. Faint cross-striations are visible along individual fibers. Coarse collagenous fibers of the endomysium run in various directions over and between muscle fibers (arrows). (Used with permission from Peachey LD, et al: *Skeletal Muscle*, American Physiological Society, Bethesda, Maryland, 1983, p 2.[214])

As seen in SEM specimens, the basal lamina can never be stripped from the sarcolemma. This reflects the tight connection between the two structures. On rare occasions the true inner surfaces are seen where patches of the sarcolemma are peeled and reflected during tissue teasing. Such surfaces are characterized by clusters of small spherical vesicles and tubules, which are somewhat regularly distributed in banding patterns corresponding to the cross-striation. This particular feature can be observed only with SEM.

Fiber Interior

Exposure of fiber interior by means of longitudinal tear permits examination of myofibrils and membranous organelles such as the sarcoplasmic reticulum (SR), tubules, and mitochondria (Figure 1-2).

Myofibrils are closely packed against each other in muscular fibers when examined by SEM. On some electron mycrographs, the network of the SR and T-tubules can be observed overlying the myofibrils.

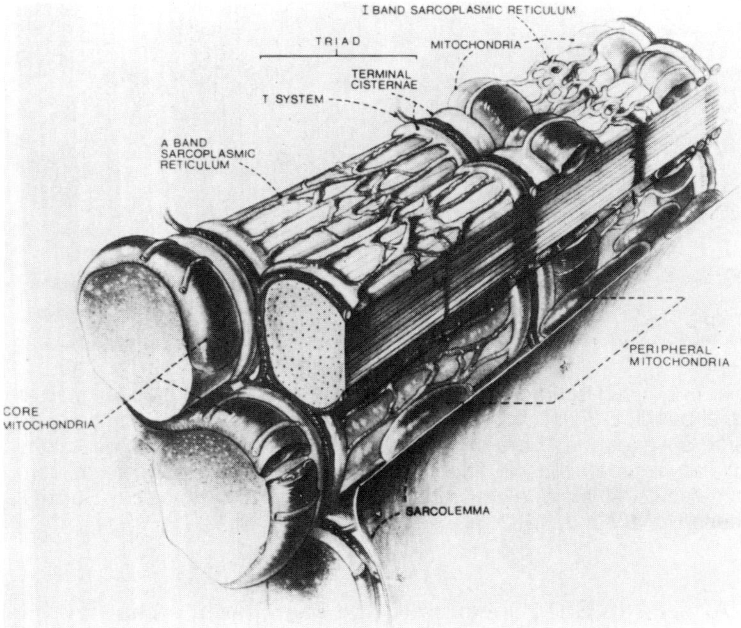

FIGURE 1–2: Schematic drawing of part of a mammalian skeletal muscle fiber showing relationship of sarcoplasmic reticulum, terminal cisternae, T-system, and mitochondria to a few myofibrils. (Used with permission from Peachey LD, et al., for Figure 1 by Eisenberg BR,[67] in *Skeletal Muscle*, American Physiological Society, Bethesda, Maryland, 1983, p 75.[214])

Electron microscopy has confirmed that the cross-striations result from internal structure of repeating subunits, *sarcomeres,* which are arranged in series along each muscle fibril. A sarcomere is the fundamental structural functional unit of contraction in skeletal muscle. Each sarcomere is composed of smaller segments or "bands" recognized by distinct refractive differences. A number of bands are known to exist in the filaments and they are well-recognized banding patterns.

T-System

The T-system of a muscle cell is a network or a series of networks of tubular invaginations (T-tubules) of the plasma membrane of the cell. The T-tubules have two different cross-sectional shapes. The more common shape is that of a flattened, or ribbon-shaped tubule. The less common cross-section is circular with a diameter approximately equal to the smaller of the two dimensions of the flattened form. These two forms are easily distinguishable from one another.

The Sarcoplasm

The sarcoplasm is a complex assemblage of organelles which provides special structural and energetic support for the upper apparatus, while serving also the general metabolic requirements of this living cellular system. It includes an elaborate endoplasmic reticulum (the sarcoplasmic reticulum), a supportive framework of intermediate and finer filaments, microtubules, a Golgi complx, variable amounts of mitochondria, few ribosomes, glycogen, and occasional lipid droplets.

Fibers that are rich in mitochondria and display fewer sarcoplasmic membranes tend to be slower due to an abundance of oxygen transporting pigment, *myoglobin*; they also have a dark appearance in the fresh state, whereas faster fibers have less sarcoplasm and are of a lighter color. In some species, the dark fibers are characteristically predominant in particular muscles and the light fibers predominate in other muscles. The two types of fibers as well as intermediate varieties are appropriately intermingled in human as well as in most other mammalian muscles.

The Sarcoplasmic Reticulum

The sarcoplasmic reticulum (SR) is formed from rough-surfaced endoplasmic reticulum and develops simultaneously with the formation of the myofibrils and T-tubules (Figure 1-3).

The SR plays a major role in controlling the state of activation of the contractile machinery of the muscle cell by regulating the concentration of calcium in the sarcoplasmic space which contains the contractile myofilaments and myofibrils. The SR first pumps calcium into its interior and holds it there, thus lowering the free calcium concentration inhibition. The pumping activity of the SR takes place continuously. The release function is triggered only when the muslce cell is stimulated. Calcium is repumped into the SR during the relaxation phase of the contraction cycle.

A property of the SR in all muscle cells which is critical for

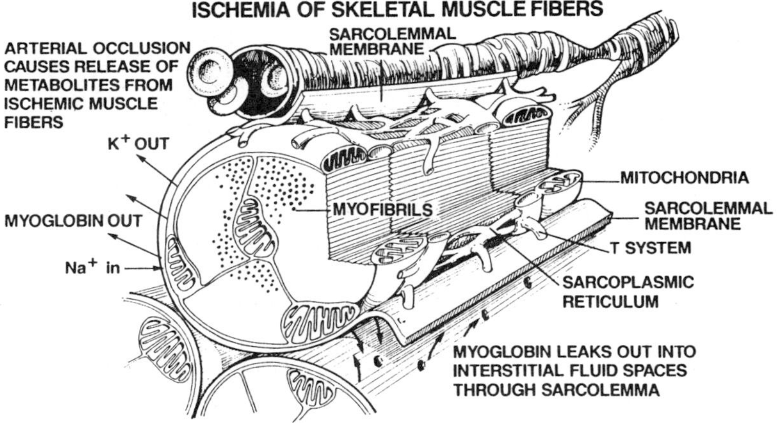

Figure 1–3: A diagrammatical depiction of arterial occlusion causing ischemia of skeletal muscle fibers. The ischemic changes consist of release of metabolites from the myofibrils. Note the sarcolemmal membrane surrounding the muscle fiber. The interior of the latter indicates the sarcoplasmic reticulum, mitochondria, T-system, and myofibrils seen at the cut end of it. Note the release of myoglobin leaking out into interstitial fluid spaces through the sarcolemma (membrane). In addition, potassium leaks out while sodium enters through the sarcolemma from the interstitial fluid spaces.

function is its division of the muscle cell into two major compartments: the internal space of the SR and the sarcoplasm outside the SR.

Mitochondria

The mitochondria of the muscle cell are found beneath the sarcolemma around the nuclei, and in the sarcoplasm between the myofibrils. In the latter location, they are generally aligned with their long axis parallel to the direction of the myofibril, although they may be found encircling the myofibril transversely, particularly in the region overlying the Z-disk. Mitochondria in muscle fibers are easily recognizable by their shape, size, and distribution. They are round, oval, or cylindrical and show smooth outer surfaces. They vary in quantity among different muscles and in different types of muscle fibers. Red muscle fibers are rich in mitochondria, often arranged in rows between myofibrils and in aggregates beneath the sarcolemma, in addition to their common distribution at the level of the I-bands. Mitochondria in white fibers are considerably reduced in quantity and localized at the level of the I-bands in mouse muscles, but are scattered and much fewer in number in frog sartorius muscle.

Cardiac muscle cells possess some morphological features of mitochondria common to red skeletal muscle fibers in quantity and distribution. Mitochondria seemed to be distributed in close relation to the sarcomere pattern of myofibrils and change their form during the contraction–relaxation cycles.

Changes During Contraction

Morphologically, changes associated with contraction have been studied both in living and in fixed muscle. In both cases, the fiber as a whole becomes shorter and broader when it contracts. Thus, each sarcomere becomes shorter and broader.

Electron micrographs of contracted muscle show an interdigitation of the thick and thin filaments throughout the length of the sarcomere, in contrast with the arrangements seen in resting muscle.

When a nerve to a mucle is stimulated, a depolarization

(action potential) spreads rapidly over the muscle cell membrane and over the membranes lining the T-tubules to the deepest regions of the cell. Presumably, a change in the membrane potential of the T-tubules induces, in some manner, a reaction in the adjacent cistern. The result is that calcium is relased from its storage place in the sarcoplasmic reticulum to enter the sarcoplasm bathing the myofibrils. Such freed calcium is necessary for the actin–myosin interaction to occur. According to one of several theories, calcium operates by invoking a steric conformational change on the regulatory protein complex of *troponins* which, in concert with *tropomyosin*, acts as a safety catch, preventing activation of myosin *adenosine triphosphatase* (ATPase) by actin (when calcium is absent). The activation occurs as soon as calcium can be bound in one part of the troponin complex and the troponin–tropomyosin assembly is warped so as to expose actin active sites to nearby adenosine triphosphatase. Adenosine triphosphate (ATP) is changed by action of the adenosine triphosphatase to adenosine diphosphatase (ADPase) with a release of energy. This energy is believed to provide the full force for contraction, perhaps by promoting banding of the flexible neck of heavy meromyosin. Apparently the phosphate group is split from ATP each time a cross bridge goes through a cycle of attachment and release at each successive actin binding site. When removal of phosphate groups from ATP stops, there is no further action of cross bridges, and muscle returns to its resting state. At the same time, calcium is withdrawn from the sarcoplasm back into the sarcoplasmic reticulum. ADP is rephosphorylated into ATP before the muscle is ready for contraction again.

Phosphorylation of ADP back to ATP can be provided by aerobic glycolysis within nearby mitochondria, or under anaerobic conditions from a storage compound, phosphocreatine. The latter is regenerated during periods of relaxation. In tonic muscles, abundant mitochondria provide ATP rather directly but somewhat slowly. By contrast, the faster muscles rely heavily and immediately on phosphocreatine stores and are adapted for long anaerobic operation.

ATP is also required to break the bonding between actin and heavy meromyosin heads. Death results in the loss of available

ATP from any source with the result that bonding persists for hours—a state referred to as rigor mortis.

Muscular Blood Vessels

The muscles as an anatomic entity constitute about 42% of the body weight. Muscular arteries play a significant role in reestablishing collateral circulation in the presence of occlusive arteriopathies. When the muscular arteries participate in the process of occlusion either by thrombosis or by other factors such as trauma, as may be the case in rhabdomyolysis, the knowledge of the arterial supply to individual groups of muscles assumes greater significance in understanding the mechanism of the pathological process. The study of the muscular arteries is divided into two major sections: (1) extramuscular arteries; and (2) intramuscular arteries.

While both groups of arteries may play a major role in the ischemia of the skeletal muscles during the occlusive process of major arteries, the intramuscular vessels may ultimately determine the viability of the tissues depending on the degree and extent of the involvement of the pathological process. Using microradiographic methods, Saunders determined the relationship between the macro- and micromesh and the capillary bed[255] (Figure 1-4A). Thus, arising at intervals from arterioles forming the micromesh, and passing off to one side or the other, one can determine the presence of small, tortuous branches. They are best designated as precapillary arterioles. By means of these studies, arteriovenous shunts or anastomoses (AVA) have been demonstrated within the muscles by Saunders by means of the techniques mentioned above. The arteriovenous shunts in the muscles do not resemble the specialized structures described in the human finger in that they do not show the so-called epithelial cells in their wall. Peripheral resistance is confined to the arterioles and capillaries. They represent the chief areas of blood flow regulation in the periphery.

Detailed description of the muscular arteries of either the upper or the lower extremity is not within the scope of this mono-

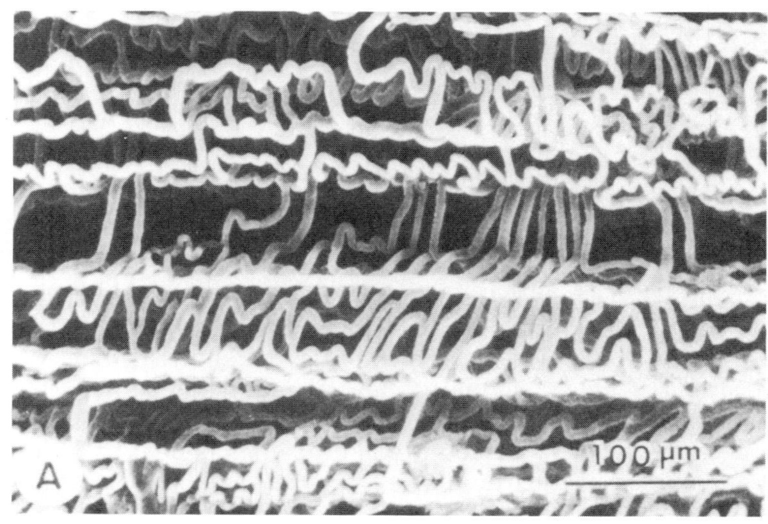

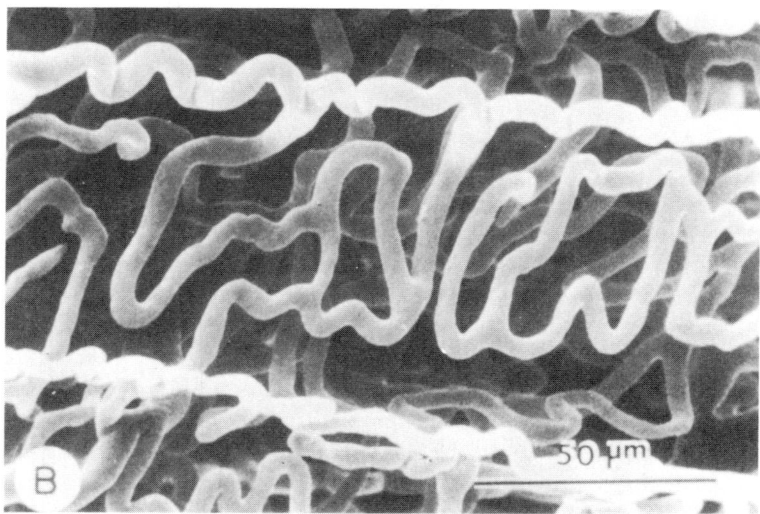

Figure 1–4: Vascular corrosion cast of mouse soleus muscle. **A:** Low-power scanning electron microscopy (SEM). **B:** High-power SEM. Capillary networks show a ladderlike pattern in this contracted state of muscle and are arranged in layers surrounding individual muscle fibers, which are dissolved away with all other tissue components. (With permission from Peachey LD, et al., for Figure 2 by Kurotaki M, in *Skeletal Muscle*, American Physiological Society, Bethesda, Maryland, 1983, p 3.[214]

graph. Such details may be found elsewhere as described by this author.[99]

Muscular Arteries of the Upper Extremity

The muscular arteries of the shoulder receive their arterial supply primarily from the axillary and brachial. Some of their branches provide the major supply while others participate to a lesser degree.

The muscular arteries of *the arm* are supplied by two major branches from the brachial artery at various levels. Again, some of the muscles receive a greater blood supply than others from different branches, which may be important in understanding some of the pathological consequences of the necrosis which may be present in certain groups of muscles.

Muscular arteries of the *forearm* and *hand* have been the focus of somewhat greater attention from both the anatomists and surgeons because of the relatively more frequent vascular involvement in this area known by the eponym of Volkmann's ischemic contracture.

One point of anatomic information is related to the variations of the arteries supplying the muscles of the hand which occur quite frequently and make it difficult to describe as unusual patterns.

Muscular Arteries of the Lower Extremity

The muscles of the lower extremity are subdivided into groups corresponding with the different regions of the limb: (1) iliac; (2) thigh; (3) leg; and (4) foot.

The muscles of the iliac region include *psoas major*, psoas minor, and iliacus. Together these muscles represent a large mass which is provided by branches from the abdominal aorta, the iliac arteries, and the femoral arteries as well. Their involvement in ischemic episodes may be responsible for rhabdomyolysis with metabolic repercussions more profound than those seen in areas where the muscular mass is much less developed. The muscles of the thigh are also a large group of muscular tissue and include the anterior medial gluteal and posterior aspects of this segment of the lower extremity. The intramuscular branches are provided by the major arteries, the iliac, femoral, and the profunda femoris. The latter artery provides 80% of this arterial supply to the quadriceps while only 20% arises from the common femoral or from the superficial at variable levels. It is beyond the scope of this monograph to detail the various branches of the major arteries supplying the lower extremity. However, due to the disparity, in general, between the upper and the lower extremity, muscle masses in the lower extremity, where the rhabdomyolytic process occurs more often, are due to the anatomical features as noted. This is not only applicable to the thigh muscular mass but also in general to the muscles of the leg, and to a lesser extent to the muscles of the foot.

The significance of the intramuscular arterial supply (Figure 1-5A, B) is that when the thrombotic or embolic or traumatic process directly involves the majority of these intramuscular arteries, the resulting pathologic changes are overwhelming and are responsible for the degree of severity of the rhabdmyolytic process. And this happens even though sometimes the major extramuscular branches have remained patent and pulsating. The ultimate prognostic factor must be looked for in the muscular arteries for an explanation of why the rhabdomyolytic process is more severe in some cases than in others.

Capillaries

The larger branches of the arteries penetrate the muscle by following the septa of the perimysium. The arterioles which penetrate the fasciculi give off capillaries at abrupt angles. The capillary supply is rich, several capillaries having proximity with each muscle fiber (see Figure 1-5B). The veins follow the arteries; even their smaller branches have valves.

Lymphatic capillaries are not found between individual muscle fibers. They are present, however, in the connective tissue septa and along the blood vessels.

The Color of Muscle

The color of muscle has long been used to classify fibers as red or white. The redness comes from the blood, in capillaries, and from myoglobin and from mitochondria in the muscle fibers. All

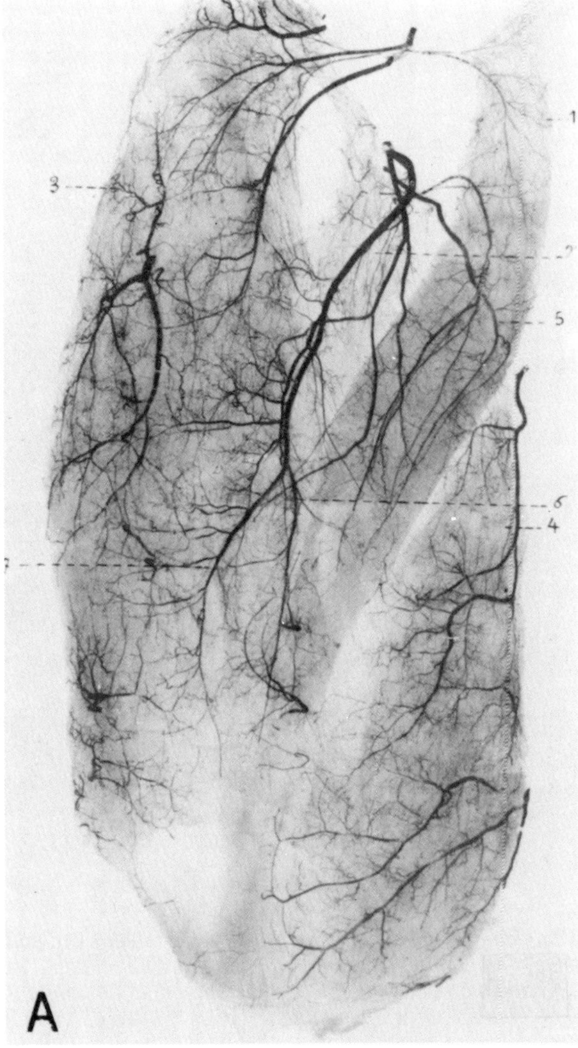

Figure 1–5A: Intramuscular arteries and their branches of the quadriceps femoris: (1) rectus femoris; (2) vastus intermedius; (3) vastus lateralis; (4) vastus medialis; (5) superior artery of the rectus femoris; (6) inferior artery of the rectus femoris; and (7) major branch of the vastus lateralis. (From Salmon M, and Dor J: Publ. Masson & Cie, Paris, 1933. From Haimovici H: Arterial circulation of the extremities. In *Structure and Function of the Circulation*, Vol. I, Plenum Press, New York, 1980, p 425.[99])

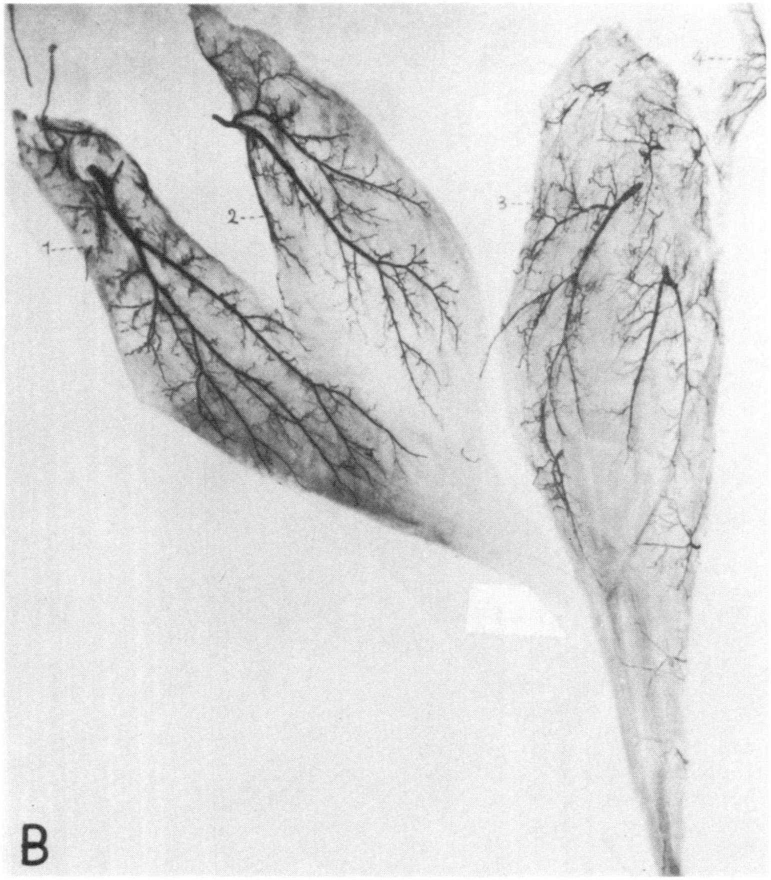

FIGURE 1–5B: Arteries of the gastrocnemius (1, 2), soleus (3), and plantaris (4). (From Salmon M, and Dor J: Publ. Masson & Cie, Paris, 1933. From Haimovici H: Arterial circulation of the extremities. In *Structure and Function of the Circulation,* Vol. I, Plenum Press, New York, 1980, p 425.[99])

three red constituents are found in large amounts in muscles with a high oxidative capacity. Although historically it was thought that all red fibers were slow twitch, type I, this is false. There are also fast twitch red fibers and so any nomenclature based on color conveys limited information about speed.

2

Muscle Biochemistry

Chemical Reactions and Metabolic Principles

Historically, in searching for the nature of the muscle machine, at the beginning of this century, thermodynamics provided a basis for the mechanical work, temperature changes, and therefore heat production during the contraction of muscles. Later, Fletcher and Hopkins[80] showed that the formation of lactate was a consequence of muscle activity and thereby launched an experimental work to demonstrate the lactate theory of muscle contraction. Later Meyerhoff[185] laid the foundations of the intermediary metabolism. The discovery that the formation of lactate in the fermentation process is exothermic fitted nicely with the prevailing lactic acid theory of muscle contraction.

The existence of a variety of hexose phosphates was recognized in muscle as was the ubiquitous role in intermediary metabolism in many types of cells. As a result, the work by Fiske and Subbarow[77a] disproved this theory of the lactic acid in the chemical energetics of muscle contracture. The discovery of an enzyme between adenosine triphosphate (ATP) and creatine resulted in the formation of adenosine diphosphate (ADP) and phosphocreatine (PCr).

Of the chemical substances that participate and produce the energetics in the muscle are ATP and CP (creatine phosphokinase). They are important in the metabolism of glycogenolysis and glycolysis, and participate in the oxidative metabolism. This class of reactions includes those of *aerobic metabolism* in the mitochondria, namely the reduction of oxygen coupled to the oxidation of substrates and the generation of ATP. Besides participating in the energetics of the muscle, ATP and CP also play a significant role related to the biochemical changes during the ischemia of the muscular tissue to be described below.

The discovery of PCr and of ATP in muscles and of enzyme catalyzing reactions in which they participate led to the conclusion that ATP is the primary and PCr the secondary source of chemical energy for muscular contraction.

Metabolic Systems

Cell metabolism is performed largely by soluble enzymes that cannot be resolved with structural techniques. However, subcellular organelles, visible in the electron microscope, are involved in metabolism and can be used as crude indices of the nature and the extent of metabolism. For example, mitochondria support oxidative metabolism (Figure 2-1) and so, the volume of mitochondria and surface area of the cristae are some measure of the oxidative metabolism of a fiber. Some cells store glycogen and lipid as reserve energy supplies. The amount of glycogen and lipid can be measured with morphometric techniques, and these measurements can also serve as an index of metabolism.

ATPases in Biological Systems

There are essentially two major groups of ATPases: one participates in the transport and the other in the synthesis of ATP. The transport type of H-ATPase resides in the plasma membrane and is frequently referred to as the plasma membrane H-ATPase. The other type, i.e., the ATPase synthetic or mitochondrial type, resides in mitochrondria, chloroplasts, and chromaffin granules.

The plasma membrane type has a single polypeptide chain of

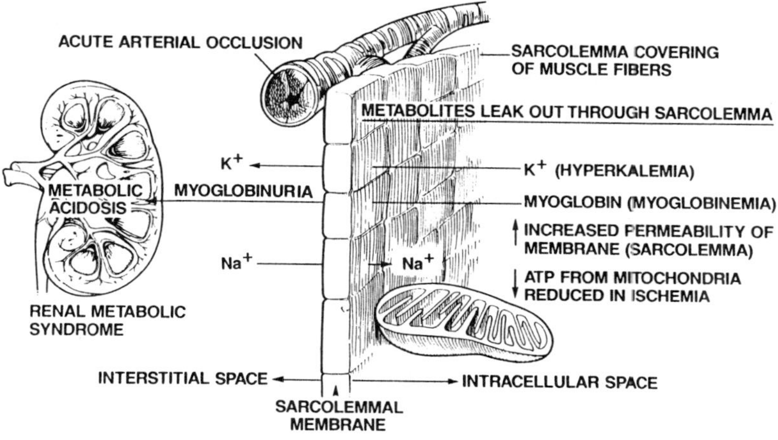

FIGURE 2–1: A schematic depiction of acute ischemia of skeletal muscle with metabolic complications. Note the sarcolemma covering of muscle fibers and the leaking out of potassium and myoglobin, which leads to myoglobinuria and hyperkalemia. Note the mitochondria and ATP being reduced by ischemia which leads to increased permeability of the membrane.

about 100 K. It is not yet known how many of these polypeptides are required for activity. However, recent work carried out by Sachs and co-workers[247a] using the technique of target-size analysis suggests that gastric H^+ K^+-ATPase may be a trimer in the membrane. It is likely that this enzyme has a hydrophilic part involved in ATP hydrolysis and a membrane part involved in H^+ translocation.

The mitochondrial type ATPase is much more complex. It consists of two separable moieties: a water-soluble head piece and a catalytic unit. It is involved in ATP hydrolysis, whereas the base piece is involved in H^+ translocation (Pederson PL: *NY Acad Sci* 402:1-20, 1982.)

Vesicular fragments of sarcoplasmic reticulum (SR) membrane constitute an advantageous system for studies of active transport coupled with ATP utilization due to a functional specificity, manifested by high enzyme activity and calcium uptake, structural specificity related to high content of calcium-dependent

ATPase in homogenous orientation of ATPase protein permitting vectorial transport of inward direction in nearly all vesicles.

This study characterization of the catalytic and transport cycle in SR ATPase indicates a fixed relationship of one forceful relation site with two calcium sites. Calcium exchanges with H^+ at the binding sites and pH has profound effects on the affinity of the enzyme for Ca^{2+} and on various tests with ATPase cycle.[135]

Metabolic Characteristics

Human skeletal muscle contains stores of glycogen and lipids in addition to the more immediate energy sources of ATP and creatine phosphate. A summary of the average values of these stores as compiled from several studies estimated from biopsy samples of the extremity muscles is presented in Tables I and II.

Glycogen Content

The average glycogen content (Table I) of human extremity muscle lies in the range from 50 to 990 mmol/kg wet weight. Part of this rather wide variation appears to be related to the diet and state of physical activity of the subject. This range is noted in the gastrocnemius, the quadriceps femoris, the triceps brachii, and the biceps brachii of man. The reason for this variation is unknown, but it may be due in part to the technical difficulties of separating the fiber from the support tissue and of accurately weighing the small tissue fragments.

Triglyceride Content

The triglyceride content of human skeletal muscle varies between 5 and 15 mmol/kg wet weight. The magnitude of the variation of the triglyceride stores between various muscles of the body is unknown (Table I).

Differences in the lipid content of the fiber types can be demonstrated when sections are stained with either Sudan black or Oil Red-O. Since mitochondrial membrane contains large amounts of lipid, stained by some methods, interpretation of the estimate of differences of triglyceride stores of individual fibers is difficult.

Table I
Human Skeletal Muscle Substrate in Vastus Lateralis Muscle

Substrate	*Mixed Muscle, mmol/g wet wt*	*Fiber Types, mmol/g wet wt*			
		ST	*FT*	*FTa*	*FTb*
Triglyceride	9.9 ± 0.6	7.1 ± 1.7	4.2 ± 1.2		
Glycogen (glucose units)	83.8 ± 18	78.8 ± 18	84.7 ± 19	83.1 ± 18	89.2 ± 2
ATP	5.0 ± 0.2	4.9 ± 0.1	5.1 ± 0.2	5.3 ± 0.2	4.9 ± 0.1
CP	10.7 ± 0.6	12.6 ± 0.2	14.7 ± 1.4	14.5 ± 1.1	14.8 ± 1.6

ST = slow twitch; FT = fast twitch; FTa = fast twitch, a type; FTb = fast twitch, b type; ATP = adenosine triphosphate; CP = creatine phosphate.

Values are means ± 1 SD and are given for triglycerides in mixed muscles (see original table for references).

From Saltin B, Gollnick P: Adaptability: Metabolism and performance, In *Skeletal Muscle*, Peachey LD, et al. (Eds), American Physiological Society, Bethesda, Maryland, 1983, p 566.

Ionic Composition of Skeletal Muscle

The various fiber types also contain different amounts of intracellular ions (Tables II and III). Sodium is low in all fibers but FT fibers contain only about 50% of that found in ST fibers. This is

Table II
Muscle Electrolytes in Healthy Subjects

Muscle	Na_m	K_m	Mg_m
		mmol/100 g FFW	
Vastus lateralis	11.6	44.7	
	(2.7)	(2.0)	
Vastus lateralis	15.9	43.1	
	(2.9)	(4.1)	
Different*	12.1	43.3	3.73
	(2.0)	(2.5)	(0.58)
Vastus lateralis	9.3	46.7	4.48
	(1.5)	(0.9)	(0.08)
		mmol/100 g dry wt	
Triceps brachii	12.7	45.0	3.86
	(5.0)	(2.0)	(0.33)
Vastus lateralis	8.9	44.9	4.12
	(2.5)	(5.4)	(0.18)
Soleus	12.5	43.3	4.07
	(3.3)	(4.7)	(0.45)
Triceps brachii			
ST fibers	13.0	44.0	3.98
FT fibers	11.6	46.2	4.15
Homogenate	11.7	44.5	3.79
Vastus lateralis			
ST fibers	8.0	42.6	4.58
FT fibers	8.9	43.0	4.76
Homogenate	8.3	44.2	4.12
Soleus			
ST fibers	9.6	42.6	4.36
FT fibers	9.6	43.2	4.52
Homogenate	10.7	41.8	4.09

Values are means with 1 SD in parentheses.

FFW = fat-free weight; ST = slow twitch; FT = fast twitch.

*In six subjects from sartorius or pectineus muscles and in six subjects from the internal oblique muscle.

Fat content averaged 8% (5–14%) of dry weight. If expressed per 100 g FFW, value should be increased by this amount.

From Saltin B, Gollnick P: Adaptability: Metabolism and performance, In *Skeletal Muscle*, Peachey LD, et al. (Eds), American Physiological Society, Bethesda, Maryland, 1983, p 571.

true for rat muscle, but special differences may exist. Campion[34] has reported slightly higher values in guinea pig muscle with no difference between ST and FT fibers. In humans, the sodium content of the muscle fiber appears to be quite low with no difference between fiber types. Species differences may also be present for intramuscular potassium concentrations. Rat and guinea pig muscle fiber types are different: the concentration of potassium of ST fibers is 140–150 mM whereas the FT fibers have a potassium concentration of 170–180 mM. In man, no difference can be detected when comparing the different fiber types, the mean value of both ST and FT fibers being approximately 160 mM (Table III).

Phosphagen

The phosphagen stores of skeletal muscle constitute 25 to 35 mmol/kg wet weight with the CP concentration being 18 to 20 and ATP 4 to 5 mmol/kg wet weight. Variations among muscles are small.

The ATP and the CP concentration in mixed fiber muscle of nonhuman species (primarily the rat) are similar to those observed in human skeletal muscle (Table I).

The glycogen and triglyceride stores of rat muscle and other species are generally present at lower concentrations than those in mixed muscle of man.

Enzyme Activities

The content and/or activities of enzymes for contraction and energy metabolism differ in the various fiber types of skeletal muscle. This can be demonstrated in a variety of nonhuman species when quantitative biochemical assays are performed on portions of muscles or whole muscles that contain only one fiber type.

The Ca^{2+}-activated myosin ATPase determined on pooled samples of a single fiber type was 2.5 to 4 times higher in the fast twitch (FT) that the slow twitch (ST) fibers.

Creatine Kinase

Major differences in creatine kinase activity of the fiber types appear to exist in all skeletal muscles. For example, in human muscle, the average creatine kinase activity has been reported to

Table III
Water Spaces and Electrolytes in Predominantly Red (SO) and White (FG and FOG) Muscles

	Predominantly Red (SO)	Predominantly White (FG and FOG)	Species
Total H_2O ml/100 g dry wt	334	310	Rat
	325	308	Rat
	350	339	Rat
	324	329	Guinea pig
H_2O extracellular, ml/100 g dry wt	72	46	Rat
	53	33	Rat
	39	35	Guinea pig
H_2O intracellular, ml/110 g dry wt	272	264	Rat
	272	275	Rat
	285	294	Guinea pig
Na in muscle, mmol/100 g dry wt	15	11	Rat
	14	9	Rat
	14	8	Rat
(Na)i, mM	13	10	Rat
	23	13	Rat
	28	19	Rat
	44	50	Guinea pig
K in muscle, mM/100 g dry wt	38	45	Rat
	42	47	Rat
	44	51	Rat
(K)i, mM	141	179	Rat
	154	169	Rat
	138	172	Guinea pig
Mg in muscle, mM/100 g dry wt	4.6	5.5	Rat

Values are means.

From Saltin B, Gollnick P: Adaptability: Metabolism and performance. In *Skeletal Muscle*, Peachey LD, et al. (Eds), American Physiological Society, Bethesda, Maryland, 1983, p. 570.

be about 222 and 333 micromole $mg^{-1}min^{-1}$ for the ST and FT fibers, respectively.

Histochemical staining of human skeletal muscle has demonstrated the existence of major differences in the metabolic profiles of the ST and FT fibers. The general pattern is for ST fibers to be well-endowed with enzymes for end-terminal oxidation and a low anaerobic potential, with the reverse being true for the FT fibers. There is not, however, a discrete relationship and enzyme activities vary considerably within each of the fiber types.

Anaerobic Metabolism

Increases in activities of some enzymes in the glycolytic pathway are small and appear to exist in only select enzymes of the system. Moreover, in some cases, the enzymes that had been reported to increase are not those whose activities are known to be regulated and which thus exert control over the flux of substrate throughout the system. Overall, the data available concerning adaptations in the glycolytic system are less certain than those for enzymes for end-terminal oxidation. An increase in the enzymes for glycolysis has an unknown role in the overall economy of the metabolic response to exercise. The suggestion was advanced that lactate per se is not responsible for terminating the exercise nor are the enzymes for metabolism significantly inhibited.

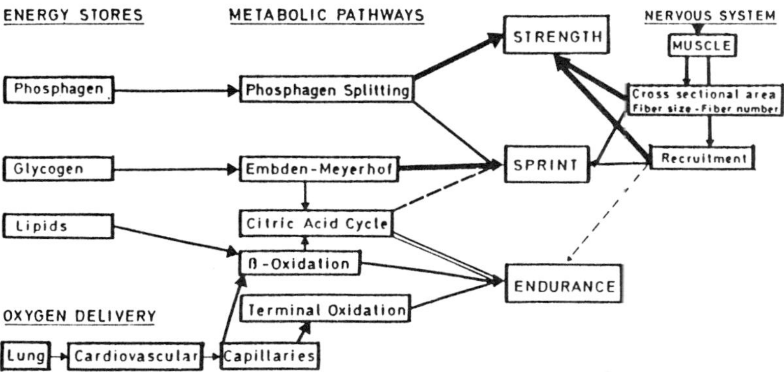

FIGURE 2–2: A schematic summary of the various energy stores and metabolic pathways for performance and strength sprint and endurance events. On the left side are indicated the energy stores including phosphagen, glycogen, and lipids. The oxygen delivery originates in the lungs, which in turn delivers it to the cardiovascular system down to the capillaries, which leads to the terminal oxidation of the tissues. This schematic summary indicates also not only how oxygen is delivered but how it interacts with the nervous system and the muscles during the various performances. (Used with permission from Peachey LD, et al. for Figure 28, in *Skeletal Muscle*, American Physiological Society, Bethesda, Maryland, 1983, p 566.)

Aerobic Metabolism

In addition to substrate levels and mitochondrial enzymes, the role of oxygen delivery is important for a discussion of the aerobic energy yield in muscle. To discuss this subject thoroughly, we need to summarize some of the adaptations that occur within the cardiovascular system as a response to various levels of physical activity. From the results indicated, it is apparent that in a maximal exercise (running or bicycling) which elicits maximal oxygen uptake, both systemic cardiac output and widening of the arterial venous difference contribute to the improved maximal oxygen uptake.

Glycogen, although stored in small amounts, is necessary to maintain blood glucose concentration as a continuous supply to the nervous system. During exercise, two regulatory mechanisms are brought into play: reduction in insulin and elevation of intracellular concentration of glucose to G-PO^4 which inhibits phosphorylation of glucose for its transport across the cell membrane.

Regulation of Calcium Release

The mechanism that regulates Ca^{2+} release from the sarcoplasmic reticulum (SR) during contractile activity has not yet been defined, in spite of a large body of experimental work. The inaccessibility of the SR to conventional electrophysiological measurements has impeded the gathering of direct information on the nature of events that cause Ca^{2+} release. Under physiological conditions, the depolarization of the surface and T-tubule membranes is the electrical signal that triggers Ca^{2+} release. There are, however, many uncertainties about the way this signal is transmitted to the SR membrane and about subsequent events at the level of this membrane.

Mechanism of Calcium Transported by Sarcoplasmic Reticulum (Ca^{2+})

The membrane potential of the SR could influence the transport of Ca^{2+} in several ways. First, the free energy change of the reaction would be dependent on the membrane potential. Second, membrane potential may alter the movement of ions, dipoles, or other charged constituents involved in the calcium uptake. In addition, changes of the ATPase induced by electrical fields across the membrane may modify the activity of the ATPase. If all of the rate-limiting intermediate reactions are voltage-sensitive, the overall rate of Ca^{2+} transport could be influenced by membrane potential.

The sarcoplasmic reticulum is a key element in the regulation of the contraction-relaxation cycle in skeletal, cardiac, and smooth muscles. Less extensively developed but functionally analogous systems in nonmuscle cells may play a similar role in the modulation of cytoplasmic movements, secretory functions, and the activity of Ca^{2+}-dependent enzyme systems. The Ca^{2+} transport of sarcoplasmic reticulum is coupled to the hydrolysis of ATP.

The rate of calcium uptake by sarcoplasmic reticulum probably accounts for the rate of muscle relaxation. The physiological role of the reversal of the Ca^{2+} pump is less clear. While it may significantly contribute to the release of activating Ca^{2+} during muscle contraction, the speed of the activation process prompts the consideration of other mechanisms (gated) as well.

Potassium Contracture

Because the action potential is an all-or-none phenomenon that can be modulated only over short ranges of amplitude and duration, studies of electrical contraction coupling (ECC) have used other means to achieve fiber depolarization.

The membrane potential in muscle fiber is practically determined by the ratio of external and internal potassium concentrations; therefore, changes in the potassium $(K)_0$ can depolarize the membrane to the desired values. The study of potassium contractures in frog single muscle fibers, initiated several years ago by Kuffler,[158] led to the elegant work of other investigators which has yielded much information of several phenomena involved in the ECC. When potassium concentration in the external medium is raised, the fiber develops tension to a maximal value, which diminishes very slowly for several seconds and then falls rapidly to complete relaxation, even though the fiber membrane remains depolarized.

Potassium Depletion

Potassium is known to be released from contracting muscle skeletal fibers and its rising concentration in interstitial fluid is thought to dilate arterioles thereby mediating the normal rise of muscle blood flow during exercise. As a corollary, if potassium release from deficient muscle were subnormal, exercise would not be accompanied by sufficient muscle blood flow and rhabdomyolysis could occur by ischemia. Knochel and Schlein[152] have examined this hypothesis by comparing the effect of electrically stimulated exercise on muscle blood flow, potassium release, and histology of the intact gracilis muscle preparation in normal and in potassium-depleted dogs. In normal dogs, muscle blood flow and potassium release rose sharply during exercise. In contrast, muscle blood flow and potassium release were markedly subnormal in depleted dogs despite brisk muscle contractions. Although minor histologic changes were sometimes observed in nonexercised potassium-depleted muscle, frank rhabdomyolysis occurred in each potassium-depleted animal after exercise.

The authors conclude that these findings support the hypothesis that ischemia may be the mechanism of rhabdomyolysis with exercise in potassium depletion.

Postscript: Future Perspective

Recently, the technique of nuclear magnetic resonance (NMR) has been applied to measurement of skeletal muscle constituents *in situ*. Additional developments have provided further information concerning the chemical composition and metabolism of both normal and diseased human muscle.

While the studies thus far published appear promising,[65a,b] it is hoped that NMR may offer in the near future noninvasive diagnosis of ischemic rhabdomyolysis and its biochemical spectrum. This may be particularly necessary for the management of many human muscular disorders, especially the ischemic rhabdomyolytic entities.

3

Myoglobin

Historical Data

Early discussions concerning myoglobin revolved around the existence and nature of the muscular pigment (Biörk,[15] see Figure 3-1). In the late 19th century, it was demonstrated that the pigment could be extracted from muscles, and that it was related to hemoglobin but the two were not identical. Later investigation confirmed the above findings by using the absorption spectrum of the muscle pigment which demonstrated that the two were indeed quite different.

At the beginning of this century, Camus and Pagniez[35] in 1902 reported that an intravenous injection of muscle juice from one dog to another caused, within 10 to 30 minutes, an excretion from the latter of a pale red urine, without any trace of blood corpuscles, giving, however, a hemoglobin spectrum. Hans Günther in 1921 presented a review of prevailing knowledge of the muscle pigment as well as his own observations on this subject.[95] Günther extracted the muscle pigment with distilled water from minced muscle of animal organs and then perfused the extract in a Ringer solution *in vivo*. This extract showed an absence of erythro-

FROM THE BIOCHEMICAL DEPARTMENT OF THE MEDICAL NOBEL INSTITUTE PROF. H. THEORELL,
THE CARDIAC CLINIC OF SÖDERSJUKHUSET (PROF. G. NYLIN)
AND THE DEPARTMENT OF PATHOLOGY AT SÖDERSJUKHUSET
(MED. DR. F. WAHLGREN), STOCKHOLM

ON MYOGLOBIN
AND
ITS OCCURRENCE
IN MAN

By

GUNNAR BIÖRCK

STOCKHOLM 1949

FIGURE 3-1: A reproduction of the title page of the book *On Myoglobin and Its Occurrence in Man* by Gunnar Biörck, published in 1949.

cytes microscopically in the capillaries. Günther[96] was convinced that the identity of the muscle pigment was different from that of hemoglobin. He is credited as being the first to apply the term *myoglobin* to the muscle pigment, thereby differentiating the two elements.

Further work, such as that by Whipple in 1926, found that there are differences in the hemoglobin content of the striated muscles depending on age, muscular strength, or functional demands.[294,295] He also found that myoglobin content in puppies was highest during the first 3 months in the heart and diaphragm, where it was proportionately higher than in adult dogs.

As a result of many other investigations, the existence of myoglobin as an independent substance was finally accepted. Ray and Paff,[233] using the spectrophotometer, found absorption values that differed from those of hemoglobin and disclosed a shift to the red end of the spectrum typical of myoglobin.

Next, a series of publications followed in which the occurrence of myoglobin and its chemical characteristics were subjected to a more comprehensive analysis. Myoglobinuria in humans had been first described by Myer-Betz in 1911.[184] This description included the clinical manifestations of muscle pain, weakness, and brown urine known later as a well-recognized syndrome due to renal tubular necrosis.

Later, in 1931, Carlström,[36] a veterinarian, showed that the so-called paralytic hemoglobinuria in horse was due to release of myoglobin when the horses were put to work again after a period of rest and heavy feeding. The myoglobin was spectroscopically verifiable in the urine, and "this myoglobinuria would, in unfavorable instances, lead to renal damage owing to the filling up of the tubuli with myoglobin cylinders." He further reported that thrombosis in the aorta abdominalis of the horse may give rise to a similar renal picture, as a result of myoglobin blockage of renal tubules.

This observation antedated the findings seen in clinical vascular cases. Indeed, myoglobinuria occurring in patients associated with renal tubular blockage is described elsewhere in this monograph in connection with acute arterial occlusions.

In the following years, 1932 and 1934, Hugo Theorell[238] at the Karolinska Institute in Stockholm succeeded in crystallizing myoglobin from horse cardiac muscle. This contribution regarding the nature of myoglobin which appeared in a series of articles reviewed the various attempts to crystallize myoglobin. With the aid of the purified preparation, he ascertained the chemical and relevant physiological properties of this substance.

Quantitative determinations of the myoglobin content in the muscle were the subject of interest by Millikan[189] in 1937 and by Bywaters[31] and Stead in 1944 in their investigations of the pathogenesis of the crush syndrome. According to the former, the soleus muscle of cat contains 0.5% of the wet weight of myoglobin, while in human muscle the latter authors found 500 mg per 100 g of muscle. Rossi-Fanelli[241] in 1948 published a method of myoglobin determination based on a different type of denaturation and decomposition in an alkaline medium of met-hemoglobin and met-myoglobin. Later, de Duve determined myoglobin on human muscle extracts by a different principle.[63] The crystallization of human myoglobin was announced as early as in 1945 by Drabkin,[59] and was also independently described in 1946 by Theorell and de Duve.[283] This latter method formed the foundation for de Duve's method[63] for simultaneous quantitative analysis of myoglobin and hemoglobin in a solution of both substances.

Chemistry of Myoglobin

Myoglobin and hemoglobin both belong to the group of hemoproteins, comprising a prosthetic group, protoporphyrin, and a protein component, namely, globin. The former consists of pyrrole rings in the center of which is an iron atom coupled to the four nitrogen atoms, thus making the porphyrin an iron porphyrin.

Hugo Theorell's work offered comprehensive knowledge of the chemistry of myoglobin. He crystallized myoglobin from the heart of horse, as previously mentioned, and was thereby able to perform a series of chemical determinations regarding the nature and the properties of this purified substance. The iron content of the myoglobin was found to be identical with that of the hemoglobin. In Svedberg's ultracentrifuge, Theorell obtained a sedimentation constant for myoglobin from horse, cattle, and cat, of approximately 2.0×10^{-13} and, correspondingly, molecular weights 34,000 to 35,000 and 68,000.

The molecular weight of 34,000 reported by Theorell was later corrected in a lecture by Svedberg in 1938 to a molecular weight of 17,200, that was also in conformity with those of Polson[225] in 1937. Considering that the myoglobin molecule probably corresponds to a fourth of the hemoglobin molecule, a molecular weight of 17,000 may be regarded as most closely representing the actual figure.

The oxygen-combining capacity of myoglobin has, of course, attracted the attention of various investigators. The earliest data were presented in 1913 by Dirken and Mook who observed a 7 to 20% lower oxygen-combining capacity of myoglobin than of hemoglobin (quoted by Biörk[15]).

Structure of Myoglobin

Myoglobin is closely related to hemoglobin and shares with hemoglobin a most important and interesting biological function, that of reversible combination with oxygen. Myoglobin consists of a single polypeptide chain of about 150 amino acid residues, associated with a single heme group. Its 1-2-4 relationship with hemoglobin, already suggested in early days by a comparison of molecular weights, turned out to be not coincidental but a fundamental structural relationship, as has now been shown by comparing the molecular models of the two proteins. Myoglobin lacks the sulfhydryl groups whose presence in hemoglobin was successfully exploited by Perutz and Ingram[221] for the attachment of mercurial agents.

The oxygen-combining capacity of myoglobin has been noted to be lower than that of hemoglobin. Hill[128] showed that the oxygen affinity and dissociation curve of myoglobin led to the estimation of the physiological function of this pigment (see below for further evidence).

From animal experiments as well as from human material, it appears that there is no constant relation between hemoglobin and myoglobin content in cases of anemia. It is possible that prolonged anemias may gradually involve a moderate reduction in the parenchymal iron, and, among others, of the myoglobin. Still, the deficiency and transport of iron that is in hemoglobin will in the first place dominate the clinical picture.

Liberation and Elimination of Myoglobin and Hemoglobin

Montagnani and Simeone[193] have reported in 1963 tourniquet experiments applied across the thigh and hip of dogs and studied the time relationships regarding the appearance of myoglobin in body fluids after release of tourniquets. After 4 to 7½ hours, myoglobin was liberated from striated muscle in both blood and lymph returning from the extremities and was excreted in the urine. It was detectable grossly in the urine within 10 minutes after release of the tourniquets. The pigment was almost always found in blood and lymph in specimens obtained 1 hour after release of the tourniquets. The peak concentration of myoglobin appeared in blood and lymph within 2 to 4 hours, while the peak urinary excretion of myoglobin occurred during the second hour after the release of the ischemia. At the end of 10 to 12 hours, myoglobin could be detected only in minute amounts or not at all. These authors felt that myoglobin is probably one of many substances liberated when circulation is reestablished in ischemic striated muscle. Evidence was presented that damage to the gromeruli or other parts of the kidney may result on a humoral basis following the release of limb ischemia.

Myoglobin and Functions of the Muscles

Knowledge of the principal properties and functions of the muscle is indispensible for our understanding of the role played by myoglobin in this connection.[189,190] As has been stated earlier, the sarcoplasm that surrounds the myofibrils in the muscle fibers contains myoglobin as well as other biochemical substances. A lot of controversy surrounded the question as to whether myoglobin is present not only in the red but also in the white muscle. It appeared, according to certain investigations, that the difference was due to the content of the myoglobin in the sarcoplasm. There is no definite knowledge available regarding whether the white musculature is generally free of myoglobin or only deficient in this substance.

The vascular supply present in the muscles is of great importance for understanding the physiological functions of myoglobin. Krogh, who pioneered this work, indicated that the muscles are provided with an immense number of capillaries, only a restricted amount of which are open in the resting condition. By contrast, the number of capillaries per unit of transverse section is greater in the muscles mostly during activity which is sufficient to allow the interchanges between blood and muscle cell. An increase in the number of capillaries was noted by Krogh both in the skeletal muscle and in the heart myocardium after a period of regular muscular exercise. Conversely, when exercise was discontinued, a successive regression of the capillaries was observed both in the heart and in the skeletal muscle.

By use of electron microscopy it was shown that the myofibrils themselves consist of still finer elements, the so-called filaments, which should represent the contracting units. Although the microstructure of the muscle and muscular contraction were not entirely elucidated, an essential point was shown, however, that under normal conditions the oxygen transmitted from the capillary blood is needed for the actual oxidation process. The oxygen is further necessary for the ultimate reoxidation of lactic acid to glycogen, which constitutes the last link in the restoration of energy reservoirs. From the data presented, it appears that the muscle is capable of anaerobic contraction while making use of its energy reserves. If these are not replenished, a deadlock is attained as represented by rigor of the muscle.

The oxygen supply to the resting muscle takes place through a limited number of capillaries where the oxygen tension in the arterial end of the capillary network equals approximately 100 mmHg, and in the venous end approximately 40 mmHg, while the oxygen saturation values are approximately 95% and 70%, respectively.

As pointed out earlier, the pressure gradient will enable the oxygen to pass from blood to muscle merely by diffusion. Its progress from the sarcolemma to the interior of the muscle cell, and its intervention in the oxidation metabolism described above, takes place along a protracted chain of intermediate links, thereby diminishing the instantaneous expenditure of energy. Part of this chain is linked to the cytochrome oxidase which reacts directly with the molecular oxygen and is reduced by the cytochrome that carry electrons in the opposite direction, being themselves reduced by other respiratory enzymes, until the final action sets in.

The myoglobin seems to be coupled parallel with the first link in the cytochrome system and the muscular system of oxygen utilization. The task of myoglobin is to act as an oxygen reservoir in the muscle. As a rule, under the condition of contractions, the muscles do not perform rhythmically like the heart.

Whatever the amount of myoglobin in the musculature, it will only suffice to execute its functions during a brief interruption in the oxygen supply, perhaps intermittent as may be assumed under the conditions that were reviewed above.

Estimation of Myoglobin in the Urine and in the Serum

It is not within the scope of this monograph to describe the various laboratory techniques that have been used over the years for detecting myoglobin in the urine and in the serum. In Chapter 22 on *Myocardial Infarction,* a number of methods have been described in connection with determining myoglobinuria and myoglobinemia. The reader is therefore referred to Chapter 22, *Myocardial Infarction,* for these methods. Although they are not described in detail in this chapter, the reference will be available in the *Bibliography* for those who wish to obtain the various details for a given method.

In addition to the above, two other methods are available: (1) "Improved estimation of urinary myoglobin by counter-immuno-electrophoresis, as compared with the double-immunodiffusion technique" by H. Hibrawl and Robert G. Blaker;[127] and (2) "Quantitative method for estimating myoglobin in the urine" by Harold Markowitz and Gary H. Wobig.[177] The reader will find these references in the *Bibliography* should one desire complete information about the technical details.

4

Membranes: Their Role in Biochemical Interchanges

Membranes

The sarcolemma of a muscle fiber is a multicomponent structure covering the entire surface of the fiber. Anthony van Leeuwenhoek[164] was probably the first to refer to a "membrane" covering individual muscle fibers, which he refers to as "flesh particles."

Sarcolemma of a muscle fiber is especially apparent in the light microscope when the fibers are damaged so that a retraction of a contractile and other internal structure in the fiber occurs. The sarcolemma has considerable strength. It can be divided into its innermost component, the plasma membrane (the true external boundary of the muscle cell), and an overlying basement membrane consisting of an inner basal lamina and an external reticular lamina. The felt-like basal lamina contains laminin, fibronectin, and collagen IV. The more fibrous reticular lamina contains fibronectin, collagen V, and another collagenous protein, high salt soluble protein (HSP).

A population of mononucleated satellite cells can be found lying between basal lamina and the plasma membrane of the muscle cell. These satellite cells are thought to be dormant myoblasts that are able to activate and participate in the fusion and differentiation of a new muscle fiber when the original had been damaged. Invasive cells, thought to originate from the circulatory system, also penetrate across the basal lamina and into the bulk of the muscle fiber but do not fuse with it.

Plasma Membrane and Caveolae

Knowledge of the form of plasma membrane in muscle cells and especially quantitative knowledge of its surface area are important in relation to impedance measurements.

Caveolae are "ellipsoidal inpocketings" of the plasma membrane connected to the exterior of vertebrate muscle fibers through a narrow neck.

Physiological Functions

During development, many small myoblast cells fuse together to form long cylindrical multinucleate muscle fibers. The fibers in young animals are loosely packed and have a nearly circular cross-section. The surface membrane of a muscle fiber was termed the *sarcolemma* by Bowman[20a] in 1840.

The ultrastructure of the sarcolemma is best viewed with the techniques of freeze fracture or scanning electron microscopy. Scanning electron microscopy allows the outer surface and the T-system openings to be seen.

The sarcolemma in a healthy muscle is homogeneous throughout its length except at its neuromuscular junction and the tendon insertions. Mitochondria are more concentrated near the neuromuscular junction.

The plasmalemma covers the peripheral muscle surface, the T-system, and the caveolae.

The entire sarcoplasmic reticulum (SR) membrane is richly studded with calcium ATPase uptakes that can be localized by immunofluorescence and are invisible in freeze-fractured replicas (see Fig. 2-1, page 19).

The Role of Phospholipids in ATPase Activity and Calcium^{2+} Transport

The ATPase and calcium^{2+} (Ca^{2+}) transport activity of SR is absolutely dependent on membrane phospholipids. Depletion of phospholipids by digestion with phospholipase, C or A, inhibits the ATPase activity and calcium transport, without major change in the steady state concentration of phosphoprotein intermediate. The inhibition of ATPase activity is accompanied by immobilization of spin-labeled fatty acids incorporated into the membrane. Inhibition of ATPase activity and Ca^{2+} transport was also observed at the extraction of membrane phospholipids cholate or deoxycholate.

The inhibited ATPase activity of lipid-depleted vesicles was reactivated after addition of micellar phospholipid dispersions of diverse fatty acid composition. Lysolecithin, unsaturated fatty acids, and neutral or acidic detergents are all effective, indicating that the lipid specificity of the Ca^{2+} transport is rather broad. On the other hand, the reactivation of Ca^{2+} transport in lipid-depleted vesicles strictly requires phospholipids. This is because in addition to the activation of Ca^{2+} transport ATPase, the restoration of the normal permeability characteristics of the membrane is also important for the retention of accumulated Ca^{2+}.

Metabolic Systems

Cell metabolism is performed largely by soluble enzymes that cannot be resolved with structural techniques. However, subcellular organelles, visible in the electron microscope, are involved in metabolism and can be used as crude indices of the nature and extent of metabolism. For example, mitochondria support oxidative metabolism, and thus, the volume of mitochondria and surface area of the cristae are some measure of the oxidative metabolism of a fiber.[80] Some cells store glycogen and lipid as reserve energy supplies. The amount of glycogen and lipid can be measured with morphometric techniques, and these measurements can also serve as an index of metabolism.

Effect of Membrane Proteins on Permeability of SR Membranes

The permeability of SR vesicles for ions, cations, and neutral molecules is far greater than that of mitochondria and surface membrane from muscle and other cells. Because the ion permeability of artificial phospholipid bilayers formed from SR lipid is very small, relatively, anion and cation permeability of SR probably reflects the contribution of membrane proteins.

Pathophysiology of Membranes

The metabolic complications resulting from ischemic skeletal muscle are due to derangement of transport processes across the membranes. The latter play a fundamental role in the biochemical functions of the various components. Changes in permeability of membranes under traumatic or simple ischemic conditions may induce severe biochemical alterations in the internal space of the sarcolemmal reticulum and outside of it (see Fig. 2-1, page 19).

The morphological components of muscle fiber are dynamic structures constantly linked to the biochemical and physiological activities.

The outer surface functions of muscle fibers interact with the DNA molecules inside the muscle fiber. The communication between the outer surface of the cell, namely the plasma membrane, represents a code that specifies its function. The plasma membrane, as mentioned earlier, is a thin flexible sac made of fatty molecules (phospholipids) among which are embedded other more complex molecules.

The physiological integrity of the membrane, which includes neural components, can be affected by decreased adenosine triphosphate (ATP). Since the latter is markedly reduced in ischemic muscle, it follows logically that an abnormal membrane permeability in the presence of reduced ATP represents the underlying mechanism of the biochemical changes. While this hypothesis is based on the decreased energy factors (ATP) regulating the membrane functions, structural abnormalities and enzymatic changes are also at the root of permeability alterations of the membrane. Direct evidence of altered membrane structure is not available. The functional interpretation is largely based on indirect assumptions.

Little is known about the exact mechanism of the interchange between biochemical substances from the muscular fiber into the interstitial space or from the latter into the retromembrane structures. The most common elements involved in this transport are myoglobin, K, Ca, Na, and a few others to be mentioned in the biochemistry of the ischemic muscle.

In brief, the dysfunction of the membrane in ischemic conditions plays an essential role in the pathogenesis of the metabolic syndrome.

5

Rhabdomyolysis

The term *rhabdomyolysis* is generally used to indicate a lesion of skeletal muscle associated with biochemical substances derived from it.

The definition of rhabdomyolysis, however, suffers from a lack of precision concerning its nature, extent, and its exact degree of morphological damage. Notwithstanding its imprecision, its definition should essentially incorporate two major parameters: (1) a muscle lesion, and (2) a biological syndrome resulting from tissue ischemia. These features are to be found in detail in the various entities described in this monograph.

Briefly, the *muscle lesions* as described in the various publications on the subject range from diffuse cell injury of variable extent to frank massive necrosis.

Three major etiologic types of rhabdomyolysis are being differentiated according to the nature of the causative factors inducing the lesions in the skeletal muscles.

1. *Acute arterial occlusions* may result in:
   a. minor or reversible muscular lesions,
   b. partial limited necrosis, and

c. massive necrosis with loss of limb and often loss of the patient's life.

2. *Traumatic*

Crushing of muscular tissues, resulting in the "crush syndrome." This occurs by direct pressure or injury to the muscle with or without involving indirectly the vessels of the traumatized region.

3. *Nontraumatic*

This group includes a wide spectrum of entities in which diffuse muscle cell injuries dominate but in which occasionally extensive muscular necrosis may also occur.

The *essential biological parameters* defining rhabdomyolysis include a host of biochemical factors of which elevated CPK and myoglobinuria often leading to renal failure are the key elements.

The following chapters will deal in detail with the major aspects of rhabdomyolysis:

- *Exertional Rhabdomyolysis: Physiopathological Implications*
- *Muscle Ischemia and Biological Functions*
- *Pathology of Rhabdomyolysis*
- *Biochemical Basis for Myofiber Necrosis*
- *Traumatic Rhabdomyolysis: Its Relation to Shock and Crush Syndrome— Experimental Studies*
- *Tourniquet Ischemia: Metabolic Responses*
- *Experimental Basis of the Myonephropathic-Metabolic Syndrome*

6

Exertional Rhabdomyolysis: Physiopathological Implications

Elevated Skeletal Muscle Creatine Kinase MB-Isoenzyme in Marathon Runners

Siegel et al.,[264] in an investigation of the above topic, have shown that mean serum creatine kinase MB-isoenzyme (CK-MB) activity in 108 trained marathon runners after competition was 98 ± 66 (SD) units/L measured by a quantitative electrophoretic technique (normal less than 5 units/L), or 7.9% of total CK activity. These levels in asymptomatic runners were comparable with peak serum values reported in patients during acute myocardial infarction. Elevated serum levels of CK-MB in runners can arise from skeletal muscle known then as *exertional rhabdomyolysis*. It is important to be reminded that it may arise also from silent injury to myocardium, or from combined tissue sources. To investigate this directly, the authors analyzed skeletal muscle obtained by needle biopsy for CK isoenzymes from 25 trained marathon runners and 10 sedentary male subjects. The MB isoenzyme accounted for 8.9% ± 1.3% (SD) of total CK activity per gram of total protein in the skeletal muscle of runners and 3.3% ± 0.7% (SD) in control tissues, a finding which is significant. Total CK activity was not as statistically different between the two groups. Similar relative concentration of CK-MB in skeletal muscle (8.9%) and serum after competition (7.9%) strongly suggests that elevated serum CK-MB activity in asymptomatic runners arises from a noncardiac or skeletal muscle source.

The authors comment on these results by emphasizing that the diagnostic specificity of serum CK-MB elevations for myocardial injury remains controversial. Using quantitatively sensitive assays such as gel electrophoresis and column chromatography, serum CK-MB activity after 5 units/L is considered normal and may increase after injury to various tissues. Chronic disorders of skeletal muscle such as dystrophies and myopathies may also display elevated serum CK-MB activity based on release of pathologically altered skeletal muscle tissue, and are not diagnostic of myocardial injury in such clinical settings.

Serum CK-MB activity is nevertheless widely regarded as a sensitive and specific marker for myocardial injury in clinical practice. Serum CK-MB level of 98 ± 66 (SD) units/L in asymptomatic runners after competition is similar in magnitude to values for patients with electrocardiographically confirmed myocardial infarction. The increase in tissue activity of CK-MB in skeletal muscle in runners is unclear. One explanation for this finding might be a selective association of CK-MB with type 1 or high oxidative fibers, which are predominant in skeletal muscle tissue of elite runners.

Appreciation of the nonspecificity of elevated serum CK-MB activity for myocardial injury in runners may avert unnecessary hospitalizations for presumed myocardial damage on the basis alone of the presumed specificity of this test. Conversely, as myocardial ischemia or infarction may occasionally develop in highly trained athletes, these complications must be fully investigated when suspected on clinical grounds and should not be discounted because serum findings may be normal in asymptomatic runners.

Siegel and Dawson published a note in *JAMA* in 1980 in

which they pointed out that small levels of the MB-fraction of creatine kinase (CK) can be detected in the undiluted sera in patients without myocardial involvement if the total CK levels are substantially elevated. Dubin, in a letter to *JAMA*, at that time concurred with Siegel and Dawson but added that these studies demonstrate that MB-fraction in noncardiac patients is typically 0% to 2% of the total CK activity if we accept the authors' assessment that about 5 units/L is the minimum detectable level of total CK activity.

Comment: It is well-known that when leakage of more than one or two metabolites occurs through the muscle fiber membrane, others, such as myoglobin, are usually also found. It is, therefore, surprising that no mention of the latter is found in their report.

Changes in CPK in Nonischemic Skeletal Muscle

Elevation of CPK has been studied by several investigators in normal individuals after recreational exercise. Thus, LaPorta et al.[161] have investigated this problem in 20 healthy male volunteers. They were divided into four groups for a period of recreational physical exercise. Standard blood chemistry determinations made before exercise and on two subsequent days have shown that CPK, SGOT, and LDH levels were transiently elevated, but the change was considered significant only in the CPK level after certain types of exercise.

These 20 normal healthy male volunteers were unselected for body build, physical fitness, or exercise tolerance and were asked to avoid physical exertion on days 1 and 2. On the morning of day 3, a fasting blood specimen was drawn in the hospital outpatient laboratory for determination of serum cholesterol, LDH, SGOT, CPK, alkaline phosphatase, total bilirubin, creatinine, uric acid, calcium, total protein, albumin, glucose, BUN, and SGPT levels.

The results of the various types of exercise have shown increases in certain serum enzyme levels compared to those of the control group. Changes in CPK were significant only for the runners and weight-lifters on the first day and for the runners on the second day. When all values are combined for the men exercising, there was a significant elevation for CPK levels for both days after exercise. Increases were also observed in SGOT and LDH levels of the exercise groups. However, concentration of these enzymes typically remained within normal limits and in only one instance did the SGOT level of a runner double. There were clinically no significant changes in other test results nor were there clinically significant elevations in the values of the control group.

In commenting on these findings, the authors state that CPK is an enzyme found in muscle, heart, and brain which catalyzes a reaction that provides high energy phosphate early in the anaerobic phase of organ function. Apparently, during strenuous exercise, especially after high intensity burst type, considerable amounts of CPK leak into the extracellular fluid and plasma as a result of changes in the membrane activity. This is due either to hypoxia, the presence of local metabolites, or direct mechanical stress. Serum enzyme levels increase several hours after exertion, occasionally in conjunction with elevated serum myoglobin level in cases where myoglobinuria has been demonstrated previously. This was demonstrated in highly standardized studies relating the increases to physical conditioning, such as the study of Olerud et al.[207]

The study of LaPorta et al.[161] demonstrates that recreational exercise, which may not be especially rigorous or exhausting, can cause clinically significant increases in CPK levels to occur that might interfere with the diagnosis of disease or with clinical investigations.

These authors believe that the effect of recreational exercise as reflected by an elevated CPK level may be found during an investigation or during a routine blood chemistry analysis. Awareness of such factors will probably increase with the present interest in sports medicine.

Ischemic Rhabdomyolysis and Creatine Phosphokinase Isoenzymes

Russell et al.[246] brought up the possibility of a diagnostic pitfall of these enzymes. It is well known that isoenzyme fraction 2 (MB-fraction) of creatine phosphokinase (CPK) is being used as a marker of myocardial necrosis. It is also well known that these enzymes or their isoenzymes have been identified in patients with various muscular dystrophies: polymyositis, dermatomyositis, and viral myositis.

The following reported case displayed high levels of serum CPK isoenzyme (MB-fraction) in connection with ischemic necrosis of an extremity. The case in point concerns a 50-year-old man who was found in the emergency room to have respiratory arrest but was immediately resuscitated. The following morning in the ICU, the patient's right leg was cold, white, and without palpable pulses. A thrombotic occlusion of the right common iliac artery was then diagnosed. Circulation was restored by insertion of a right aortofemoral bypass graft.

Severe edema developed in the right calf over the next 24 hours, with an associated foot-drop. Urine was burgundy-red; analysis showed a myoglobin level of 4800–9000 mg/liter (normal being less than 4000/liter). The patient was returned to the operating room, where a fasciotomy of anterior and posterior compartments of the leg was performed, relieving the compressed ischemic muscles.

The total CPK level rose rapidly from less than normal on the first day to 400 times normal on the third day when the urine was burgundy-red and the right leg notably edematous. The CPK (MB-fraction) appeared on the third day and disappeared by the fifth day, when the total CPK level had fallen to one-fifth of its peak level.

The lactic dehydrogenase (LDH) values exhibited a similar contour, rising from just above normal, peaking on the third day, and falling subsequently. LDH fractionation disclosed the expected LDH_5 isoenzyme elevation consistent with skeletal muscle necrosis. The LDH-1/LDH-2 remained less than one unit throughout the hospital course. The SGOT determinations also showed a rapid increase by the third day; the subsequent decline occurred more slowly. The patient's clinical status improved gradually over the following month. He was last seen as an outpatient walking well with the assistance of a foot brace.

The significance of this finding, CPK isoenzyme MB-fraction, in a patient with an acute arterial occlusion was due to rhabdomyolysis in the absence of any clinical and electrocardiographic changes consistent with myocardial infarction.[102] This underscores the fact that caution is needed in the use of CPK as a marker of myocardial infarction since this may be found in rhabdomyolysis in an acute arterial lesion.[102]

This case further underscores the fact that metabolic complications associated with acute arterial occlusions not commonly recognized may lead to incorrect diagnoses. The fortunate fact was that leg compartments syndrome was promptly treated by fasciotomy, which is often a limb-salvaging procedure. This case calls further attention to the revascularization syndrome which was not sufficiently emphasized in the original article, since the primary scope was to correlate the findings with myocardial infarction and thus failed to pay attention to the presence of rhabdomyolysis of the leg.

This case was included in this section as an example of differential diagnosis between myocardial infarction and rhabdomyolysis based on these enzymes.

7

Muscle Ischemia and Biological Functions

Introduction

Metabolic acidosis is one of the important components of the metabolic syndrome induced by muscle ischemia. While the pH provides precise information concerning the metabolic acidosis, this factor does not in general quantitate the physiological impairment at the cellular level. Acute ischemia results in general in a severe tissue anoxia leading to a profound deterioration of the structures that are indispensable to the biotic function of the tissues in which the lactic acid is only a witness to the biological changes.

Lactic Acid

Lactic acid is a metabolite which is part of the cycle of glycolysis. This cycle includes first an anaerobic phase, leading to the formation of pyruvic acid then to an oxidation phase of the pyruvic acid leading to the acetyl-coenzyme A, which is part of the Krebs cycle, which leads to the liberation of the CO_2, water, and energy. The lactic acid is situated in this chemical phenomenon between the two phases, anaerobic and aerobic.

Lactic acid is in equilibrium with pyruvic acid and this chemical reaction is coupled with the transformation of nicotinamide-adenine-dinucleotide or an abbreviated form, $NADH_2$. This chemical reaction requires the intervention of the enzyme called lactic dehydrogenase (LDH). This reaction takes place at the cellular level in the cytoplasm. Lactic acid at the normal pH of the organism results in a serious disturbance due to its excess of the acid-base equilibrium.

The lactates are metabolized in the liver, skeletal muscle, and the myocardium. The liver metabolizes a third of the lactate produced by the organism. The lactate is transformed into pyruvate which, depending on the case, will participate in the aerobic glycolysis (Krebs cycle) or will be resynthesized into glycogen.

With regard to the skeletal muscle, there is a resynthesis of the glycogen from the 4/5 of the latter. The myocardium consumes three times more lactate than glucose. The kidney eliminates the lactates depending on the concentration of the arterial renal blood.

It is clear from the biochemical changes taking place at the tissue level that formation of the lactic acid is an important factor leading to metabolic acidosis.

Huckabee[131] has shown that the lactate-pyruvate equilibrium allows cases of hyperlactacidemia to be differentiated from those that are not as severe. It appears, therefore, according to Huckabee, that at a constant concentration of H^+, an increase in the concentration of the lactate may be due either to an augmentation of the concentration in pyruvatae or to an elevation of the ratio $NADH_2/NAD$ or even an increase of these two factors. When the lactic acid is not in equilibrium with an equivalent amount of pyruvate, the phenomenon is known as excess lactate. This situation then reflects directly the seriousness of the metabolism.

Enzymes

In general, the lesion of a normal tissue results in the increase of enzymatic activity by liberating into the plasma the enzymes present in the involved cells of the corresponding tissue. This fact was particularly well established in myocardial infarction and in certain muscular lesions, in particular during acute ischemia.

The Transaminases

One of the responsible enzymes connected with transamination was isolated from muscle extracts. The comparison of various tissues has shown that the intensity of transamination was highly variable: the muscular tissue and the myocardial tissue have a very great transaminase activity. Increase of transaminases translates the presence of muscular necrosis especially in the acute ischemia of the extremities.

Creatine Phosphokinase

It was thought for a long time that a muscular contraction was deriving its energy directly from the degradation of the glycogen. The muscle contains another source of energy which is constituted by the adenosine triphosphoric acid (ATP) and through the phosphagen and creatine phosphate. ATP plays an essential role since it is directly responsible for the phenomenon of muscular contraction.

During acute ischemia of the extremities in the venous blood, there is a great elevation of creatine phosphokinase and creatinine.

Lactic Dehydrogenase and Its Isoenzymes

LDH is the enzyme which completes the anaerobic oxidation of glucose through the glycolytic cycle. As already mentioned, in this reaction, there are changes from pyruvic acid to lactic acid. This enzyme is present in all the tissues, particularly in the myocardium and skeletal muscle, the kidney, the liver, the red blood cells, and the pulmonary tissue.

The isoenzymes are different through their electrophoretic mobility. There are five LDH isoenzymes with different normal values. Distribution of the LDH isoenzymes is well known. The muscle fraction (M) is predominant in the skeletal muscle while the H is more predominant in the myocardium, the brain, the kidney, and the red blood cells.

The tissue necrosis, the ultimate stage of anoxia, will flood the blood stream with byproducts of cytolysis: the biochemical elements, including the minerals (potassium, phosphorus), the amino acids and their catabolites, and their enzymes.

In general, all of the above elements are more or less increased in the venous blood which drains the ischemic limb. At the initial determinations, they reflect the extensive tissue necrosis, with a minimal chance of functional recovery.

During the revascularization, these biochemical elements continue to increase. Their prognostic significance varies with each one of them individually:

Potassium may become a problem either as hypokalemia or hyperkalemia. In the former, it may induce, together with myoglobinuria, a more or less marked rhabdomyolysis and in the latter, if elevated, hyperkalemia may be fatal by inducing a sudden heart arrest.

Phosphorus in itself as an isolated element offers no particular hazard, except when combined with other elements.

Enzymes usually increase after the revascularization. Of those, two are most significant metabolically: the CPK and the LDH.

The *CPK*, depending on its level, is always an index of muscle ischemia with variable degrees of necrosis. At or about 1,000 IU/L, it translates into major muscular necrosis, very likely associated with important damage of the arterial vessels. The prognostic index of this level of CPK reflects irreversible necrotic changes, leading to amputation.

LDH, like CPK, reflects tissue necrosis. The study of its isoenzymes allows assessment of the gravity of the tissue necrosis. If LDH is increased, and especially if LDH_1 and LDH_2 are decreased at the expense of LDH_4 and LDH_5, the functional prognosis is poor. The increase of LDH_5 is not surprising since it determines preferentially anaerobically the passage of pyruvic acid to lactic acid.

Depending on their concentrations, LDH and CPK may indicate the direction of the functional prognosis of the ischemic limb. There seems to be no quantitative relationship between lactic acidosis and the enzymatic changes.

8

Pathology of Rhabdomyolysis

Introduction

The evolution of ischemic changes in skeletal muscle has not always been reported in terms of duration of the ischemia and especially the morphologic changes as seen sequentially. It is, however, important from a therapeutic point of view to obtain a sequential picture of what happens to the morphologic alterations at the time of onset of ischemia as well as at different post-ischemic stages. The nature and the course of these changes are therefore significant for the assessment of the picture of the immediate and subsequent post-ischemic lesions.

Because the ischemic picture resulting from the human muscular lesions do not lend themselves to this sequential analysis, there has been an attempt to gain this knowledge of muscle ischemia from animal experiments. This study will be divided into (1) animal, and (2) human data.

Pathology of Experimentally Induced Ischemic Muscle

Fishback and Fishback,[76] using the rabbit as an experimental animal, reported muscle degeneration from ischemia due to bacterial, traumatic, or heat and cold injuries and found the response to all these types of muscular injuries to be similar. They divided the course of events into the following stages: (1) slight granular clouding with dimming of cross-striations; (2) edema of fibers with prominent longitudinal fibrils; (3) vacuolization; (4) true granular degeneration, such as albuminous or fatty; and (5) waxy degeneration with further lumpy or granular disruption. They proposed the term "acute molecular degeneration of striated muscle" instead of waxy degeneration. Subsequently, the same authors, using a more standardized experimental model of traumatization similar to the methods used earlier (in 1918) by W.B. Cannon consisting of blows induced with a hammer to the rabbit muscle, made observations ranging from 4 hours to 28 days after the injury. From the data obtained in this experimental model, they found that the course of repair is toward regeneration. The completeness of this latter process appears to depend upon the course of the lesion and not upon the extent or severity of fiber degeneration.

Legros-Clark and Blomfield,[165] investigating the possibility of intramuscular collateral anastomoses after devascularization of different types, described similar degenerative and regenerative changes seen in the muscle tissue. Their description did not seem to differ in essentials from that given by the previous investigators.

Harman,[120] using rats and rabbits as experimental subjects, studied ischemia for 1 to 96 hours by ligation of vessels and application of tourniquets. The animals were sacrificed and investigated at the end of the period of ischemia. The findings in this investigation showed on the normal, control side, a sincitoid structure of the muscles, while on the ischemic side after 2 to 4 hours, the fibers were individualized, in which longitudinal striations disappeared, and cross-striations became a conspicuous cytological feature. After longer periods of ischemia, abnormal anisotropic disks appeared and involved the muscle fibers in increasing numbers up to 18 hours of ischemia. Weakness or absence of contractility preceded and accompanied the appearance of these disks. Their presence and extent of involvement served as a clear indication of nonviable fibers and constituted a morphological manifestation of cell death in skeletal muscle.

The same investigator,[121,122] in another experiment, using the same animals and the same model of ischemia, produced complete arterial occlusion in one leg of these animals. The results obtained were studied by histology and angiography. Irrespective of the duration of the ischemia, it was possible immediately after release of the tourniquet, to palpate the pulse in the leg. Harman summarizes as follows the main conclusions of this investigation:[122]

> 1. By means of direct palpation and visualization of pulsation and with supplementary angiography, spasm of arteries was excluded as a major factor in the pathogenesis of ischemic necrosis of skeletal muscle.
>
> 2. The angiographic studies and histologic lesions indicated that the condition was not caused by venous obstruction.
>
> 3. In view of the manner of movement of the dye bromphenol blue into and out of ischemic muscles and the histologic picture of stasis, it was most likely that the principal cause of the ischemic necrosis was the persistence of initial ischemic damage of the intimate vasculature.

Moore, Ruska and Copenhaven,[195] using electron microscopic studies on the post-ischemic changes in muscle induced by tourniquet application, expressed the view that discoid, granular, and hyaline degenerations are not different stages in the development of this process. They found that the form of degeneration depended on whether the muscle is stretched or not and its content of mitochondria of the fiber. Thus, discoid degeneration was seen in stretched muscle, and hyaline degeneration was seen in unstretched muscle rich in mitochondria. The authors postulated then that "the extent of degeneration was not a function of ischemia time, there being both nearly normal and severely damaged fibers at 20 minutes and 16 hours after the release of tourniquets."

Dahlback and Rais,[49,50] using rabbits as an experimental

animal and producing ischemia by Esmarch's bandage applied from the foot to midway up the thigh and producing ischemia for periods of 30 minutes through 6 hours periodically, have studied these animals after gross examination and primarily by histologic evaluations.

Essentially, these investigators found that the edema following application of the compressing bandage was most marked in the subcutaneous tissues in the interspaces between the muscle bellies and around the tendons. The most massive edema is usually noted around the Achilles tendon but the muscle itself seemed to be edematous as well. Edema was recorded as early as 1 hour after the end of ischemia and generally reached its peak after 1 to 2 hours. It would appear, therefore, that the edema was more or less marked but did not confine itself to the muscle alone. The severity of degenerative changes beyond 30 minutes of compression were related to the duration of the ischemia. They were slight to moderate and regressed rapidly when the circulation was restored.

Reznick[236] in 1967 described the microscopic alterations occurring during ischemia. After 24 hours, edema is formed in the interstitial spaces associated with hemorrhagic foci, fibrin exudation, and discrete nuclear infiltration. The muscular fibers present as granular swelling of the sarcoplasm. The longitudinal striations become irregular at the same time that they become more accentuated. Almost all the nuclei are pyknotic and disappear rather rapidly. After 48 hours, a number of fibers completely lose their structure.

After 72 hours, regeneration phenomena are visible at the border of the necrosed tissue adjacent to the level of the intact muscular zone. Thus, little by little, muscular regeneration fills in the destroyed muscle. Fibrous organization of a scar-type formation develops, especially in the incompletely regenerated muscular area. By means of electron microscopy, it was demonstrated that the ischemia induces fragmentation of the mitochondria. The intermyofibrillar spaces are enlarged and the muscular nuclei of the ischemic zone undergo pyknosis, occurring at the same time as the alterations of the mitochrondria. The contractile elements undergo important alterations which occur usually after the degeneration of the mitochondria and nuclear pyknosis. In the presence of ischemia, it is not unusual or rare that the glycogen is a little more abundant than normal. Later it disappears completely at the level of necrosed fibers. Important cellular infiltrations accompany the ischemic necrosis of the fibers where polynuclear macrophages exist.

Veress et al.[287] described three phases of muscular necrosis based on studies that included both human and rats. The human material used necropsy and biopsy specimens and inflammatory myosytis cases. The three phases are:

1. During the first phase, the degenerative process of the structure of the muscular fibers resulted in disappearance of the striations. At the same time, isolated myofibrils became visible and were increased in diameter. During the beginning of necrosis, the proteins were precipitated in the fibrils.
2. During the second phase, a discoid degenerative process occurs, the fibrils become fragmented and are visible only as isolated segments. This phase corresponds to what is described as a floccular degenerative process.
3. During the third phase, there is a complete disorganization of the structures of the fibers of the necrosed muscle.

Phases 2 and 3 are irreversible and fibrosis developed at the site of the disrupted fibers.

This brief review of the literature relating to experimental studies indicates some of the factors responsible for the ischemic changes of the skeletal muscle. An attempt was made to point out the time relationship between ischemia and the degree of degenerative changes. Some of this knowledge acquired in the experimental laboratory in dogs[260] provides a possible basis for the human pathological findings, as they may relate to acute arterial occlusions, traumatic vascular lesions, and other allied conditions.

Pathology of Human Ischemic Skeletal Muscle

Scully and Hughes[259] published a detailed description of early changes in muscles of the extremities following damage to major peripheral arteries based on material available on the Korean battlefield. Comparatively scant attention had been paid to the striking changes that take place in devascularized tissues, especially in ischemic skeletal muscle.

In view of the above, they decided to focus their investigation based on the changes of skeletal muscles secondary to specific vascular lesions: (1) obstruction of the arterial blood flow alone; (2) obstruction of both the arterial and the venous blood flow; and (3) pure venous obstruction.

What follows is, in part, based on Scully and Hughes' observations. My personal macroscopic and microscopic findings in acute ischemic muscle may be found in Chapter 14 on *Arterial Embolism,* Chapter 18 on *Vascular Trauma,* and later in this chapter as well.

Obstruction of Arterial Blood Flow

Early in the course of more or less complete arterial occlusion, ischemic muscles are known to go into a temporary state of contracture, simulating "rigor mortis." Eventually, a permanent contracture, not unlike Volkmann's contracture, may supervene in humans. "In the end-stage of severe arterial ischemia, the muscle is hard and is composed of yellow or greenish-yellow infarcts separated by scarred tissue."[259]

In less complete arterial obstruction, foci of infarction may occur. Following restoration of circulation, Scully and Hughes[259] noted striking changes consisting of the appearance of tense swelling, capillary engorgement, edema, hemorrhage, acute inflammatory exudation, and release of myoglobin. Harman and Gwinn,[122] who experimentally produced essentially complete interruption of arterial flow by means of a tourniquet, described a sudden increase in the rate of muscle fiber damage upon release of the tourniquet. They noted the appearance of two new types of degeneration that were not seen in unrelieved total ischemia. (*Note:* these changes not known at that time of those experiments seem to be consistent with the post-revascularization syndrome and the reperfusion in which free radicals are involved.) Harman, quoted above, had further presented evidence that muscle capillaries and the possibly finer arterioles and venous channels were damaged in ischemia, and that following restoration of circulation, blood flow through them was sluggish. "Such vascular damage may account, at least in part, for the severe changes occurring in ischemic muscles upon resumption of their arterial flow." (This again is a remarkable intuition of the present concept of the reperfusion syndrome.)

Obstruction of Both Arterial and Venous Blood Flow

Claims that simultaneous ligation of veins in cases of arterial occlusion lessens ischemia failed to be confirmed.

Pure Venous Obstruction

Effects of obstruction of the entire venous outflow of the muscle, with arterial supply intact, leads to the swollen dark blue blood tissue. Microscopically, hemorrhage, necrosis of fibers, and marked neutrophilic infiltration were noted. Later, while a proliferation of fibroblasts takes place between individual muscle fibers, contracture is produced constantly. Working with the entire limb instead of isolated muscles, Fontaine and de Sousa-Pereira[81] showed that complete ligation of the venous system was necessary before gangrene could be produced. This refers to venous gangrene and has little relevance here. (See "Ischemic Venous Thrombosis," Haimovici.[103])

Results of Muscle Changes During the First 2 Days After Arterial Injury

Many of the specimens may exhibit artifacts or changes properly attributable to trauma rather than to ischemia. According to Scully and Hughes,[259] "the more common of these were blurring and patchy fragmentation of cross-striations, retraction of fibers from the sarcolemmas and separation from one another, swelling and thus obstruction of sarcoplasm, and nuclear shrinkage or swelling. Certain of these changes are considered artifactitious only when they appeared in relation to the cut edges of the specimens."

Muscle changes during the first 2 days after surgical repair of arterial injury presented a striking clinical feature of swelling occurring only hours after vascular repair. Fasciotomies done to relieve the tension within the muscle compartment disclosed swollen muscle bulging through the incisions. In some instances, bloody fluid exuded. In addition to swelling, all muscles exhibited changes suggestive of severe ischemia, with rare exceptions in which the muscles were not swollen and appeared normal at operation.

Microscopic Appearance of Muscles, As Seen in a Few Cases

The specimens of "severely ischemic" muscles, on the other hand, exhibited diverse and sudden changes. A variety of lesions were found, such as: (1) In one advanced necrosis characterized by disruption and loss of structure of fibers, and extensive neutrophilic infiltration, such changes were different from those observed in purely ischemic muscle, and appeared secondary to contusion. (2) In another case after repair of a lacerated superficial femoral artery, an anterior tibial compartment developed. A fasciotomy done 34 hours postoperatively revealed a swollen muscle that was severely ischemic. A biopsy of a specimen showed changes consistent with early ischemia, namely exaggeration of cross-striations, congested small vessels, and numerous hemorrhages. (3) Following relief of spasm of the common femoral artery in another case, pulsations became palpable in the foot but disappeared later as the calf muscles began to swell.

Late Stages of Ischemia: Gross and Microscopic Pathology of Muscles

A wide range of pathological changes characterized the later stages of muscle ischemia. Essentially four types of muscle were seen. Categorized in order of decreasing damage, there were: (1) more or less completely necrotic muscle with little or no evidence of inflammation or repair; (2) muscle showing patchy and usually extensive necrosis, accompanied by inflammatory reactions in the reparatory process; (3) severely damaged muscle with small foci of complete necrosis, but notable for widespread survival of stroma and muscle regeneration; and (4) essentially normal or minimally damaged muscle. Although borderline forms existed among these four categories, and although one portion of the given muscle might fit into one category and another portion into a second, by and large an entire muscle or a part of it is uniform in its pathological appearance.

In one case of group 2, the muscle peripheral to the area which had undergone complete necrosis, a variety of changes was seen. Early bands of disintegrating neutrophils characterized this zone. Later histiocytic invasion of sarcolemmic tubes with digestion of degenerated sarcoplasm and the appearance of chronic inflammatory cells were prominent features. Proliferation of capillaries and of fibroplasms with limited muscle cell regeneration was still noted. Only minimal penetration of fibroblasts, capillaries, and regenerating muscle fibers into the areas of completely necrotic muscle could be seen. Among these cases, in one instance the myoglobin content of a pale yellow muscle belonging to this category was analyzed and was found to be half its normal value.

Discussion

A comparison of clinical and pathological observations in humans with experimental findings is of importance and will be mentioned here.

Contracture. An inconstant early manifestation of muscle ischemia in humans is contracture. This phenomenon is not to be identified with a permanent Volkmann's contracture, although it is possible that the former represents an initial, reversible stage in the development of the latter (see Chapter 20 on Volkmann's Syndrome). In this series, no instances of permanent contracture were encountered. No structural basis for early ischemic contracture was discovered in the human specimens. In the earlier cases where the muscles involved appeared otherwise normal at operation, microscopic examination of the same was unremarkable. In later cases where the muscles exhibited other evidence of ischemia at surgery, the specimens taken for biopsy showed changes similar to those seen in ischemia without accompanying contracture.

Swelling of ischemic muscles occurs in humans with arterial injury as well as in experimental animals. In humans this may take place in instances of unrelieved ischemia; however, *it is more frequent and more severe following surgical restoration of circulation*. This is an example of post-reperfusion edema, a well-recognized phenomenon.

Regeneration. Extensive muscle regeneration and reconstitution in small experimental animals may occur even when the degree of arterial ischemia had been so great that necrosis of interstitial tissue had taken place. However, a similar degree of regeneration would appear unlikely in humans, because of the bulk of the muscles.

Depigmentation. Liberation of myoglobin from muscles upon release of ischemia, as visible depigmentation, has not been described as a phenomenon of experimental ischemia. In humans, severe and widespread loss of pigment may occur not only in muscles that show large areas of necrosis but also in those exhibiting regenerative changes. Thus, the appearance of the "fish-flesh" cream or pale yellow coloring in a muscle does not necessarily indicate that it is irreversibly degenerated.

Pathologic Findings in Acute Arterial Occlusion

The data described below relate to personal observations of skeletal muscles in patients with acute arterial embolism or thrombosis.

In this group of civilian, i.e., non-military, cases, the degree of ischemic damage to the skeletal muscle following acute arterial occlusions should offer the possibility for determining the degree of muscular lesions somewhat sequentially at various stages of the post-occlusion time. Surprisingly, only scant information is available concerning these pathological changes taking place in the acutely devascularized muscle. As already stated earlier in the beginning of this chapter, to supplement some missing information concerning the sequential early and late stages of rhabdomyolysis, experimental investigations were helpful in providing these data.

On the basis of personal human observations in arterial embolism as seen during and at various stages after thromboembolectomy, sequential observations were indeed possible.

The *gross appearance* of the muscles, displayed by pallor and swelling of moderate intensity, is seen intraoperatively hours after an acute arterial occlusion. These changes become more pronounced within 24 hours, when the swollen, pallid muscles take on an appearance described as "fish-flesh." Beyond 24 hours, the muscles appear grossly congested, purple, and hard. Upon fascial incision, if still viable, they turn pink and herniate through the opening of the fasciotomy. If unrelieved by decompression of the involved area, the edema usually further increases after additional revascularization of the limb. Beyond this stage, the muscle may also display variable degrees of necrosis ranging from focal to extensive areas (see Chapter 14, *Arterial Embolism*, and Chapter 26, *Role of Free-Radicals in Post-Ischemic Skeletal Muscle Reperfusion Injury*).

Microscopically, some fibers show initially well-preserved outlines. In some areas, absence of some nuclei is noted and the cytoplasm is slightly coagulated and granular (Figure 8-1). Such findings are characteristic of early anoxic changes. Within 24 hours, individual fibers display swelling and foci of loss of striation and of sarcolemmal nuclei of muscular fibers.

Specimens from amputated limbs may show a mixture of degeneration of muscular fibers, ranging from slight to moderate changes to actual necrosis. The muscle cell lesions are translated into biochemical alterations and metabolic complications (Figure 8-2). As is well known, the sarcoplasm contains a large number of chemical substances and enzymes, including myocin and actin.

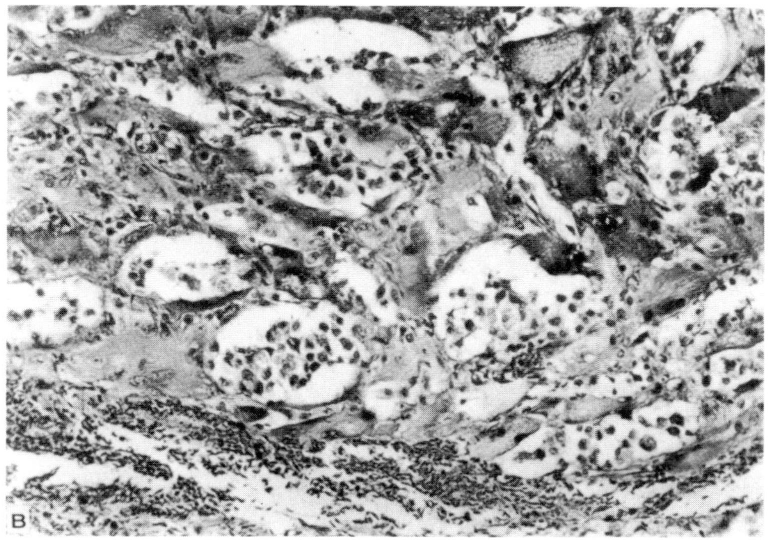

Figure 8-1: Photomicrograph showing muscle necrosis with loss of sarcoplasm. Note cellular infiltrates with histiocytes and occasional leukocytes (Hematoxylin and eosin: ×250). (From H. Haimovici.[98])

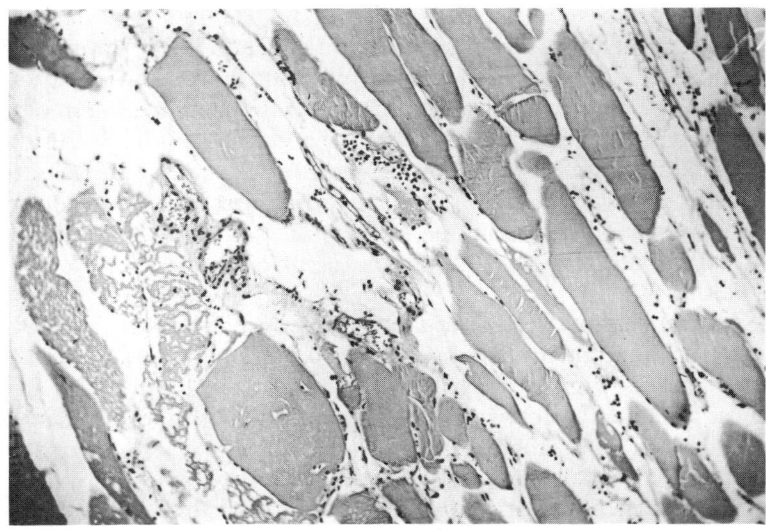

FIGURE 8-2: Muscle biopsy specimen resulting from acute arterial embolic occlusion during fasciotomy indicates the loss of sarcolemmal nuclei, homogeneous appearance of cytoplasm with loss of striations, interstitial edema, and infiltration of polymorphonuclear and mononuclear leukocytes. (Original magnification × 100). (From H. Haimovici.[109])

The normal relationship between myoglobin, myocin, and actin is disrupted as a result of loss of adenosine trisphosphate (ATP) and the changes of other muscular enzymes, all of which are attributable to altered permeability of the muscle cell membrane.

In connection with the muscular enzymes, following leg amputation for foot necrosis, it should be mentioned only briefly in this chapter that ATP is decreased in the muscles especially distal to the level of amputation, but it is elevated in the serum, along with LDH and its isoenzymes.

Conclusion

The histopathological findings in ischemic skeletal muscles noted in the two groups of patients are not entirely identical due to the different environmental conditions. Both groups, however, are in greater need of systematic evaluation of the sequence of muscular changes in relation to ischemia time.

9

Biochemical Basis for Myofiber Necrosis

The main feature of a myofiber necrosis as distinguished from that of atrophy, is death of the muscle cell. Autolysis is a central feature of necrosis, but in muscle fibers this phenomenon may be quite variable in extent, and to a microscopist, sometimes the clearest indication that necrosis has occurred is the presence of phagocytes in the muscle fiber.

Muscle fiber death and necrosis result from severe cellular injury and may have many causes, either exogenous or endogenous.

Examples of exogenous injuries are crushing, severe heat or cold, drugs, or venoms.

Examples of endogenous injuries are those that result from absence or alteration of an essential enzyme as may occur in muscular dystrophy, the glycogenoses, and other muscle diseases. Among the endogenous factors are the arterial lesions primarily of an acute nature. In some cases, the injury may not be lethal, and the cell may adapt to it through structural or functional modifications. This situation, where a muscle fiber survives or adapts to an injury and does not become necrotic, represents a third category of muscle fiber breakdown.

Although the cellular response to injury of any sort may be variable (Figure 9-1), it appears that myofibrils react in one of at least three ways: (1) complete disintegration of the regular myofilament array so that misaligned nonpolarized thick and thin filaments fill the bulk of the fiber; (2) preferential dissolution of one band of the fibrils so that the fiber becomes filled with individual segments of myofibrils; (3) severe overcontraction resulting in areas empty of myofibrils alternating with dense contraction clumps. Of some common observations in necrotic fibers, one includes chromatin clumping and lysis of nuclei, rounding off of mitochondria, particle deposition between cristae, swelling and vacuolization of sarcoplasmic reticulum, and the appearance of local discontinuities in the plasma membrane. Usually necrosis in which myofibrils are completely disorganized and have lost their regular alignment with respect to the longitudinal axis of the fiber is usually confined at an early stage to the central core of the fiber.

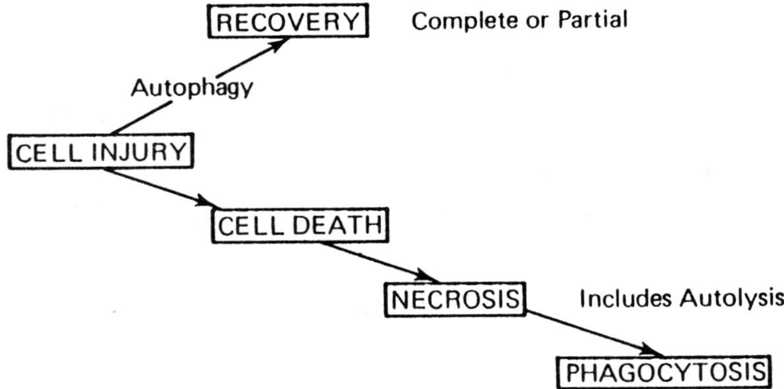

Figure 9-1: Shown are the five types of disruption of the normal structure of muscle and the types of myofiber breakdown. Essentially, the figure lists alternative histopathological events after cellular injury. At the bottom, following cell injury, the events would lead to cell death which ends up in necrosis and finally includes autolysis. In the contrary event, the disease process through autophagy of damaged cells through a scavenging process would lead to a complete or partial recovery. (From Cullen MJ, et al: *Ann NY Acad Sci* 317:440–463, 1979.[47])

There is a sharp boundary between the area of necrotic muscle and the advanced line of the inflammatory cells. Certain changes in the cellular milieu have to occur or do occur before the phagocytes can invade a necrotic area. This necessary condition may be the achievement of ionic equilibrium between the dying muscle cell and the extracellular space, a suggestion that is supported by the obvious swelling of the fiber in the necrotic area.

Role of lysosomes is an essential part of the armamentarium of macrophages and other phagocytic cells that digest necrotic areas of muscle. Any contribution by lysosomes originating in the muscle to its own breakdown is probably very small, because the activity of lysosomal enzymes in muscle compared with other tissues is known to be low and, also, when conditions have been reached at which lysosomal enzymes may escape to the general cell cytoplasm, other more drastic events are likely to have overtaken the muscle fiber.

Possible role for calcium ions in myofiber breakdown. Calcium is generally known to have been termed as the "molecular assassin" in injured muscle fibers. This expressive phrase stems from calcium's central role in the muscle contraction-relaxation cycle such that any disruption in the normal distribution of calcium ions would have drastic and, probably, irreversible effects on the muscle.

In normal relaxed mammalian muscle, the calcium ion concentration in the sarcoplasm is about 10^{-7} to 10^{-8} M, which is three to four orders of magnitude lower than in the extracellular space. Muscle sarcomeres contract in the presence of ATP when the calcium ion concentration in the sarcoplasm is elevated to 10^{-5} to 10^{-6} M, which removes the troponin-tropomyosin inhibition and allows actin and myosin to interact. Therefore, when the calcium ion concentration in muscle sarcoplasm reaches equilibrium with that outside the muscle cell, the sarcomeres will contract and, unless the calcium ions are removed, will stay contracted.

Cullen et al.[47] suggest that a structural defect in the plasma membrane that allowed an uncontrolled entry of extracellular fluid could be a primary event in the course of muscle fiber breakdown (Figure 9-2). A recent x-ray microanalytic study of elemental concentrations in normal and diseased human muscles has shown some possible ionic changes in the diseased muscle. An elevated calcium to phosphorus ratio was found in both myonuclei and

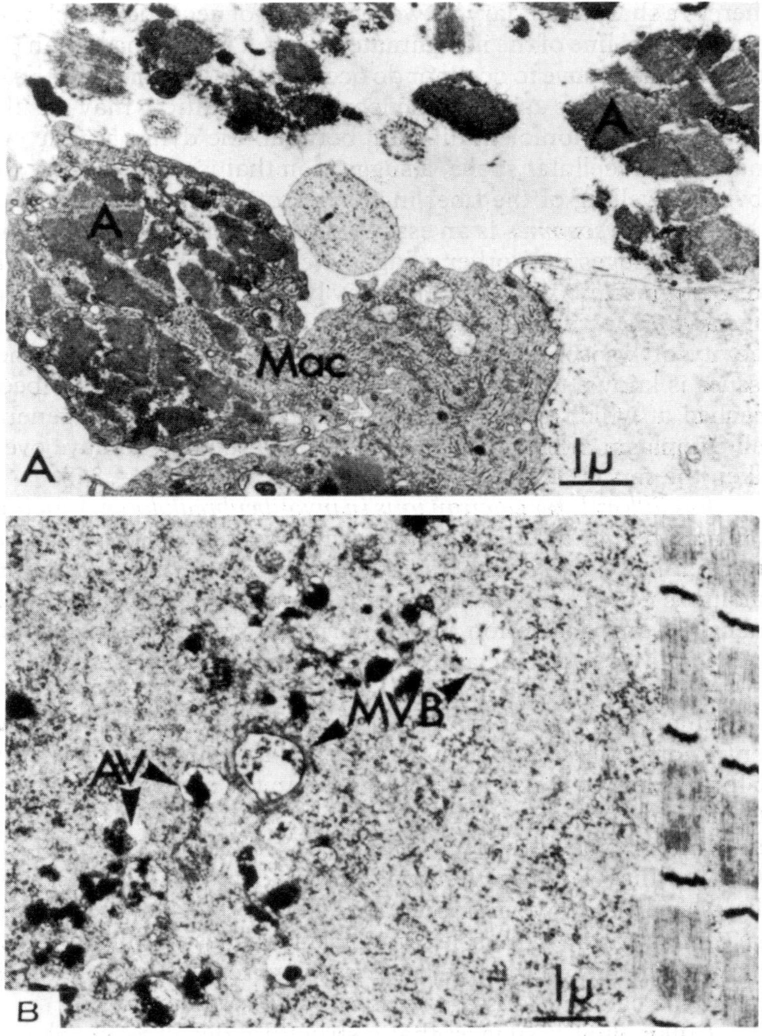

FIGURE 9-2: A: Indicates macrophages in a necrotic muscle fiber in which the myofibrils have broken down. **B:** Longitudinal section through part of the soleus muscle of a rat 7 days after injury. To the right, the structure of the fiber is normal, while to the left is an area of extensive disruption that contains multivesicular bodies (MVB), autophagic vacuoles (AV), and other secondary lysosomes. (A: × 90,000, B: × 10,000). (From Cullen MJ, et al: *Ann NY Acad Sci* 317:440–463, 1979.[47])

interstitial cell nuclei in the diseased muscle compared with normal muscle.

A hypothesis that suggests that muscle cell necrosis is a result of an increased influx of calcium and subsequent organelle overloading has been proposed by Wrogemann and Pena.[301] They suggest that a plasma membrane defect allows an increased net influx of calcium into the cell. This excessive calcium is sequestered by mitochondria, but massive overloading caused functional and structural damage to these organelles. Elevation of the free cytoplasmic calcium levels will thus occur, causing overcontraction and cellular death.

Based on the foregoing data, Cullen et al.[47] conclude that there is good morphological evidence for the presence of lysosomes (in the form of autophagic vacuoles, lipofuscin granules, and multivesicular components broken down in these lysosomes). These authors therefore support the suggestion that in an atrophic muscle, the myofilaments are probably first disassembled by a calcium-activated extralysosomal protease, before being further hydrolyzed in muscle lysosomes.

Supporting this suggestion, several lines of evidence show that calcium ion concentration rises significantly within the fibers in necrotic muscle. This rise may result from an alteration in muscle cell membrane. The consequences may be twofold: an uncontrolled overcontraction of the myofibrils and/or activation of the sarcoplasmic protease capable of disassembling the filaments. The subsequent breakdown of muscle contractive proteins is largely accomplished by inflammatory cells, and any contribution by lysosomes that originates in the muscle is probably minimal.

10

Traumatic Rhabdomyolysis: Its Relation to Shock and Crush Syndrome—Experimental Studies

Traumatic Rhabdomyolysis

A primary consideration in experimental study of natural phenomena is that the reproduction of the phenomena under controllable conditions shall resemble as closely as possible the occurrences in nature. This is a consideration which has been largely neglected, it seems to me, in experimental investigations of shock.
(Walter B. Cannon, Traumatic Shock, *1923, p 142)*

In 1923, Walter B. Cannon[33] in his classic book *Traumatic Shock* stated: "None of the theories thus far discussed has offered a satisfactory account of the *initiation* of secondary shock. The problem still requires the demonstration of some factor, naturally related to the onset of shock, which may so operate in the body that, when hemorrhage and infection are ruled out, the persistent low blood pressure characteristic of the shock state will become gradually established" (Figure 10-1).

In 1918 Cannon, while working with Bayliss, explored the question of whether a toxic substance develops in injured tissues which might be a contributory factor in the production of shock as seen in man.

To that effect "in order to bring about in lower animals a traumatization similar to that giving rise to shock in man, thigh muscles in the anesthetized cat, while being supported by an iron block, were repeatedly struck with a blunt wedge-shaped hammer or crushed by compression." After crushing the muscles in one hind leg of the cat, "for about 20 minutes (and still longer in the dog), the pressure would begin to fall; after about an hour the pressure has usually fallen to 80 mmHg or even lower, that is, to a shock level. There it persisted for several hours. In other words, a general bodily condition resembling shock was produced by duplicating circumstances which induced shock in man." The only notable difference was the presence of anesthesia. "That this is not a determining factor was shown by use of a controllable anesthetic, such as ether, which may be lightened as the animal falls in deeper and deeper insensibility. The lessening of the ether concentration under these circumstances did not improve the circulation."

In order to rule out the possibility of the fall of blood pressure as due to the loss of blood in limbs by damaged tissues, Cannon and his associates have tested this point by removing *post mortem*, symmetrical segments of the two hind legs, one normal and the other injured, and then weighing them. The difference of weight, which in some instances was only 10% of the estimated blood volume, "was not considered to represent enough extravasated blood to account for the fall of pressure." It was then surmised or admitted, however, that loss of blood by extravasation, even when slight, may play a role in the subsequent development of the low pressure. To further rule out the possibility of a neurogenic cause of the shock resulting from the trauma to the nerves of the limb, the section of the spinal cord or of the nerve had been carried out and it was clear that there was no essential relation between the production of shock and excessive stimulation of the central ner-

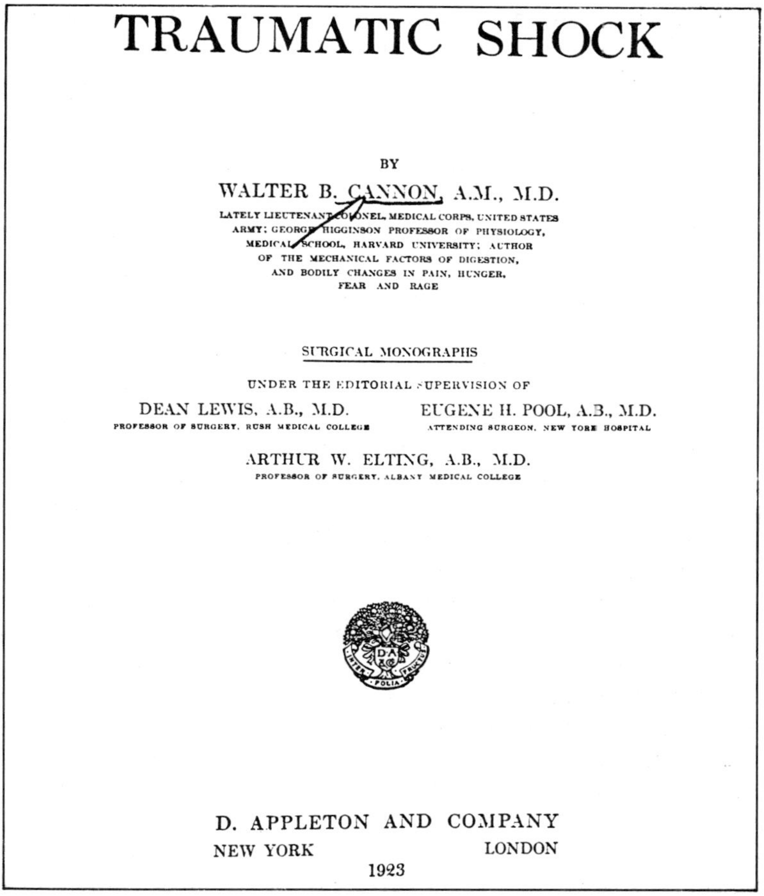

TRAUMATIC SHOCK

BY

WALTER B. CANNON, A.M., M.D.

LATELY LIEUTENANT-COLONEL, MEDICAL CORPS, UNITED STATES ARMY; GEORGE HIGGINSON PROFESSOR OF PHYSIOLOGY, MEDICAL SCHOOL, HARVARD UNIVERSITY; AUTHOR OF THE MECHANICAL FACTORS OF DIGESTION, AND BODILY CHANGES IN PAIN, HUNGER, FEAR AND RAGE

SURGICAL MONOGRAPHS

UNDER THE EDITORIAL SUPERVISION OF

DEAN LEWIS, A.B., M.D.
PROFESSOR OF SURGERY, RUSH MEDICAL COLLEGE

EUGENE H. POOL, A.B., M.D.
ATTENDING SURGEON, NEW YORK HOSPITAL

ARTHUR W. ELTING, A.B., M.D.
PROFESSOR OF SURGERY, ALBANY MEDICAL COLLEGE

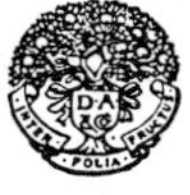

D. APPLETON AND COMPANY
NEW YORK LONDON
1923

Figure 10-1: This is the title page of the book *Traumatic Shock* by Walter B. Cannon, published by Appleton in 1923.[33] This book includes, among other problems, the methods of production of shock by crushing of the muscles as indicated in this text.

vous system. In addition, other factors such as fat embolism and acapnia were ruled out and the cause of shock further narrowed to the trauma of the soft tissues, namely skin, subcutaneous tissue, and specifically to the muscles. This conclusion was confirmed by Cannon[33] and Bayliss by producing shock by muscle injury without acapnia, while breathing was kept uniform by artificial means.

"If the low pressure resulting from local trauma was not due to loss of blood into the injured region, or to fat emboli, or acapnia, or to effects of the nervous system, the connection between the general bodily states and the local damage was reasonably looked upon for the remaining great connecting system, the circulation."

Having ruled out the various possibilities, it still had to be proven that from the traumatized tissue a factor was carried by the circulatory system to the rest of the body proving to be toxic and disturbing to the control of the blood pressure. This idea was then readily tested.

"The blood vessels of the leg (iliac artery and vein) were tied, and the muscles were then crushed. In the experiment thus carried out, the blood vessels of the leg were tied before the muscles were smashed and the ligatures were left in place for 33 minutes after the trauma. The record showed that there was no drop of blood pressure during this period although in the cat the arterial pressure usually begins to fall about 20 minutes after the injury. As soon as the blood flow was restored, however, the pressure promptly fell to a low level"[33] (from Figure 16 in *Traumatic Shock* by W.B. Cannon; see Figures 10-2 and 10-3).

"This phenomenon could be explained on the assumption that the pressure-lowering substance passes from the traumatized region to the rest of the body by way of the circulation when the blood flow" was again restored. The inference just set forth receives support from experiments in which the muscle was injured and, while the pressure was falling, the vessels of the leg (the iliac artery and vein) were closed. As soon as this was carried out, there was a progressive rise of pressure to the normal level (Figure 15 in Cannon[33]). If the injury is not great, the blood pressure, after falling for a while, may be spontaneously restored. However, the evidence indicates that whatever may be the substance originating in the damaged tissues, it was fairly promptly changed in the body or eliminated so that the effect was not permanent. Further confirmation of the inference that the pressure-lowering material is given off from injured tissues was obtained by massage of the traumatized region. The result was a further drop in pressure."

Figure 15 from his article indicates a fall of blood pressure after muscle injury though the nerves to this injured limb had been cut (Figure 10-4). Rise of blood pressure to the original level after placing a clip on the blood vessels to and from the injured region is obvious in this experiment.

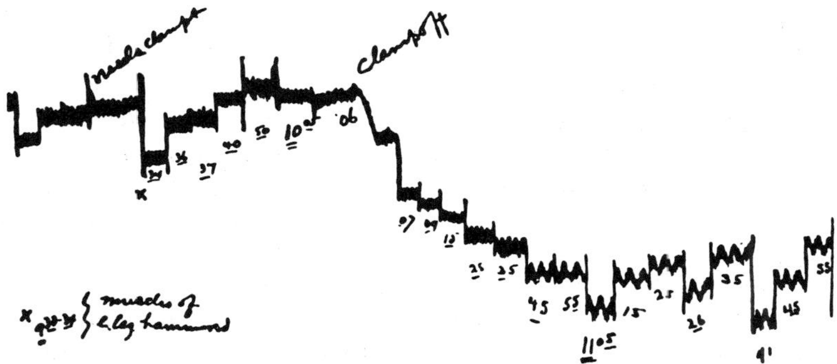

Figure 10-2: This graph depicts the results of an experiment in which Cannon recorded "failure of blood pressure to fall at the usual time after muscle injury if the blood vessels to the injured region have been tied. On restoration of the blood flow (at 10:07), the pressure promptly falls." (From *Traumatic Shock*, by Walter B. Cannon.[33])

The conclusion arrived at by Cannon and Bayliss at the time was that following trauma of the soft tissues of the hind limb of the cat or dog, a toxic substance is produced which is subsequently carried by the blood vessels into the systemic circulation and induces a fall in blood pressure and a consistent state of shock as seen in humans. However, if the blood vessels shortly after the production of the shock are tied or clamped, there is a restoration

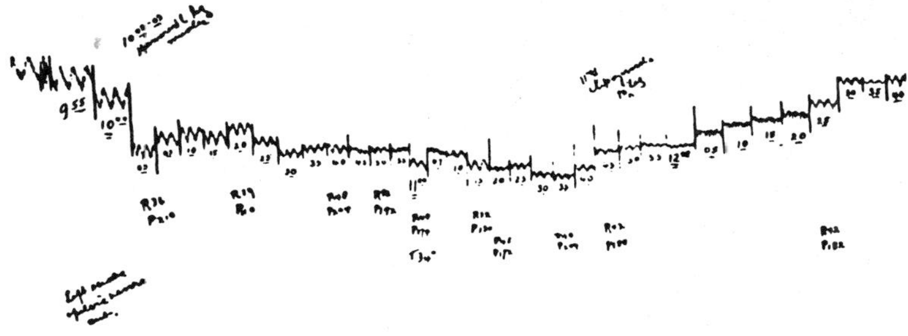

Figure 10-3: This figure depicts the fall of blood pressure after muscle injury (at 10:02–03) though the nerves to the injured limb had been cut, and the rise of blood pressure to the original level after placing a clip (at 11:41) on the blood vessels to and from the injured region. (From Cannon WB: *Traumatic Shock*. Appleton, New York, 1923.[34])

of the blood pressure to the pre-trauma level which would indicate that the release of the toxic substance into the systemic circulation had been stopped.

Further evidence supporting the inference that damaged tissue itself induces shock has been obtained by McIver (personal communication to Cannon and quoted by him[33]). This experiment consisted of a cross-circulation between two animals, A and B. He crushed the muscles of the hind legs in animal A; after an interval varying from 20 to 30 minutes, the blood pressure began to fall in animal B and continued onward until it reached the shock level. Similar experimental work has led to the same conclusion by Cannon and Bayliss.

Clinical Observations

The shock-producing effect of substance(s) which may arise from the injured or crushed muscles in humans was the subject of investigation during World War I. The above-mentioned experiments performed by Cannon which supported the view that the injured striated muscle played a major role in inducing shock appeared to be corroborated by the experiences acquired on the battlefield.

Indeed, paralleling Cannon's experimental studies, during the same period clinical observations by Quenu,[231] a French surgeon, together with his team of surgeons, reached similar conclusions regarding the toxic factor in shock. They demonstrated clearly the association of shock with extensive damage of muscles or multiple wounds scattered over the body. Their clinical observations, among other findings, led to three important conclusions: (1) everything that favors absorption of substances at the site of injury favors the development of shock; (2) conversely, anything that delays or prevents absorption from the injured region delays its development; and (3) if there is a sudden removal of the device which checks absorption such as a tourniquet, serious results followed, leading to "toxemia" and death. As long as the tourniquet remained in place above or proximal to the injured area, such phenomena failed to develop. But, shortly after its removal, by accident or unawareness of its significance, patients would go into shock and die within a matter of a few hours.

Another observation of great significance made during this

period was that if removal of the injured lesion is not too long delayed, avoidance of shock could be achieved. Thus, when a quick amputation of a lacerated muscular region was possible, the operation was commonly followed by a remarkable improvement, so rapid and striking that it appeared to be a direct sequel to the removal of the damaged limb. The time interval between the muscle injury and the removal of damaged tissues was of great import. Thus, mortality was only 11% when the amputation was performed in the first 3 hours, close to 37% if there was delay of between 3 and 6 hours, and 75% in the eighth and ninth hours. These figures, reported by the French team, as Cannon stated, vividly illustrated what was reasonably to be expected if time was given both for disintegration of damaged tissue and the absorption of toxic material.

Civilian Skeletal Muscle Ischemia

The history of acute skeletal muscle ischemia following injuries in civilian and war conditions most likely has remained unreported until the beginning of this century. Thus, von Colmer[42] is credited to have been the first in 1909 to have described civilian crushing injuries as a result of traumatic lesions during the Messina earthquake of December, 1908. In his report of 1909, although describing what appears to be a crush syndrome, he failed to mention anuria associated with the trauma. Later, Frankenthal[82] in 1916 was first to report muscle necrosis in soldiers, buried due to mine explosions, and noted bloody discolorations of the urine in two of the cases.

During the same period, Minami[191] summarized the experience observed in Germany by several military surgeons concerning renal damage and urinary discoloration associated with severe muscle injuries.

Civilian casualties resulting from traffic accidents were initially reported in 1937 by Husfeldt and Bjering.[134] They were described as renal lesions due to traumatic shock. Shortly afterward, McClelland[180] also reported three cases of anuria after mining accidents.

Despite these isolated cases, this syndrome did not become well known until Bywaters[31] and others published a larger clinical experience with such cases during the "Battle of Britain" in 1940–

1942. Gilmour[89] is generally credited for having suggested in 1941 that the urinary pigment noted by many investigators of patients with crush syndrome was myoglobin. Shortly thereafter this was confirmed spectroscopically by Bywaters and co-workers to be in fact myoglobin.

The description of the crush syndrome and the nature of the urinary pigment brings us back to World War I in connection with Cannon's work on "traumatic shock."

Bywaters,[31] in his classic paper of 1944, "Ischemic Muscle Necrosis," reflecting on the findings in the "crush syndrome," states perhaps intuitively and philosophically "was this not the same 'shock' that had been seen in World War I when Cannon and his associates described cases with hemoconcentration?" As has been reviewed earlier in this monograph, Cannon's experimental method for inducing "shock" consisted indeed of "crushing" (his word) the skeletal muscles and recording their effects on blood pressure and other hemodynamics. An important conclusion by Cannon was that the "traumatic shock" induced by the crushing of the muscles was *not* due to loss of blood but possibly to a "toxic factor," the nature of which remained not entirely elucidated at that time.

Without further analysis of the historical role of a traumatized or crushed skeletal muscle in inducing "shock" as seen during World War I and the clinicopathological manifestations of the "crush syndrome" as seen since World War II, it is overwhelmingly obvious that *the acute ischemia of the muscle is at the center of the pathogenesis of these entities*.

The lessons from these experimental and clinical observations from World War I reported by Cannon and other physiologists and surgeons had been rather forgotten during World War II when the crush syndrome was described. Of course, the identification of the biochemical factors and the metabolic changes secondary to the trauma of the striated muscles leading to renal complications described in 1940–1942 provided the current basis of the pathogenesis for this complex syndrome.

The original experiments carried out during WWI have largely been unnoticed or ignored by subsequent investigators during WWII and after. The fundamental difference between the WWI experiment and that of the WWII was that the toxic substance suspected by Cannon and by others could not be identified biochemically, while during WWII several biochemical substances were identified. Myoglobin, one of the first to be recognized, was not in itself the "toxic" factor responsible for shock. Indeed, from the traumatized muscle were released other substances which could account for the lowering of the blood pressure. These were clarified later, after World War II, when these biochemical studies had delved into areas other than the myoglobin released from traumatized muscular fibers. The nature of the toxic factor remained elusive. One fact appeared clear, however, that the so-called toxic substances released from the traumatized muscle were the cause of the lowering of the blood pressure to the shock level. In modern times, in spite of the fact that these had not been entirely identified or elucidated, it is quite clear that the traumatized muscle was the source of these hemodynamic alterations following its crushing.

Because of the persisting controversies over the mechanism of traumatic shock, it is important to point out that Cannon's major goal, as he himself clearly described earlier, was to identify the toxic factor responsible for the *initiation* related to the onset of shock. The subsequent events were to involve multiple organs due to the interaction with many other biological factors. As recently as 1983, Blaisdell,[18] in trying to define the toxic factor of traumatic shock, felt that the damaged tissue itself constitutes the toxic factor in traumatic shock. He further felt that fragments of damaged tissue enter the blood stream and through other mechanisms set off additional manifestations of the late phase of traumatic shock.

Later Laboratory Experiments

Confirming and expanding this problem to a large extent were the studies by Duncan and Blalock[62] who, in 1942, have shown that uniform production of experimental shock can be readily induced in crushing large muscular masses. The goal of this study was an attempt to reproduce experimentally the so-called crush syndrome which had been observed during 1941 and 1942 in the Battle of Britain. The laboratory method consisted of compressing the extremity of the dogs used in this experiment. After various attempts, they adopted the use of a press which exerted an even pressure resulting in a consistent greater injury to the tissues of the thigh by means of a 500-pound pressure applied for a period of 5 hours.

Results

The results of the experiments were divided into: (1) crush for a period of 5 hours of compression of the extremity; (2) the period following release of compression, with no therapy being employed (half of the experiments); (3) the period following release of compression with pressured therapy (half of the experiments).

During the *crush period*, there was no significant change in blood pressure in any of the animals. The significant findings were: an average fall in plasma creatinine of .69 mg %, and an average increase of plasma creatine of .48 mg %. Nonprotein nitrogen values increased an average of 4.05 mg %. Microscopic examination showed red blood cells in the urine in every case within 2 to 3 hours after the press was applied. The *benzidine reaction* became positive in 2 to 3 hours. Albumin was present in the urine in 2 to 4 hours. Except for the urinary findings, the alterations in most of the functions were minimal.

Release of Crush Without Therapy

In 19 experiments after release of the press, the animal was observed but no therapy was applied. All animals died except one.

Upon removal of the press, there was a sudden sharp decline in blood pressure to 50 to 60 mmHg with subsequent progressive decline. Hemoconcentration of red blood cells occurred as soon as the press was removed with an average rise of 44% over the control values from 2 to 6 hours. The average survival in this group was 7.55 hours. Urinary changes were significant. It usually became grossly bloody within an hour after the press was removed, with an output during a 2 to 6 hour period averaging 3.3 cc. Although granular and red blood cell casts were frequently found, the dark variety described in clinical cases of crush injury were not observed. In three dogs of this group, in which blood and urinary chemical changes were present, plasma creatine, creatinine, and nonprotein nitrogen were all increased while urinary creatinine decreased.

A Release of Crush with Therapy

There were 21 experiments in which, following the removal of the press, a pneumatic rubber cuff was applied to the injured thigh at a pressure of 40 mmHg. When the cuff was applied for a period of 13 hours, three of six animals died. When the time of application was increased to 18 hours, three of 15 died. The average survival time of these six animals was 26.3 hours. The average fall in blood pressure of the entire group in the first 4 to 6 hours was 16.9 mmHg. Hematocrit volumes increased in this same period an average 28.5% over the control values.

Just as in the untreated group, the urine became discolored and showed gross blood within 1 hour after the press was removed. The average urinary output for the same period of time was 36.2 cc. On microscopic examination of urine, several animals showed granular and red blood cell casts and then occasional hyaline casts. The two animals of this group showed in the urine large dark brown granular casts which were similar in appearance to those described in clinical cases of crush injury. The urinary creatine output averaged 3.67 mg per cc. The creatinine output showed an average decrease of 0.27 mg per cc. Plasma creatine increased an average of 3.60 mg % and plasma creatinine, an average of .57 mg %.

Pathological Changes

The pathological changes in the treated group of animals which ultimately succumbed were as a rule more marked than those of the untreated group, probably because duration of life was longer and there was a longer period of time in which anoxia could exert all its effects. Among the visceral involvements, it is significant that microscopic examination showed engorgement of the glomerular capillaries with extravasation of blood into Bowman's capsules. The collecting tubules in many areas were dilated but empty and the lining epithelium was flat. No large brown casts were found. The injured extremity revealed massive swelling of the thigh and to a lesser extent of the leg and foot.

Discussion

The injury that occurred was a crush of large masses of skeletal muscles. Shortly after the release of that compression, signs of shock with renal failure developed. Evidence of plasma loss was demonstrated by the marked increase in concentration of red blood corpuscles which invariably occurred.

In the animals that were successfully treated by application of the pneumatic cuff, there was comparatively little swelling of the injured extremity at the time of removal of the cuff after 13 or 18 hours. In the animals that died in spite of treatment, comparison of the weight of the injured and uninjured side showed a fluid loss as great as that of the untreated group. *The beneficial effect of the pneumatic cuff would appear to be due chiefly to its role in lessening local fluid loss into the extremity.*

The urinary changes in these experiments are of interest. Blood was present on microscopic examination of the urine, within 2 to 3 hours after the press was applied. Gross blood was present in the urine within an hour after the press was removed. A peculiar brownish discoloration of the urine was often noted during the period following removal of the press. Oliguria was observed in all experiments and was most severe in the untreated animals and in those that died in spite of treatment, that is to say, those animals in which shock was most profound. The oliguria was due at least in part to the physiological imbalances accompanying shock: diminished blood volume and flow, depression of blood pressure, and hemoconcentration. Granular and red blood cell casts were frequently found and occasionally hyaline casts were noted, but in no animals of the untreated group and in only two of the treated group were large brown granular casts observed. In these two animals histologic examination did not show selective tubular changes and the casts which had been described in clinical cases of crush injury. Had the length of life been greater, it is possible that this observation would have been made more often. Urine benzidine reaction was negative in the control animals and positive within 4 to 6 hours after the press was removed. It was positive *in all* of these animals with positive presence of albumin.

Elevated blood creatine levels and the creatinuria had been observed in several types of muscular diseases. Aub and Wu[7] have reported an increase in blood creatine following injuries to muscles. The values obtained in the present experiments are high and are suggestve of severe muscle damage. Marked disturbance of creatine–creatinine ratios in blood and urine were observed. The levels are higher in the plasma of the untreated group than in that of the treated group, and higher in urine of the treated group than in that of the untreated group. These observations may indicate failure of excretion of excessive creatine because of diminished renal function. Destruction of renal function in itself would produce an elevation of blood creatine. Further evidence of diminished renal function in tissue injury is presented by the progressive rise in nonprotein nitrogen seen in all experiments.

In the conclusion of this interesting experimental study of traumatic shock, the authors state: "Whether the experimental conditions have any relationship to the crush syndrome as observed in patients remained to be proved, but it can be stated that the use of this method results in a more uniform production of traumatic shock than any with which we have worked."

Comment

In this author's opinion, the results revealed by this experimental study had more significance than that of a simple technique for reproducing shock, as originally assumed by the investigators. One of the highlights hardly underscored was the fact that the urine contained, in addition to red cells, a benzidine-positive pigment which was later identified as being characteristic for myoglobin. They attributed the latter positive test only to hemoglobin. Had the authors pursued the biochemical identification of this pigment, they probably would have been among the first to show the biochemical characteristic of the substance observed in the urine. As far as the renal tubules are concerned, their observations were perhaps not sufficiently long to allow them to induce renal tubular necrosis as one of the complications of the traumatic shock or crush syndrome.

Subsequent studies—both clinical and experimental—provided sufficient evidence for the underlying biochemical aspects of the crush syndrome described by Bywaters during WWII, as well as the hemodynamics and pathological findings described by Cannon during WWI.

11

Ischemic Muscle Necrosis: The Crush Syndrome

The Crush Syndrome

In 1940, during the air blitz of Great Britain, particularly in London, a great number of patients with a history of burial beneath debris for several hours were seen as a result of compression of a limb by fallen masonry. While a number of these patients showed mild or relatively insignificant symptoms, others developed oliguria and died in uremia with pathological changes seen primarily in the kidneys. The original impression from these cases was that the patients presented a clinical entity akin to "shock." It was found out shortly thereafter that the clinical syndrome of shock was only a part of several other components which set in motion multi-organ complications.

While such accidents were seen occasionally in civil practice, this condition seen during the Battle of Britain seems to have been unrecognized up to that point in the English-speaking countries. Thus, in Germany during World War I, this condition was recognized and in 1916 Frankenthal[82] described muscle necrosis in soldiers buried as a result of mine explosions. Similar observations were also recorded by von Colmers[42] in 1910 in civilian accidents that occurred during the Messina earthquake. It appears probable that this condition occurred in World War I but was not recognized as such except for the traumatic shock described by Cannon as previously discussed.

Bywaters[31] gave a comprehensive description in his 1944 paper published in *JAMA* indicating that the patients, after release from the compression, developed a syndrome which since then has been known as crush syndrome. Indeed, soon after the patients had been freed from the masonry debris, it was noted that their limbs became swollen and hard. Of interest was that no subcutaneous pitting edema was present since most of the fluid was almost entirely beneath the deep fascia. It became obvious subsequently that this extravasation of plasma or blood was confined primarily to the muscular masses. As a result of the leakage of plasma and blood to the damaged blood vessels, particularly to the capillaries and to the extravascular tissue spaces, was a major pathological finding which explained to a great extent the hypotension in which these patients were found at that moment. Indeed, the blood pressure fell to levels of 60 to 80 mm systolic or even lower and the blood was found concentrated with hemoglobin levels of 140% to 160% per 100 cc. This level of low blood pressure due to oligemia was consistent with shock as described previously. Restraining the local loss by bandaging or by plaster as shown by several authors and especially by the experimental evidence as shown by Duncan and Blalock[62] as described above. While such measures may have halted the plasma leakage after several hours, recovery of the loss of plasma and blood necessitated plasma transfusion in order to maintain blood pressure at the normal level for the first day and for the same purpose a continuous infusion was necessary.

At the level of the injury of the limb, edema increased either spontaneously or following intravenous fluid. Occasionally, fasciotomy was carried out along the course of the artery resulting in much serous fluid seeping from the wound and showing the pale necrotic muscle bulging out.

Of great significance from a pathological and prognostic point of view was the condition of the renal function in these patients. On admission, the urine pH was as low as 4.6 and displayed dark brown sediment of acid hematin granules. This pigment was not hemoglobin and after centrifuging the urine, the latter showed benzidine-positive urine as has been demonstrated by Duncan and Blalock in their experiments. The urinary output decreased progressively in the very seriously injured patients to the point that at the end of the first week, only 25 to 50 cc in 24 hours were being passed. Subsequently, evidence of severe tubular dysfunction became obvious. The exact mechanism of the tubular necrosis was not evident at that point in the description of the renal damage.

In conjunction with the general condition of the patient, it is important to note that there was marked retention of nitrogen and that the patient had become drowsy, occasionally anxious and apprehensive. These symptoms were characteristic of shock as well. Among other findings, the serum carbon dioxide combining power was low after release from the compression as a result of the liberation of lactic and other acids from the damaged muscle. The outcome of the severely injured patients was that one-third of these casualties went on to recovery while two-thirds died toward the end of the first week. Death was sudden and preceded by cardiac arrhythmias. Of interest was that the T-waves were increased indicating what was later known to be due to hyperkalemia. Insulin and dextrose were given to those patients with raised blood potassium and increased T-wave height. The therapeutic lowering of potassium levels may be found useful in cases where there are indications of improving renal function, such as an increase in output in urea concentration.

From a pathological point of view, Bywaters stresses the essential lesion of crushing injury in the muscle to be necrosis. This may be due to the ischemia of direct compression or it may be due to the ischemia from interference with the main arterial supply, by sudden spasm, thrombosis, rupture, or obstruction.

The treatment of these cases was somewhat similar to what is being done today in shock or the crush syndrome. It consisted of administration of fluid and alkali, such as sodium bicarbonate, the treatment of shock consisting of hydration and alkalinization as already mentioned above in order to overcome the "oligemic shock" although the blood pressure remains normal for a time because of vasoconstriction. Local treatment of course of the injured limb should be kept cool if possible with ice bags as this will decrease the rate of autolysis and also allow living tissue to survive on a low margin of blood supply. Immobilization may prove to be a useful measure especially if fractures are also present. Amputation was also considered if the leg was severely damaged and was the source of the metabolic changes that they noticed. The value of tight bandaging is uncertain while it will decrease the severity of shock by limiting fluid loss as shown by Duncan and Blalock; observations have yet to be made of its effect both on the kidneys and on the residual local lesions. This was the statement made earlier by Bywaters and it may have gained some validity in certain cases in the later concept of treatment of these patients. Regarding treatment concerning cases with established renal failure, insulin and dextrose proved to be of some value in some cases where hyperkalemia was present but did not help too much without hemodialysis of the present-day therapy in such cases.

The contributions made by Bywaters and the British team working at the same time deserve credit for having obtained evidence of the biochemical changes as a result of skeletal muscle damage. As stated earlier, the evidence produced by "traumatization" that Cannon and Bayliss have obtained in their experiments in which they produced shock is to some extent similar to what Bywaters and the British team have observed from the injuries of the skeletal muscles observed in the Battle of Britain. It is difficult to differentiate biologically what was meant by traumatic shock as described by Cannon in the initial stages of this process and that of crush syndrome seen also in the initial symptoms and signs that were seen subsequently during the blitz on London or other parts of Great Britain. The biochemical findings of the crush syndrome have been of great impetus in the study of traumatic shock and other conditions that had been observed in civilian patients, such as acute arterial occlusions and vascular trauma, as well as other nontraumatic lesions in which the rhabdomyolytic process dominated as the initiating cause of these changes. The pathogenesis of myoglobinuria and other biochemical changes which occur as a result of the traumatic lesions of the muscles remain to be analyzed and explained. The next few sections will attempt to answer these questions.

Observations on the Liberation and Elimination of Myohemoglobin and of Hemoglobin After Release of Muscle Ischemia

Without going into a detailed history of this syndrome, the first civilian casualties demonstrating the crush syndrome were described by Husfeldt[134] in 1937, the entity having been called then "traumatic anuria." Shortly afterward, McClelland,[180] Glenn,[88] and later Bywaters and others used the same terminology. Despite some isolated cases reported earlier in World War II, this syndrome did not become well known and well understood until a large clinical experience had accumulated from casualties trapped beneath masonry and rubble during the Battle of Britain in 1940. It was Gilmour[87] who suggested in 1941 that the urinary pigment observed by numerous investigators in patients with the crush syndrome could be myoglobin. Bywaters and co-workers demonstrated then spectroscopically that the pigment in the urine from such casualties was in fact myoglobin. Few investigations were carried out to elucidate the mechanism of liberation and excretion of this pigment.

Montagnani and Simeone[193] have reported experiments in 1953 describing in detail the time relationships regarding the appearance of myoglobin in body fluids after release of limb ischemia.

The experiments were carried out in dogs, using rubber tube tourniquets placed across the thigh and hip either in unilateral or bilateral studies. The tourniquets were released after a period of ischemia lasting from 4 to 7 ¼ hours.

In summarizing their findings and conclusions, the authors stated:

"1. After release of arterial tourniquets which maintaned limb ischemia for 4–7 ¼ hours, myoglobin is liberated from striated muscle into both blood and lymph returning from the extremities and is excreted in the urine.

2. Myoglobin is detectable grossly in the urine within 10 minutes after release of the tourniquets. The pigment is almost always found in blood and lymph in specimens obtained one hour after release of the tourniquets.

3. The peak concentrations of myoglobin appeared in blood and lymph within 2–4 hours after release of the tourniquets.

4. The peak urinary excretion of myoglobin occurred during the second hour after release of the ischemia.

5. No evidence was obtained to suggest that diminution of renal function accompanies application and release of the tourniquets on a reflex nervous basis in the anesthetized experimental animals.

6. Myoglobin is probably one of *many* substances liberated when circulation is reestablished in ischemic striated muscle. Evidence is presented that damage to the glomerulus or other parts of the kidney may result on a humoral basis following the release of limb ischemia."

Therapeutic Attempts to Reduce the Effects of Myoglobinuria in Experimental Crush Syndrome in Dogs

Thompson and Campbell[284] have devised an experimental model in order to "wash out ischemic lower limbs with intra-arterial dextran immediately prior to release of the muscle ischemia in an attempt to obviate the egress of products of ischemic muscle injury into the general circulation."*

The experimental model consisted essentially of two phases:

1. The femoral vessels, artery and vein, were dissected bilaterally and polyethylene cannulae were placed in the femoral vein and artery also bilaterally. A heavy wire tourniquet was slipped under the femoral vessel cannulae and the two ends of the tourniquet were twisted as tightly as possible with pliers. The circulation was occluded to both hind extremities for a period of 4 hours.

2. At the end of this time, the clamps that were placed on the cannulae were removed from the femoral tubing and blood was allowed to circulate through the leg via the cannulae and the femoral vessels. The wire tourniquet was left in place. A similar

*Washout of ischemic limb (perfusion) was also used by Stipa[276] in 1967 and more recently by Esato[73] and other Japanese (1985) investigators.

number of control dogs were used except that the control group received a washout with dextran solution for a period of up to 4 hours.

Without going into the details of these experiments, it is of interest to review their results. It is also important to state that the experiment consisted of attempting to isolate a muscle mass supplied by a single major arterial trunk, the femoral artery, and drained by a single major vein, the femoral. To a considerable extent, this has been achieved successfully in this model.

Using the tourniquets as a crushing agent, the experimental crush syndrome revealed the following:

1. The degree of myoglobinemia;
2. The rise of plasma hemoglobin;
3. The urinary excretion of myoglobin; and
4. The urinary excretion of hemoglobin.

All of these four events following release of limb ischemia are significantly decreased by the perfusion technique.

The scope that the investigators set out to achieve was to wash out the involved extremity with crush of the muscles and the biochemical responses. Although they had not been able to achieve a total washout of the myoglobin or hemoglobin, they had been able, however, to reduce considerably this metabolite of muscle ischemia. Whether this kind of management in patients with rhabdomyolysis and the production of myoglobin and myoglobinuria can be achieved in clinical work is a question of debate. This has not been attempted, however, to my knowledge in clinical work.

In another set of experiments, Synder and Campbell[267] have attempted a different experimental model. This consisted of a cross-circulating set-up between two dogs. Of the many biochemical findings in the perfused animal, it is of interest to note the condition of the kidneys in five dogs expiring after ischemic muscle perfusion revealed hydropic tubular degeneration, and numerous protein casts and peritubular and glomerular vascular engorgement. The kidneys of the surviving dogs 2 weeks postperfusion were normal histologically except for occasional areas of tubular regeneration. The factors that are responsible for tubular damage and crush syndrome were not completely understood. Many authors believed anoxia secondary to renal ischemia was a primary etiological factor, although Powers and his co-workers[229] felt that tubular changes associated with increased vascular resistance and crush syndrome were responsible for the damage and stated that the increased vascular resistance and tubular damage could be obviated by either denervation of the renal pedicle or administration of a ganglionic blocking agent. This was not consistent with findings of Corcoran and Page[43] who have shown that precipitation of hemoglobin and myoglobin in the renal tubules was the etiological factor in renal damage associated with crush syndrome. They produced renal impairment by the injection of bovine myoglobin into aciduric dogs. It is our opinion also based on our histologic data that the findings by Corcoran and Page correspond to what we have obtained in our cases. The overall results of this cross-circulation showed that five of 16 dogs died with hypotension and hyperkalemia, while the kidneys of these dogs showed hydropic tubular degeneration and numerous protein casts. The 11 surviving dogs exhibited a transient impairment of glomerular filtration rate and effective renal blood flow which returned to normal within 2 weeks.

It appears, therefore, from these results that the crush syndrome as produced by the experimental model was not adequate to release enough myoglobin to induce renal changes as anticipated.

Briefly, Thompson and Campbell, and Snyder and Campbell, using the experimental models as described, have reproduced essentially the crush syndrome of declamping hypotension, hyperkalemia, and acute tubular degeneration of the kidneys. Also in the earlier experiments they have shown that by "washing out" the ischemic limbs prior to release of the damaged muscle, they could decrease significantly the degree of myoglobinemia, myoglobinuria, and hemoglobinuria.

More recent studies carried out by Biglioli et al.[14] and Trazzi et al.[285] have shown that the renal function is altered in proportion to the severity of the degree of induced ischemia after revascularization in dogs in which ischemia was induced by a tourniquet applied around the groin or hind limbs.

12

Tourniquet Ischemia: Metabolic Responses

Tourniquet Ischemia

Application of a tourniquet around an extremity for the purpose of temporarily obliterating the arterial and venous flows may induce, among other effects, complex vascular changes associated with metabolic and morphological alterations of the muscles. Recent experimental and human studies have attempted to clarify these features.

Initial Physiopathological Effects

The time safety of tourniquet ischemia, which is a major factor, may be variable in animal experiments as well as in clinical conditions. As a rule, in routine surgical applications, 2 hours of complete tourniquet ischemia have traditionally been considered as safe (Bruner,[25] Chiu et al.,[39] Mullick[198]) except in advanced cases of limb ischemia. If tourniquet ischemia time is extended in certain microsurgical procedures, its safety may also be jeopardized. In such cases its safety could be assessed by the cellular responses, including those of the nerves, vascular bed, and skeletal muscles.

Among the physiopathological effects during the initial ischemic phase, a fall is routinely found in temperature of the skin and muscles of the limb, which become pale and pulseless. In 2 hours, the conventional critical time of tourniquet ischemia, the venous pH falls from 7.4 to 6.9 in a linear fashion to reach a value that is close to that of the intracellular pH. At the same time, the venous PO_2 falls from 45 mmHg to 4 mmHg and the venous PCO_2 rises from 35 to 104 mmHg. As the critical period becomes irreversible, in addition to muscle fatigability, striated muscles rendered ischemic show not only evidence of metabolic changes but also concurrent cell damage alterations. Additionally, there is atrophy of muscle tissue, consisting of a decrease in the content of myosin, water soluble protein, and nonprotein nitrogen.[198]

Prolonged tourniquet ischemia beyond 2 hours of hind limbs of normal anesthetized dogs usually results, after 5 hours, in increased volume of the extremities reaching 100%.

After *release of the tourniquet*, following a 2-hour ischemia, there is a transient increase in the blood flow of the post-ischemic limb, as well as a hyperemic blush irrespective of the length of ischemia. As the pulse returns, the temperature of the skin rises. The venous PO_2 tends to remain equal to the arteriolar PO_2 for a variable period before returning to normal, suggesting little or no diffusion of oxygen across capillary beds. Bypassing of many capillary beds by metarteriolar shunts in the extremities results in little or no capillary filling and even arteriovenous shunting, which is a possible explanation of the hyperemic blush. As the venous pH slowly returns to normal, the blood goes through a hypercoagulable to a hypocoagulable state, with a pH below 7.2, the clotting time being markedly prolonged.[198]

Protection against the effects of prolonged tourniquet ischemia may be obtained conventionally by cooling the limb for half an hour prior to tourniquet application and by administration of heparin just prior to the application or just prior to removal of the tourniquet.* The protective effect of cooling is caused by reduc-

*For more recent developments, Chapter 26, *Role of Free-Radicals in Post-Ischemic Skeletal Muscle Reperfusion Injury*.

tion of tissue metabolism, more rapid restoration of circulation and the equilibrium between the oxygen supply and the oxygen requirement of the tissues. The beneficial effects of hypothermia and heparin, however, are insignificant when the tourniquet is used for a period of 2 hours or less.

Experimental Vascular Responses to Tourniquet Ischemia

These responses have been studied in dogs as well as in smaller animals such as rats. Strock and Majno[275b] have used rats weighing 150 to 250 grams for the experimental use of tourniquet ischemia. In their experiments they maintained the tourniquet for 33 minutes to 8 hours, and the rats were studied after the release of the tourniquet. A marked decrease in capillary filling was observed when the ischemia lasted for 1½ hours. The vessels involved were especially those of the superficial network. With longer periods of ischemia, deeper vessels were also affected. The muscles were much more severely affected, traces of no-reflow being apparent after an ischemic period that was as short as 15 minutes; an ischemic period of 30 minutes created substantial areas of no-reflow, which increased to a maximum after 1 hour of ischemia.

In general, edema of the limb was considerable. In the skin, water content after an ischemia of a 30-minute duration rose to 72.7% and it reached a maximum of 86.5% after 4½ hours. If the ischemic period was any longer, the amount of edema began to decrease. Some edema also developed in the contralateral limb, although it was not grossly noticeable. The edema was less in the muscle and none developed in the contralateral limb. Normal muscle contains 76.5% water; an ischemic insult of 2½ hours caused a small increase to 80.1% and maximal edema developed after an ischemic period of 5½ hours, i.e. 85.4%. At this stage, the edema was grossly obvious.

Histologic changes were minimal since these studies were limited to early stages. Extensive degranulation of mast cells was observed at the time of removal of a tourniquet in place for 30 minutes. Of interest was the observation of very few platelet thrombi in small veins. The size of injury in muscle fibers became apparent after one-half hour of ischemia and less than 5 minutes of re-flow. However, there were scattered areas of muscle necrosis in sections taken 5 hours after a 2½ hour ischemic insult.

Muscle Metabolism During Ischemia

In the muscle upon release of the tourniquet after 2½ hours, there is no re-flow at all, only the major vessels of the limb were found patent. Fifteen minutes later the injected carbon reached the small arteries and arterioles as well as occasional capillaries. At 30 minutes, some areas of no re-flow persisted together with areas of good perfusion; at 2 hours, the results were essentially the same. Heparin was found to be of little or no value in preventing post-ischemic injury. Thus, in post-ischemic muscle, the blood flow is so sluggish in many areas that the capillaries become more susceptible to microembolization where vascular leakage is a relatively minor problem.

Metabolic changes may be noted within approximately 2 hours, which is the critical period of ischemia. In assessing the ischemic damage during the tourniquet application to skeletal muscle by CPK levels in the femoral venous blood, Chiu et al.[39] have shown that its elevation becomes apparent within 2–3 hours of the occlusion. These results were obtained in anesthetized dogs, with a pneumatic tourniquet applied to a hind limb for 1, 2, or 3 hours.

After tourniquet release, resulting ischemic damage to skeletal muscle was assessed by the level of creatine phosphokinase (CPK) in femoral venous blood. Skeletal muscle injury, as measured by the level of venous CPK elevation, becomes apparent after 2 to 3 hours of occlusion, but can be prevented by short periods of recirculation. This experimental finding may have a clinical application during the use of a tourniquet during surgical procedures.

During human operations, Haljamae and Enger[114] have shown that CPK levels in the muscle decreased by 40% within 30 to 60 minutes and by 60% after 60 to 90 minutes. In prolonged tourniquet ischemia, restoration of flow may remain impaired especially due to thrombosis in the microcirculation of the muscle which may account for distal gangrene in spite of patency return to the main arterial tree.

Focusing their investigation on the energy metabolism during and after complete tourniquet ischemia, they have shown that cellular deterioration and its reversibility on human skeletal muscle occur as determined by needle biopsies during operations in a bloodless field. The tissue levels of high energy phosphates and glycolytic metabolites were analyzed after various times of tourniquet ischemia and compared to contralateral control extremity levels. In the ischemic extremity, the phosphocreatine (CrP) levels decreased by 40% within 30 to 60 minutes and after 60 to 90 minutes a 60% reduction was found. No significant ATP changes occurred. Lactate levels increased by 225% after 30 to 60 minutes and by 300% after 60 to 90 minutes. The glucose and the G-6-P levels increased slightly and indicated glycogenolysis. The rate of the metabolic changes decreased with ischemia time. In the control leg, no significant metabolic changes could be seen. After the release of the tourniquet there was a rapid restoration of the phosphagen content, and clearance of lactate in the ischemic leg. Near control levels of these substances were seen already after 5 minutes.

In addition to metabolic changes, histochemical alterations in skeletal muscle fibers and motor nerve terminals were demonstrable as long as up to 10 to 15 days later. The post-ischemic period showed interference with the microcirculation and nerve function. Therefore, it appears that "*acute* metabolic data on skeletal muscle cannot be used as a sole and direct evidence for a wide 'margin of safety' since there is a possibility of delayed post-ischemic reactions." Delayed post-ischemic studies are, therefore, necessary (see Chapter 26).

The results from these investigations show that clinical tourniquet ischemia of up to 90 minutes' duration produces less pronounced metabolic alterations than those seen in working muscle. However, these results are additional important data of metabolic responses in skeletal muscle, but are somewhat more complex than those obtained following direct arterial occlusion.

Role of Membrane Function During Ischemia

The changes in tissue metabolism, which occur during ischemia, do not give any information about the extent to which, or if at all, cellular membrane function is affected. Therefore, it is necessary to measure the ability of cells to maintain a normal transmembrane gradient for various electrolytes. For an evaluation of the direct effects of ischemia on cellular membrane function, membrane potential registrations of single cells give some information about the net disturbance in electrolyte distribution across the cell membrane.

Membrane potential changes occur during complete tourniquet ischemia. Under resting conditions, the mean membrane potential level of muscle cells is about −90 mV and during ischemia there is a progressive decrease to a mean level of −54 mV after 3 hours of ischemia.

The observed membrane depolarization occurring during ischemia could be due to lack of energy, inhibition of membrane Na^+-K^+ ATPase activity, or changes in the membrane permeabilities of sodium and potassium. The membrane potential changes occurring during tourniquet ischemia in skeletal muscle also seem to be intimately correlated to changes in extracellular-free potassium concentration.[115]

The *restitution of membrane potential* levels in skeletal muscle is complete within 1 hour after the release of the tourniquet. The restitution in membrane potentials is parallel to the normalizations in tissue pH, tissue lactate, and in the extracellular potassium concentration.

Conclusion

This review of ischemia-induced changes in skeletal muscle distal to a tourniquet shows that there is an increasing metabolic deterioration with increasing tourniquet times. Of significance are the data showing that there is a relatively complete cellular recovery within 1 hour after the release of the tourniquet if the period of complete ischemia does not exceed 3 hours. However, on the basis of such data, it may be questioned whether clinical tourniquet ischemia times can be routinely extended to 3 hours, if needed. Monitoring of the biochemical parameters may be essential in such cases.

13

Experimental Basis of the Myonephropathic-Metabolic Syndrome

The Myonephropathic-Metabolic Syndrome: Experimental Reproduction

The experimental reproduction of this syndrome has been attempted by two main methods: (1) by inducing ischemia using direct acute muscular injury, and (2) by acute arterial occlusions of major vessels of the extremities. The former methods, although they may reproduce some of the hemodynamics, biochemical, and renal consequences of the muscular-induced ischemic lesions, do not meet, however, entirely the clinicopathological criteria of the myonephropathic-metabolic syndrome. The results obtained with those methods provide essentially similar data to the crush syndrome. In view of some analogous aspects with those resulting from acute arterial occlusions, these experimental studies have been reported for comparative reasons in other chapters in this monograph (Tourniquet Ischemia: Metabolic Responses, Crush-Induced Syndrome).

In the present chapter, the main focus will be dealing with experimental acute occlusion of major arteries exclusively.

This study will be divided into two phases: early and recent experimental data.

Early Studies

The early studies were of a different scope and were concerned only with hemodynamic and metabolic complications encountered as a result of cross-clamping of the major arteries, mostly of the infrarenal abdominal aorta. The sudden decrease in blood pressure and variable degrees of transient metabolic changes following the declamping of the aorta have been the subject of extensive experimental laboratory investigations. Similar human studies of declamping phenomena of the aorta were reported in conjunction with reconstructive arterial surgery.

Originally, the reported experimental laboratory investigations were dealing only with the above-mentioned phenomena after isolated aortic clamping. The results observed were far from providing sufficient information comparable with the clinical observations.

Later, it became obvious that duplication approaching clinical responses to the declamping phenomena required combined aortic clamping with multiple interruptions of its branches. But in spite of the greater number of exclusion of the branches and collaterals of the aorta, the duration of the hemodynamic and metabolic effects, although more pronounced, were still transitory. One of the main reasons was the relative short clamping time.

Since these early experiments induced only temporary and transient changes, a more profound degree of ischemia appeared necessary to achieve results which would parallel those in clinical situations in which the skeletal muscles were affected. Thus, a greater number of branches had to be excluded from the vascular tree. In addition, the arterial occlusion time had to approach that of human ischemia duration. With use of these two major prerequisites, reproduction of the myonephropathic-metabolic syndrome appeared to offer a greater consistency with the above clinical findings.

Recent Experimental Data

Several investigators in the late 1960s, using the above criteria, have reproduced hemodynamic and metabolic complications following temporary exclusion of the aorta and its major branches. Of the many studies attempting to reproduce this condition, only a few will be referred to in more detail as information for the repercussions following arterial interruption of a large vascular territory to the extremities.

1. Stipa's Investigations

Stipa et al.,[276] using a very extensive arterial exclusion technique for an ischemic duration of 10 hours, obtained results approaching the severity of massive ischemia with corresponding metabolic responses similar to those in the myonephropathic-metabolic syndrome.

The experimental method was carried out on 50 mongrel dogs in whom a standardized exclusion technique for inducing ischemia was used. This technique consisted of ligating the last two lumbar arteries, the sacral and internal iliac arteries, and the deep femoral arteries. The common femoral arteries were temporarily occluded and, in addition, a rubber band was tightened around the base of the limbs in order to occlude also the collateral circulation. The completeness of ischemia was checked by measurement of the temperature in the muscles, which approximated very rapidly the room temperature, and by measurement of the pH in the venous blood of the limbs which reached levels between 6.40 and 6.50.

After 10 hours, the circulation was reestablished by releasing the occlusion of the common femoral arteries. This technique, when applied to five dogs, resulted in death of these animals within 3 hours. In 20 dogs, anesthetized during the entire experiment, the ischemia of only one limb was sufficient to cause death. Small quantities of mannitol and dextrose in water were infused to the dogs during the experiment.

After the return of the circulation, the urine was heavily loaded with hemoglobin and myoglobin. It was evident from the biochemical studies that these dogs developed hyperkalemia, hyponatremia, and high levels of lactic and pyruvic acid. The increase of these acids was responsible, at least in part, for the severe metabolic acidosis, documented by progressive decrease of base excess and standard bicarbonate. But, at the same time, the pO_2 diminishes and the pCO_2 increases, clearly showing respiratory acidosis.

Several groups of animals, treated in different ways, were studied using the same parameters as in the control group, followed for 24 hours, and then sacrificed.

The main results highlighting this experimental study are as follows:

In the control group, without treatment, recirculation after 10 hours of ischemia was accompanied by progressive acidosis, at least a 50% increase of the limb volume, shock, and death within 15 minutes to 3 hours.

Four groups of animals were given treatment after 10 hours of ischemia:

1. Amino buffer, THAM (tris hydroxymethyl aminomethane), was infused in the ischemic limb before recirculation until the venous blood was frankly alkalotic.
2. A quantity of THAM sufficient to maintain the pH within the normal range was infused into the general circulation after the reestablishment of the blood flow.
3. Rheomacrodex was infused into the ischemic limb to obtain a 50% increase in its volume and THAM was added to reach a high pH. Rheomacrodex and THAM were infused in the general circulation.
4. The ischemic limb was perfused with a small heart–lung apparatus filled with Rheomacrodex. The pH of the entire system was adjusted with THAM to a high volume.

From this study, it appeared that the best results were achieved in the third group of dogs in which the Rheomacrodex and THAM were infused in the general circulation. As a result, there was a 24-hour survival, and acid-base status, lactic and pyruvic acid, blood pressure, cardiac output, and urinary flow were all improved.

It is of interest to note that in the last group of dogs (the fourth group), the authors used a small heart–lung machine to wash out the limb circulation before the return of blood flow. The machine had a capacity of 500 ml, the flow being set at about 150 ml/min, and the pH in the circuit was adjusted with adequate doses of THAM. The extracorporeal circulation lasted 30 minutes and the dogs were later treated in the same way as the previous group. The purpose of this extracorporeal circulation procedure was tried in order to wash out a great quantity of toxic metabolites which could otherwise escape from the interstitial tissues and the cells.

The sacrifice of these animals after 24 hours was a deliberate act after having obtained the necessary physiological information based on the method for producing this syndrome. It would have been, of course, desirable to have a longer term observation for survival of these animals in order to be able to judge the ultimate efficacy of the treatment applied to these cases.

While this study was carried out in 1966, subsequent experiments which may differ to some extent in the modalities of the procedure had nevertheless a similar number of criteria for the evaluation of the metabolic changes and their biological behavior as a whole.

2. Winninger's Investigations

In 1969, A. Winninger[300] published a detailed experimental study on the consequences of the revascularization after acute ischemia of the extremities. Before undertaking the description of his experimental results, he reviewed a number of typical clinical observations from the literature that clearly indicated the basis upon which to build the experimental studies to follow. He based the presentation of this syndrome on my classification of the clinicopathological manifestations into two phases: the devascularization and the post-revascularization phases.

His experimental study consisted essentially of determining the effects of temporary experimental muscle ischemia in 32 dogs weighing between 25 and 37 kg. For that purpose, he used two ischemic procedures: (1) clamping of the aorta after median laparotomy with subsequent ligation of all lumbar arteries; and (2) clamping of the aorta after transverse laparotomy widened with ligature of the spinal muscles, leaving the lumbar arteries intact. After 1 hour of clamping, arterial hypotension and acidosis were evident. Therapeutic reversal of these effects was possible by injecting THAM and a dilute vasoconstrictor substance (Levophed) into the arterial bed immediately before releasing the clamp.

Morphological Changes

In agreement with Malan,[175] who in 1963 described the morphological changes of the tissues due to acute ischemia, Winninger emphasized that after 6 or 7 hours of acute occlusion of the arteries, complete recovery of the revascularized limb cannot be anticipated.

During the *devascularization* stage, the tissues suffer progressive changes varying in extent and degree according to the individual fibers. In the *revascularization* stage, the pattern of the lesions changes in various ways; some muscular fibers become necrotic and then fibrotic, while others lose some of their cytoplasmic contents and appear discolored under the light microscope. Tissue edema appears also concomitantly.

The *revascularized* edematous limb shows a reactive rash characterized by compressive edema, hyperthermia, vasomotor disturbances, and focal variegated muscle lesions (rhàbdomyolysis). The edema involves the tissues of the entire limb, and hence the development of blisters may be observed in the warm part of the limb which is receiving blood. The rhabdomyolytic foci are surrounded and concealed by the surface manifestations of hyperthermia. This phenomenon may be related to some extent to the opening of physiological arteriovenous anastomoses.

The dominant physiopathological aspect in the *revascularization* phase is represented by the muscular lesions. It is difficult to estimate how long the evolution of these muscular ischemic lesions will take before healing could occur. The course varies from one fiber to another, but most of them are characterized by necrosis followed by fibrosis, depigmentation, followed by either recovery or necrosis and, finally, interstitial lesions.

Due to lysis of the striated fibers (rhabdomyolysis), the waste products of anaerobic metabolism (lactates, pyruvates), the products of tissue lysis (potassium, myoglobin, creatine, ATP, histamine), and certain toxic factors synthesized by the muscles pass into the blood stream.

Hemodynamic Changes in the Revascularization Stage: The hemodynamic changes consist mainly of a severe drop of the arterial pressure when the clamp is released and the circulation is restored to the ischemic limb. In 20 aortic cross-clampings in the dog, Winninger constantly observed this phenomenon. Taking into account the nature of the experiment, the pressure drop varied from 12% to 69%. Injecting a weak vasoconstrictor into the arterial bed immediately before releasing the clamp enabled him to prevent both this pressure variation and the paradoxical rise in pO_2 in the venous blood. On the other hand, it is important to point out that this therapeutic effect of the vasoconstrictor substance may be hazardous in patients with severe arterial disease for which reconstruction was carried out.

The post-ischemic arterial hypotension is produced by a number of factors which were reactive hyperemia, opening of arteriovenous anastomoses, loss of plasma, and circulatory absorption of hypotensive substances produced within the ischemic muscles.

Biochemical Changes in the Revascularization Stage: A wave of acidosis appears immediately after the circulation has been restored to the ischemic limb, a well-known phenomenon previously reported. The drop in arterial pH after experimental aortic cross-clamping is a function of the transitory ischemia in the muscle mass, the duration of the clamping, and the pH level at the moment of unclamping. The author was able then to correct his drop in arterial pH by injecting 150 ml of THAM into the abdominal aorta immediately before releasing the clamp. This phenomenon had been noticed previously as well as subsequently by other investigators.

In the majority of cases reported by Winninger, neither vascular accidents nor acidosis appeared following the injection of THAM. It is of interest to point out that myoglobin appears in the blood together with acid metabolites. Acidosis favors the fixation and precipitation of myoglobin at the level of the renal tubuli, as already mentioned previously in this monograph. The respiratory effects of THAM or bicarbonate can be avoided by injecting the drug directly into the distal arterial bed during the operation.

A drop in arterial pH after revascularization of a limb has

been noted as well as significant variations in blood electrolytes. Thus, there is an elevation of potassium levels that may be significant and fatal if it is high following revascularization.

As final conclusions from his experimental study, the author states that the sudden return of the circulation in an ischemic territory may provoke vascular phenomena with arterial hypotension and local edema, metabolic repercussions on various viscera, particularly renal insufficiency, and even psychic disturbances due to acute circulatory insufficiency. Coagulation of blood disturbances were also noted and were attributed to a syndrome of microembolic dissemination, at the level of the lungs. The suddenness of the "arterial rush" inundating the muscular fibers which are already fragile may lead to further anoxia, and anaerobic metabolism which finally aggravates considerably the extent of the ischemic necrosis already present. Then a muscular post-revascularization lysis appears as a complication of the above hemodynamic studies.

Note: It is interesting to consider these observations in the light of the free radicals superoxide changes that were not known at that time, but can be used today for the explanation of these superimposed necrotic changes after revascularization noted by Winninger.

3. Cassar's Investigations

Cassar,[37] in an excellent study on the metabolic disturbances secondary to acute ischemia of the extremities, is concerned also about the experimental study of the revascularization syndrome: although he personally had not performed any specific experimental investigation in the animal laboratory, he attempts to summarize what appeared in the literature at the time of his report (1974).

After reviewing the various experimental studies of the myonephropathic-metabolic syndrome, he is able to define the manifestations that characterize the post-revascularization phase. The following major parameters characterize this syndrome, as seen by Cassar: (1) arterial hypotension, constantly present, to be distinguished from the original arterial fall in blood pressure; (2) the metabolic acidosis, constant biological disturbance, is related to the toxemia emerging from the rhabdomyolysis as a persistent phenomenon due to the lysis of the muscular mass. Once the rhabdomyolytic tissue, source of the toxemia, is excised, either by amputation or ablation of the muscular mass, metabolic acidosis is easily controlled; (3) as a result of these metabolic changes and biochemical disturbances, renal post-revascularization shutdown occurs; (4) coagulation disturbances; and (5) psychic problems.

Although Cassar's important study on this subject had focused primarily on the clinical aspect of the syndrome, he nevertheless had also directed part of his attention to the experimental observations made by a large number of other investigators.

4. Esato's Investigations

The problem of acute arterial occlusions of the extremities resulting in severe and complex metabolic derangements continued to stimulate further interest in this subject. Thus, recent publications emerging from the Japanese literature have provided a further basis of experimental studies for the myonephropathic-metabolic syndrome, its pathogenesis and treatment.

Esato et al.[73] published in 1985 an experimental study in which the emphasis is on the methods of suppression of this metabolic syndrome. Although little new had been added to it, there are a few points that have been reemphasized and seem to be of great actual interest as seen by a group of Japanese vascular surgeons, and serve as a reminder of their persistence.

The experimental study was carried out in dogs weighing 7 to 15 kg in whom the infrarenal abdominal aorta was occluded by cross-clamping and maintained in this condition for 48 hours. The experimental animals were anesthetized only during the procedures of aortic cross-clamping and its release. He divided his experiments into three groups:

(1) *Control Group:* Simple occlusion of the infrarenal abdominal aorta with release of the clamp 48 hours later without any therapeutic measures.

(2) *THAM Group:* This buffer was administered intravenously 1 hour after the occlusion at a dosage calculated for pH correction. Just prior to release of the occlusion, the previously injected amount of THAM was administered twice in all these animals.

(3) *Perfusion Group:* A peripheral washout was performed immediately before release using 30 ml/kg of lactated Ringer's solution. The washout solution was injected into the aorta just distal to the occlusion and sampled through a catheter inserted in the infrarenal inferior vena cava. The author underscores the fact that no intravenous fluids or blood transfusion were administered during the experiment.

The important biochemical parameters studied were serum glutamic oxalacetic transaminase (SGOT), blood urea nitrogen (BUN), serum creatinine, serum creatine phosphokinase (CPK), lactate dehydrogenase (LDH), lactic acid, pyruvic acid, aldolase, and serum sodium and potassium in venous blood samples obtained before and 1 hour after the occlusion extending from 1 to 48 hours after the release of the occlusion.

The results of this experimental study indicate that a 48-hour cross-clamping is consistent with a very advanced ischemia of the tissues when deprived of vascularization by the aorta and its branches. The parameters serving as criteria of ischemia of the tissues are quite different in the control and treated series of dogs.

In the control group, which is the untreated group, SGOT levels increased significantly, reaching the highest level within 12 hours after the release of the occlusion. They decreased thereafter, but remained higher than the pre-occlusion level up to 48 hours. On the other hand, SGOT levels in the THAM and in the perfusion groups remained near the control values even after release of the occlusion. There were statistically significant differences between the untreated and the THAM groups at 1, 3, and 12 hours before release of the clamp, while significant differences were seen at 1 and 3 hours between the untreated and perfusion groups.

Serum creatine phosphokinase (CPK) levels in the untreated group rose significantly following the release of occlusion, recording the highest mean value of 16,749 ± 11.409 units at 12 hours, while the other two groups remained near the pre-occlusion levels throughout the experiment (Figure 13-1). There were statistically significant differences from 1 to 24 hours after the release between the untreated and treated groups. It appears that aldolase was somewhat similar to CPK in its changes to the occlusion. THAM did not significantly help the prevention of aldolase increase, nor was the perfusion as significantly prophylactic as it was in the CPK

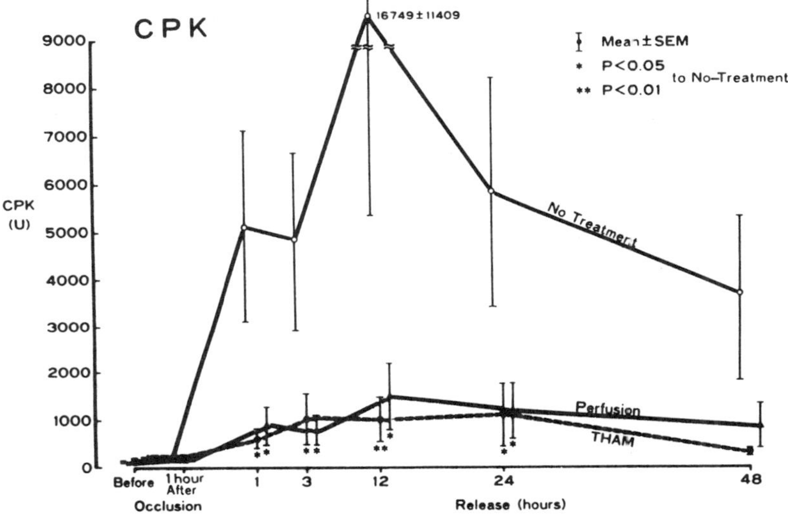

FIGURE 13-1: This diagram depicts changes in serum creatine phosphokinase. Serum creatine phosphokinase level in the non-treatment groups rose significantly after the release of the occlusion. There were statistically significant differences between the non-treated groups after the release. CPK = creatine phosphokinase. (From Esato K, et al: Methods of suppression of myonephropathic metabolic syndrome. *J Cardiovasc Surg* 26:473–478.[73])

study. Of interest in this particular study is that serum sodium and potassium levels remained at the pre-occlusion levels in all three groups, which is somewhat surprising.

It is also surprising that the authors have not studied the response of myoglobin to the ischemia because they felt that the measurement of this metabolite is not always simple, since the evaluations of the ischemia by the measurements of SGOT, CPK, aldolase, and some other enzymes were sufficiently useful as indicators so that they had no need to study the fluctuations of myoglobin. (*Note:* it is possible that the methods used by this group of Japanese investigators were not sufficiently sensitive and simple enough to use in order to obtain the consistent results that are claimed by ourselves and most European investigators who have studied myoglobin in connection with acute arterial occlusions.)

As to the method of controlling the metabolic derangements that develop after the reperfusion, their use of THAM seems to have resulted in survival after the 48 hours of prolonged limb ischemia, but failed to indicate the later survival rate, unless the dogs were all sacrificed at the end of the experiment. In agreement with my own statements in previous publications, they felt that large amounts of buffer substances were necessary to neutralize the metabolic acidosis that develops after devascularization. They accomplished this with THAM which they consider to be an ideal buffer if the dosage is well titrated. However, it is not always easy to determine which is the ideal dose in a particular experiment. They add, however, that due to the fact that the increases in the various parameters such as CPK, SGOT, and aldolase were only minimal in the THAM-treated group, they consider the dose of utilized THAM to have been effective for suppressing the metabolic acidosis developed during the 48-hour occlusion.

The important points in this study suggest that even with a 48-hour cross-clamping of the aorta and its main branches, a reversal of the ischemic changes could be achieved, with or without the use of perfusion of the limb before the declamping of the aorta. The combined intravenous injection of THAM and peripheral washout of the ischemic site with lactated Ringer's solution immediately before release of the occlusion appeared to offer an effective method of management in certain difficult cases.

The use of washout of peripheral ischemic limbs by Esato, mentioned earlier by the European surgeons (Stipa), was also applied by Kusaba and other Japanese surgeons for treating the ischemic limb prior to revascularization. It is possibly a useful therapeutic method, but it is quite cumbersome and sometimes time-consuming. The results published by a few authors claimed in certain cases to be useful in conjunction with other methods.

While this study had specifically focused on the usefulness of THAM, it failed to indicate what was the status of the muscular tissue in the 48-hour cross-clamping of the aorta. It might have been of interest to know how much of the damage had been inflicted by this prolonged ischemia and what was the status of the nongangrenous or markedly ischemic tissue. Similarly, failure to indicate the status of the kidney is an important omission in the context of this prolonged and severe ischemia.

5. Ikezawa's Investigations

Use of a new scavenger of superoxide free-radicals was recently reported to me personally by Teruo Ikezawa.*[140a] His study deals with an experimental investigation of the cause and treatment of myonephropathic-metabolic syndrome with alpha-tocopherol. The premise of this investigation concerning the cause of rhabdomyolysis is focused on the lipid peroxidation by the active oxygens or free-radicals of superoxide nature and, therefore, he felt that a prophylactic effect of alpha-tocopherol (vitamin E) on the healing of rhabdomyolysis was indicated. He divided his experimental study into three groups: (1) the control group in which simple laparotomy was performed; (2) a second group, a 6-hour occlusion group in which the terminal abdominal aorta was clamped and then released 6 hours later; and (3) a third group in which a 6-hour occlusion was carried out plus alpha-tocopherol treatment in which 500 mg of this drug was given intravenously just before declamping.

All experiments were carried out in dogs. The method of occlusion of the aorta and its branches was quite extensive and included the infrarenal abdominal aorta, the lumbar arteries, the caudal arteries and branches (Figure 13-2). This canine model produced ischemia of both hind limbs. The biochemical studies in this model were done after declamping at 3 hours, as well as at 6 hours, and every subsequent 6 hours until 48 hours after the completion of the experiment. A catheter inserted into the inferior vena cava just below the renal veins served as a source of blood samples for the study of serum CPK and serum LPO (lipid peroxidase). These were determined as indexes of rhabdomyolysis and lipid peroxidation due to active oxygens, respectively. In addition, serum alpha-tocopherol was also determined in the venous blood.

The results obtained indicate that CPK levels increased rapidly immediately after declamping and continued until 48 hours later. However, the CPK level in group 3 did not increase as much as in group 1. There was a significant difference between

*This contribution was presented during the XVII Japanese Congress of Cardiovascular Surgery, May 1–2, 1987, where I presented the key address of the Myonephropathic-Metabolic Syndrome.

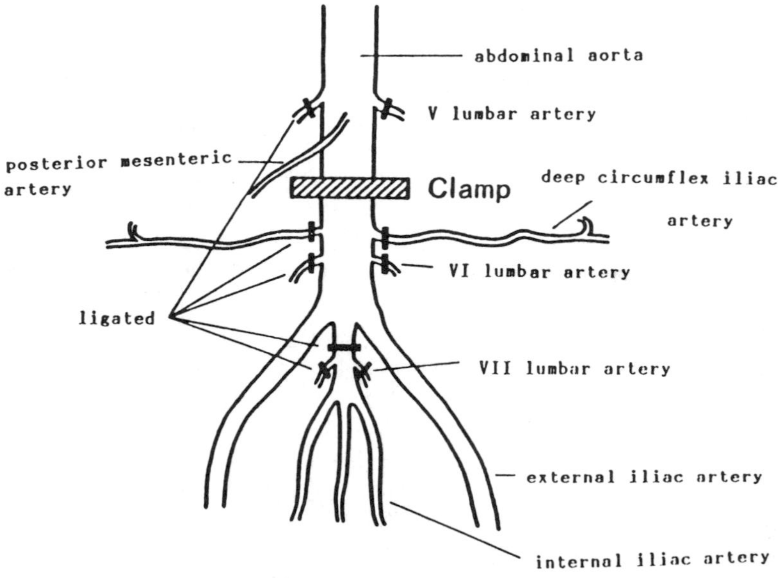

FIGURE 13-2: A canine model for producing ischemia of the hind limbs by cross-clamping the aorta and multiple arterial ligations. (From Teruo Ikezawa, presented at the XVII Japanese Cardiovascular Surgery Congress; Personal communication.[140a])

group 2 and group 3. As far as LPO is concerned, its values varied according to the group. In group 2, the peak level of serum LPO ranged between 19.8 nmol/ml and 76.3 nmol/ml. There was a significant difference between the level of serum LPO before clamping and individual peak level of LPO.

In group 3, after 6-hour occlusion and tocopherol administration by intravenous route just before declamping, the LPO level decreased and fell to a minimum 6 hours after declamping. There was no significant change in the serum level of alpha-tocopherol in either group 1 or 2, although it increased in group 3.

It is of interest that serum CPK and LPO both increased after declamping which indicated that rhabdomyolysis had resulted from the peroxidation of lipids, the main component of the membrane by active superoxide radicals. The levels of serum CPK and LPO were subsequently regulated through administration of alpha-tocopherol. The author considers that the peroxidation of the lipids was regulated by the radical scavengers such as the alpha-tocopherol and that the progression to extensive rhabdomyolysis was blocked by this administration of the drug.

This study appears to be quite novel in this area and it is of great interest for those who wish to have a new scavenger administered before releasing the clamps or during the revascularization phase.

Conclusion

The study of experimental myonephropathic-metabolic syndrome as presented by the few investigators mentioned in this chapter is of great interest in relation to the pathogenesis, clinical aspects, and possible treatment to overcome the various metabolites resulting from the ischemia of the skeletal muscle. Some of these studies had been done previosly, but they had not advanced perhaps as much as in the past few years, when the initial observations made clinically and then experimentally reemphasized that the major source of the metabolic syndrome is the ischemic skeletal muscle. The newer understanding of the superoxide radicals and the management of these metabolites by the scavengers is still new and little has been used in the study except as mentioned in Chapter 26 of this monograph entitled *Role of Free-Radicals in Post-Ischemic Skeletal Muscle Reperfusion Injury*. Further investigations in this area are obviously necessary before establishing more firmly the role of these free-radicals and the use of the scavengers which are at the present time being investigated by a number of pharmaceutical companies, and by a number of cardiovascular surgeons.

II

Clinical Entities

14

Arterial Embolism

Introduction

The most common conditions of acute arterial occlusions associated with a metabolic syndrome secondary to rhabdomyolysis include:

1. Arterial embolism;
2. Acute spontaneous thrombosis of
   (a) Abdominal aorta (nonaneurysmal)
   (b) Abdominal aortic aneurysm;
3. Acute graft thrombosis;
4. Arterial cross-clamping;
5. Arterial cannulation during cardiopulmonary bypass;
6. Arterial trauma.

Metabolic complications associated with acute ischemia of an extremity have received scant attention in spite of countless publications dealing with arterial thromboembolism or trauma. Although considerable progress has been and is being achieved in the management of acute ischemic syndromes, limb loss and mortality rates still leave much to be desired in a significant percentage of such cases. In these instances, the immediate outcome of limb and patient survival may depend on many factors, one of which may be a metabolic syndrome secondary to ischemic myopathy.

Although the importance of the biological response of striated muscle to a variety of acute pathological conditions has long been known to biomedical investigators,[5,7,15,33,49,50,90,302] their clinical significance in acute ischemia of an extremity was not fully appreciated until recently. This is reflected in the paucity of reports on the role of rhabdomyolysis in the pathogenesis of the metabolic syndrome, and its therapeutic implications in sudden arterial interruptions. A critical analysis of a number of acute vascular entities that display a similar rhabdomyolytic process will be attempted to provide a unified concept of their pathogenesis by pointing out their common as well as their divergent features.

Arterial Embolism

Before describing in detail the pattern of arterial embolism associated with the metabolic complications, a brief review of an uncomplicated pattern of arterial embolism may serve as a background to this problem. Arterial embolism is a well-known complication of a preexisting cardiopathy or proximal arterial lesion or the result of a cardiovascular procedure. The site of the most common cardiogenic embolism is the left heart. The published relative incidence of intracardiac thrombosis associated with arterial embolism varies from 60% to 90%. The majority of cases of arterial embolism result from detachment of thrombi from the heart or proximal major arterial tree.[70,101] However, exceptional cases may be related to bacterial endocarditis, atrial myxoma and tumor of other than atrial origin, atheroembolism, bullet embolism, or echinococcus cysts, all of which may be suspected in the absence of a typical cardiac lesion.

Clinical manifestations associated with an embolic occlusion of a main limb artery, although usually characteristic, need reemphasis in some aspects. Although arterial embolism is characterized by sudden onset of pain or numbness and coldness in about 81% of the patients, by contrast, in a small percentage there is a progressive onset, or even a silent one, of the symptoms. Acute pain signals the initial manifestations of the region of impaction of an embolus. The nature of this pain was controversial for a long time. It was generally accepted that it was due to the stimulus or impact set up in the arterial wall by the embolus. At variance with this concept, Lewis suggested that the pain of embolism is the result of ischemic muscle and that its appearance does not indicate the moment of lodgement of the embolus. It is likely, however, that the initial pain is due to the impaction of the embolus into the artery and that the later pain which is situated distal to the site of occlusion is rather ischemia of the limb, due to muscular ischemia, as suggested by Lewis.

All the other signs such as numbness, coldness, tingling, and absence of arterial pulsations, are well-known and need not be emphasized in this brief overview. However, the degree of ischemia resulting from an arterial embolism is not uniform.[100] Its grading previously emphasized is based on the degree of spontaneous restoration of the circulation in a series of untreated cases,[100] and was classified as follows:

Grade I: *Moderate* ischemia with early pulse return resulting in an anischemic embolism (29.5%).

Grade II: *Advanced* ischemia with only partial late recovery: *chronic post-embolic ischemia* (22.2%).

Grade III: *Severe* ischemia leading to variable degrees of gangrene often with metabolic complications (28%).

Grade IV: *Very severe* ischemia with early fatal outcome of the patient (11.3%).

From this classification of the grading of the severity of ischemia, it appears that Grade III and especially Grade IV are those cases which are associated with metabolic complications that might explain not only the local severity of the lesion but also the metabolic complications systemically.

One of the factors that determines the outcome of the degree of ischemia and its metabolic complications is the location of the arterial occlusion. Thus, in the lower extremity, the main locations are the aortic bifurcation, the common iliac, and the bifurcation of the femoral artery. More rarely are those of the popliteal and tibial vessels.

The occlusion of the major vessels such as the aortic bifurcation and the iliac artery involve, in general, large masses of skeletal muscle ischemia which would account for the greater potential of metabolic complications (Figure 14-1).

The prognostic factors governing the results of treatment of an arterial embolism are the *duration* of the occlusion, the *degree* of ischemia, the *location* and *extent* of the occlusion, and above all, the degree of skeletal muscle ischemia. It is generally recognized today that perhaps the more threatening factor in the prognosis of

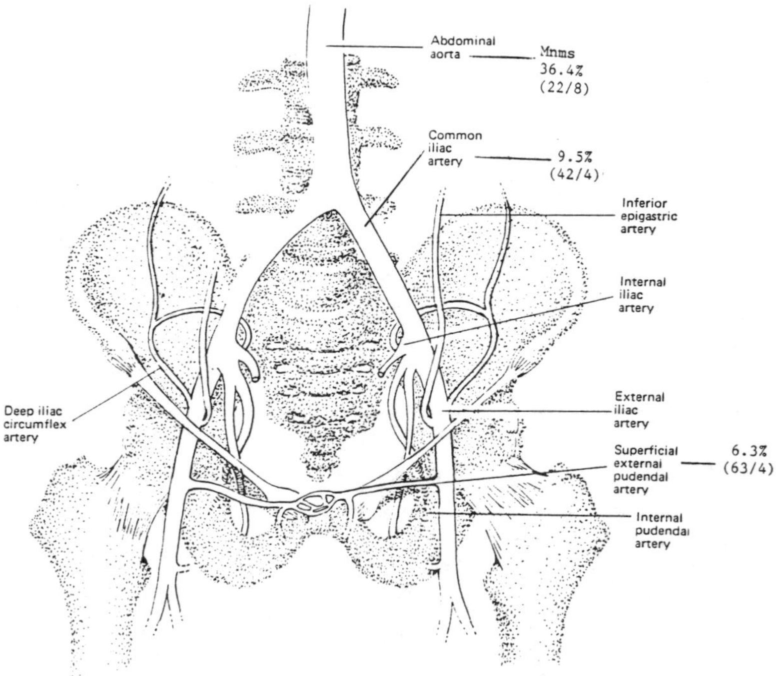

FIGURE 14-1: This diagram depicts the aortoiliac-femoral arterial tree. Acute occlusion of these segments vascularize large masses of skeletal muscle. As a result, the myonephropathic metabolic syndrome is more prone to occur in these areas. As indicated in this diagram, this syndrome occurred in 36.4% of the cases in the abdominal aorta, in the common iliac in 9.5%, and in the femoral in 6.3%. These figures seem to relate to the muscular mass irrigated by the various segments.

an arterial embolism is the presence of severe muscle ischemia with possible necrosis. Lack of awareness of this factor and the presence of myoglobinuria with release of other metabolites from the necrotic muscle may lead to loss of not only the limb but also the life of the patient if these complications are not recognized in time and vigorously treated (see below).

Myonephropathic-Metabolic Syndrome

Since my original report[98] in 1960, and further personal experience as well,[102105,109,110,113] an increasing number of publications have confirmed the fact that a certain percentage of cases of arterial embolism may be associated with a syndrome of severe and often fatal metabolic complications.

Incidence of this group of cases as it relates to the overall experience with arterial embolism is difficult to assess because of few reports dealing with the importance of the potential of metabolic repercussions of these cases. Since the clinical picture is sometimes obscured by the often present cardiovascular manifestations, the persisting high rates of morbidity, amputations, or mortality are rather erroneously attributed to a cardiac origin.

In a retrospective study based on a compiled series of 1,601 cases of acute arterial occlusions (which includes embolism and thrombosis), Cormier and Devin[44] reported an overall mortality of 27.9% (447 cases), mostly as a result of cardiovascular factors (heart, cerebrovascular, visceral infarcts, pulmonary embolism, etc.). Of these 447 cases, it is significant that in 112 (25%) of the fatal cases or 7% of the total group of 1,601 cases, the cause of death was attributed to the metabolic syndrome. They failed to mention if there were survivors with the metabolic complications.

Gutierrez Carreño[97] reported four deaths (44.4%) and five successful results in a total of nine cases, but failed to indicate the overall experience with acute arterial occlusions.

Francisco,[83] on the other hand, provided more data on this subject. Of the total 210 embolectomies in 194 patients, 17 had the myonephropathic-metabolic syndrome, or 8.7% of the patients and 8.1% of the embolectomies. In 16, the syndrome occurred after the embolectomy and in one was present prior to surgery. The overall mortality was 76.4% (13 patients). The average ischemic period in this group was 21.1 hours and the location of the embolism was 9 aortic, 4 iliac, and 4 femoral. This great delay of operation and the high location account for the high percentage of mortality.

Cassar[37] studied a series of 23 cases of acute occlusions of which 15 had embolism and eight had acute thrombosis. Ten or 43.5% were successful, 10 died as a result of the myonephropathic-metabolic complications, and three died from unrelated causes.

In a personal study based on over 200 acute arterial occlusions, there was an overall incidence of 7.5% of both fatal and recovered cases associated with this syndrome.[109]

Kagen[144] reported on 16 patients who underwent open heart surgery. Of these, six (37.5%) developed the syndrome with myoglobinuria and mortality of one patient.

Kugimiya[159] in 420 patients undergoing open-heart surgery encountered eight cases (1.9%) of the syndrome.

From the above few reports, it is clear that the overall incidence of the myonephropathic-metabolic syndrome is relatively small (Table I). However, morbidity and mortality in these cases are usually very high. Their early recognition is obviously essential, for to be beneficial, immediate intensive therapeutic measures should be applied without delay.

Clinical Manifestations

The clinical manifestations are of unusual and extreme severity both locally and systemically. These are in sharp contrast with the common form of arterial embolism as described above. They may be observed: (1) initially during the acute ischemic or devascularization phase; (2) after the revascularization of the ex-

Table I
Incidence of Myonephropathic-Metabolic Syndrome (2,447 Patients)

Range %	Average %
7.0–37.5	13.7 (178 Patients)

tremity; and (3) during the reperfusion of the ischemic tissues. The clinical and metabolic manifestations differ in degree and extent in the three phases. Recognition of the early phase is of paramount significance, as was pointed out previously.

Ischemic or Devascularization Phase

The clinical picture in this phase is most characteristic and dramatic, as it is quite different from the usual form. In all instances the clinical onset is ushered in by *excrutiating pain*. Any attempt at mobilizing or examining the extremity is accompanied by its exacerbation. The *profound ischemia* of the tissues is characterized by coldness, waxy pallor mixed with cyanotic mottling, and sensory anesthesia. The severity of the ischemia is due to massive obstruction of the main arterial axis and its collateral network which is translated into extensive rhabdomyolysis (Figure 14-2). The most striking characteristic feature of this clinical syndrome is the *rigidity of the extremity* (rigor mortis). Muscular contracture and stiffness of the joints appear so pronounced that their presence in an acute embolism or thrombosis should evoke the possibility of ischemic myopathy associated with myoglobinuria. Indeed, limb rigidity was found in all cases and may be considered an "alarm signal" heralding the metabolic syndrome. The joints, especially the distal ones such as the ankle and the knee, appear to be "frozen."

Edema of the extremity is nonpitting, which is unlike that of a venous thrombosis. Massive swelling occurs within 12 to 24 hours and usually involves the entire extremity, although the swelling of the thigh may be more pronounced than that of the leg. The swollen limb is usually tender, tense, of woody consistency, and nonpitting. The edema is mostly in the muscles. The association of coldness and cyanosis may lead to confusion with phlegmasia cerulea dolens. However, unlike its distribution in venous thrombosis, the edema is most pronounced in the muscles and less pronounced in the subcutaneous tissue.

Because of the pain and the metabolic disturbances, the patient often appears to be agitated, confused, and disoriented. The so-called neuropsychiatric manifestations are probably the

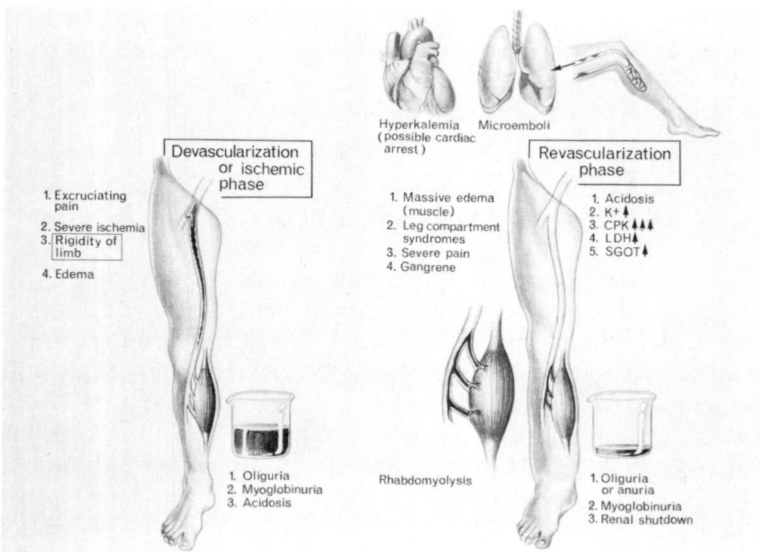

Figure 14-2: This illustration shows the two clinical phases with the corresponding major muscular, renal, biochemical, and morphological alterations. During the acute *devascularization phase*, the dominating features are: (a) severe ischemia and rigidity of the limb (muscle contracture), and (b) oliguria, incipient myoglobinuria, and acidosis. During the immediate *post-revascularization phase*, the dominating features are: (a) edema and leg compartment syndromes, (b) rhabdomyolysis, and (c) renal shutdown. The *reperfusion phase*, not depicted here, is associated with ischemic muscles, due to free-radicals ischemia and superimposed necrosis.

result of the combination of azotemia and the effects of other metabolites upon the brain function as well.

Indeed, during this ischemic phase, variable degrees of metabolic acidosis, together with incipient azotemia and hyperkalemia, are already present, all of which, if uncorrected, may lead to serious complications or even death of the patient. The significance of recognizing this early phase cannot be overemphasized.

Revascularization Phase

Restoration of arterial flow to a previously acutely and severely ischemic extremity has been reported sporadically in the past to result in a syndrome of pain, edema, and tenderness of the muscles. However, the metabolic complications in these cases were rarely noted or fully appreciated. At present, a fair body of experimental and clinical information is available on the revascularization phase and its metabolic repercussions.[98,109]

The clinical picture varies according to the degree of the ischemia. In *severe* cases, the pain may increase in intensity in spite of revascularization, due to incomplete reperfusion of the distal tissues. Edema of the limb becomes more pronounced than it was prior to the operation, while the muscular contracture and rigidity subside. Leg or forearm compartment syndrome are nearly always present. While the overall tissue perfusion may become adequate, ischemia may remain severe in the distal portion of the limb. The prognosis of this phase depends essentially on the extent of the muscular mass involved and its degree of necrosis.

Microemboli containing platelets and fibrin may invade the pulmonary circulation following revascularization as a result of embolectomy, thrombectomy, or the declamping of the aorta.[18] While this complication may not represent a truly metabolic phenomenon, there is little doubt that it is a direct effect of a post-occlusion coagulability disturbance. As such, it should be mentioned in the context of the revascularization syndrome.

Metabolic Syndrome

Most of these patients display metabolic manifestations that may be transient or prolonged, shortly after onset of the arterial occlusion, and especially after the limb revascularization.

Metabolic acidosis. This may be of variable degree and it is always present. It is the response to the accumulation of acid metabolites. Tissue hypoxia or anoxia leads to a decrease of aerobic oxidation through the Krebs cycle, followed by an increased anaerobic glycolysis of the Embden-Meyerhoff pathway, resulting in lactic acid and pyruvic acid. Both lactate and pyruvate increase initially; lactate later increases more than pyruvate, producing an increased lactate to pyruvate ratio.

Blood pH and carbon dioxide (CO_2) content fall. There is a decrease in bicarbonates and the difference in the number of cations and anions increases considerably. The pH of the venous efflux of the involved extremity before revascularization of the limb varies with a degree of the metabolic acidosis already present. If the initial pH is below or equal to 7.20, the prognosis appears to be very poor, especially if it subsequently falls even further. In such instances, the treatment of the metabolic acidosis requires a considerable amount of buffer substances (sodium bicarbonate or THAM) to neutralize the fresh appearance of the H ions after revascularization. If the fall in pH persists, management of the acidosis becomes extremely difficult and it must be fought rigorously. In the milder cases, 15 minutes or longer may be needed before the pH returns to a normal range following restoration of arterial flow.

Electrolytic Changes

The serum sodium has been found to be within normal limits in the majority of cases, both before and after the revascularization phase. Before restoration of the arterial flow, *serum potassium* is normal in the venous blood from both the ischemic limb and the systemic circulation. By contrast, after restoration of the arterial flow, serum potassium levels are variable and depend on the level of ischemia. In *milder cases,* the serum potassium is within normal limits and in some cases, hypokalemia may be noted. In the *severe* cases, hyperkalemia is noted in the venous efflux from the ischemic limbs, the concentration of potassium usually being proportional to some extent to the duration of the arterial occlusion and the resulting degree of ischemia. Hyperkalemia represents a poor prognostic factor which translates the significance of muscle cytolysis. Its sudden release at the time of the declamping of the artery may lead to cardiac arrest, as reported in some cases of revascularization.

The venous PO_2 of the ischemic limb is significantly lower than in the systemic venous blood. The venous PCO_2 of the ischemic limb is higher than that of the systemic blood. After restoration of the arterial circulation, the venous PO_2 and PCO_2 may return to normal within a variable period of time depending on the degree and duration of the ischemia.

Enzymatic Changes

The serum creatine phosphokinase (CPK) concentration is usually slightly elevated in the systemic blood before revascularization. However, it is far higher in the venous blood from the ischemic limb. After restoration of the arterial flow, the average CPK volume rises even further, in most cases. Elevation of the enzyme concentration is direct evidence of damaged striated muscle. Indeed, high values of the enzyme usually reflect advanced muscle necrosis. Preservation of intact skin in such cases may be misleading since it is not always an index of viability of the underlying muscles. In mild cases, the serum level of CPK may decrease within several hours or 1 or 2 days after revascularization. In moderately severe cases, it may increase over a period of several days to 1,000 or 2,000 units and then progressively to a normal level within 10 to 12 days. However, in very severe and fatal cases, as the CPK keeps increasing progressively, it may reach 20,000 units or even higher.

Lactic acid dehydrogenase (LDH) and glutamic oxaloacetic transaminase (SGOT) are also elevated in all forms of acute arterial occlusions displaying this syndrome. The transaminases (SGOT, SGPT) are increased in proportion to the degree of ischemia. In mild and moderate muscle damage with minor infarction, the serum level decreases within a matter of a few days to a normal level. By contrast, in patients with very severe muscle damage, persistence of high levels of transaminase indicates irreversible changes of the tissue.

Lactic acid dehydrogenase (LDH) is increased shortly after revascularization in at least half of the cases, becoming more pronounced within a few hours of about 80%. In recent years, determination of total LDH and of total CPK activities has been found in a wide spectrum of diseases of which myocardial infarction is a most frequent entity (see Chapter 22, *Myocardial Infarction*). Since patients with severe occlusive disease may also have myocardial damage, it is essential to identify the specific LDH and CPK isoenzymes in the blood. Thus, of the five isoenzymes of LDH, LDH 1 and 2 are usually significantly increased in myocardial infarction, while LDH 4 and 5 are more specific for striated muscle damage. Likewise, isoenzymes of CPK, fraction 2, MB-fraction, is indicative of myocardial necrosis, while CPK-MM is found predominantly in skeletal muscle. There is still, however, some controversy about the specificity of isoenzymes. All these enzymatic changes are found in large amounts, especially in the first 3 to 4 days, as seen in our own cases. They may persist beyond 1 or 2 weeks, depending on the degree of muscle necrosis. Decrease of, or return to normal blood levels of these enzymes may reflect resolution of muscle damage. Interpretation of these serum enzymes (CPK, LDH, SGOT) carries a number of pitfalls due to the wide spectrum of diseases in which they are positively identified. It is, therefore, important to correlate properly these chemical changes with the clinical and operative findings.

Myoglobinuria

Within a few hours after onset of the occlusion, the urinary output is usually decreased and the urine displays a dark cherry-red or burgundy-red color, due to myoglobin. Myoglobinuria may reach a peak within 48 hours and may last several days depending on the extent and severity of the rhabdomyolysis. Occasionally, myoglobinuria may escape detection due either to laboratory mishap or to delay in testing the urine.[136] Its presence can be determined as a guaiac- or benzidine-positive or orthotolidine-positive pigment in the urine containing no red cells, especially if the serum is clear. The most common mistake in diagnosis in myoglobinuria is hemoglobinuria. Berman[14] suggested that a naked-eye look at the plasma may suffice to suspect myoglobin by application of this rule: "Red plasma plus red urine equals hemoglobin; clear plasma plus red urine equals myoglobin." Of course, the specific chemical tests available described above for detecting these pigments in the urine provide the final accurate diagnosis. The methods available for estimating myoglobin are chemical, spectrophotometric, and immunologic (see Chapter 3, *Myoglobin*).

Most of these tests are primarily qualitative in nature. Recent methods have been described for quantitative investigation of myoglobin in the urine, thus making possible earlier and more accurate detection of myoglobin of the serum and urine as well.

Myoglobinemia

It is possible that among the pitfalls of detecting the myoglobin in the urine is the delay or small amounts of myoglobin which are cleared through the kidney and therefore the latter is difficult to demonstrate. However, the myoglobin in the serum or plasma may and should be tested because it may be easier to identify it in the blood before it reaches the urine through the kidney clearance.

This test has not been used often in these cases and therefore in a number of these instances myoglobin in the urine had been missed. One has to think in terms of myoglobinemia, especially in those patients in whom the rhabdomyolysis due to ischemia is highly suspected.

Hypocalcemia and Hypercalcemia

Hypocalcemia with concurrent hyperphosphatemia and oliguria is noted in more than half of the patients, especially in those that I have been able to follow. Conversely, hypercalcemia has been reported in 22–25% of the patients with nontraumatic rhabdomyolysis during the diuretic phase. The mechanism of alteration of the calcium to phosphorus ratio in the oliguric phase is attributed to the overall sarcolemmal membrane permeability changes. Thus, in normal muscle, the calcium ion concentration is three to four times lower than in the extracellular fluid. If the calcium ion concentration in the muscle sarcoplasm reaches equilibrium in the extracellular space, contraction of the muscles will be increased, which may explain their rigidity. On the other hand, the presence of hypocalcemia in acute renal failure may account for the twitching and the seizures noted in some patients.

Rhabdomyolysis: Acute Muscle Devascularization

The degree of ischemic damage to the skeletal muscle is of central significance since it determines the viability of the limb and to a great extent the metabolic syndrome. Surprisingly, scant attention has been paid to the pathological changes taking place in the acutely devascularized muscle in arterial occlusions. In an effort to provide some missing information concerning this phase of rhabdomyolysis, a number of experimental investigations have produced a substantial body of data. These data have been based on the effects of acute ligations or tourniquet ischemia and therefore bear only limited resemblance to the human findings. Their significance, however, derives from the chronological evaluation of damaged muscle fibers and thereby indicates the various stages of the histopathological changes, as related to the duration and extent of the ischemia.[49,50,70,120,195]

On the basis of personal human observations, the gross appearance of the muscles of pallor and swelling of moderate intensity are seen intraoperatively hours after an acute arterial occlusion. These changes become more pronounced within 24 hours, when the swollen, pallid muscles take an appearance described as "fish-flesh." (Figure 14-3A). Beyond 24 hours, the muscles appeared grossly congested, purple, and hard. Upon fascial incision, if still viable, they turn pink and herniate through the opening of the fasciotomy. If unrelieved by decompression of the involved area, the edema usually further increases after further revascularization of the limb. Beyond this stage, the muscle may also display variable degrees of necrosis ranging from focal to extensive areas (see Chapter 26, *Role of Free-Radicals in Post-Ischemic Skeletal Muscle Reperfusion Injury*).

Microscopically, some fibers show initially well-preserved outlines. In some areas, absence of some nuclei is noted and the cytoplasm is slightly coagulated and granular. Such findings are characteristic of early anoxic changes. Within 24 hours, individual fibers display swelling and hyalinization (Figure 14-3B). At a later

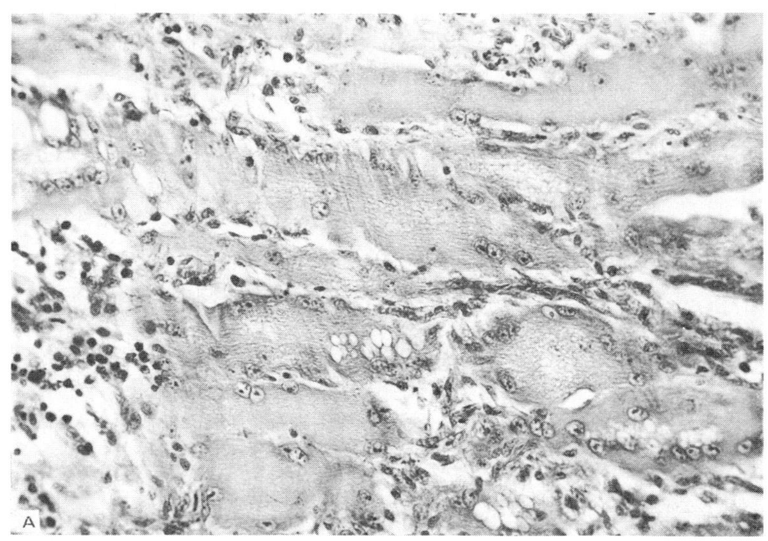

Figure 14-3A: Muscular necrosis with sarcolemmal proliferation and regeneration of muscular fibers ($\times 400$). (From H. Haimovici.[98])

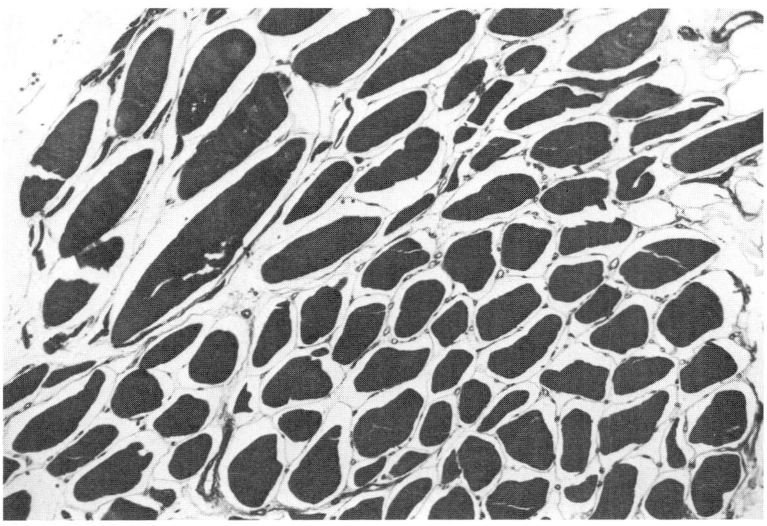

FIGURE 14-3B: Photomicrograph showing swelling of individual muscular fibers and their hyalinization. (Hematoxylin and eosin, × 250.) (From Haimovici H: Myonephropathic-metabolic syndrome. *J Cardiovasc Surg* 14:589, 1973.[108])

phase (48 to 72 hours), the lesions consist of foci of loss of striation and of sarcolemmal nuclei of muscular fibers (Figure 14-4). Specimens from amputated limbs may show degeneration of muscular fibers, ranging from slight to moderate degenerative changes to actual necrosis (Figures 14-5 and 14-6). The muscle cell changes are translated into biochemical alterations and metabolic complications. As is well known, the sarcoplasm contains a large number of chemical substances and enzymes, including myocin and actin. The normal relationship between myoglobin, myocin, and actin is disrupted as a result of loss of adenosine triphosphate (ATP) and the muscular enzymes, all of which are attributable to altered permeability of the muscle cell membrane.

Acute Renal Failure

The acute renal impairment usually varies with the degree of muscle ischemia, acidosis, and myoglobinuria. In mild or moderately severe cases, renal function is temporarily impaired and

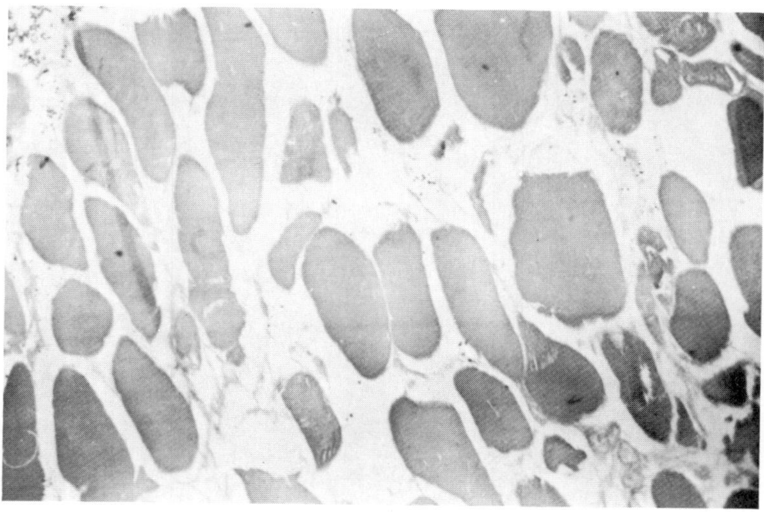

Figure 14-4: Anterior tibial muscle biopsy specimen indicating the loss of sarcolemmal nuclei, homogenous appearance of the cytoplasm with loss of striation, interstitial edema, and infiltration of polymorphonuclear and mononuclear leucocytes (× 100.) (From Haimovici H: Muscular, renal, and metabolic complications of acute arterial occlusions. *Surgery* 85:461, 1978.)

completely reversible. Urinary output may be decreased during the devascularization phase and may be further impaired after the revascularization. Most patients display either oliguria or anuria. Their BUN and creatinine rise to very high levels quite rapidly after the renal impairment is detected clinically. In cases with severe complications, prolonged myoglobinuria in the presence of acidosis, if not treated promptly with vigorous peritoneal dialysis or hemodialysis, leads to irreversible shutdown and usually to the death of the patient.

Post-mortem examination usually shows the kidneys to be of normal shape and consistency. The capsule can be stripped with ease. One may find focal infarctions even though some of the renal glomeruli appear to be entirely patent. Histologically, the renal tubules contain casts of myoglobin, with reactive epithelial cells occasionally indicating their regeneration (Figures 14-7 and 14-8).

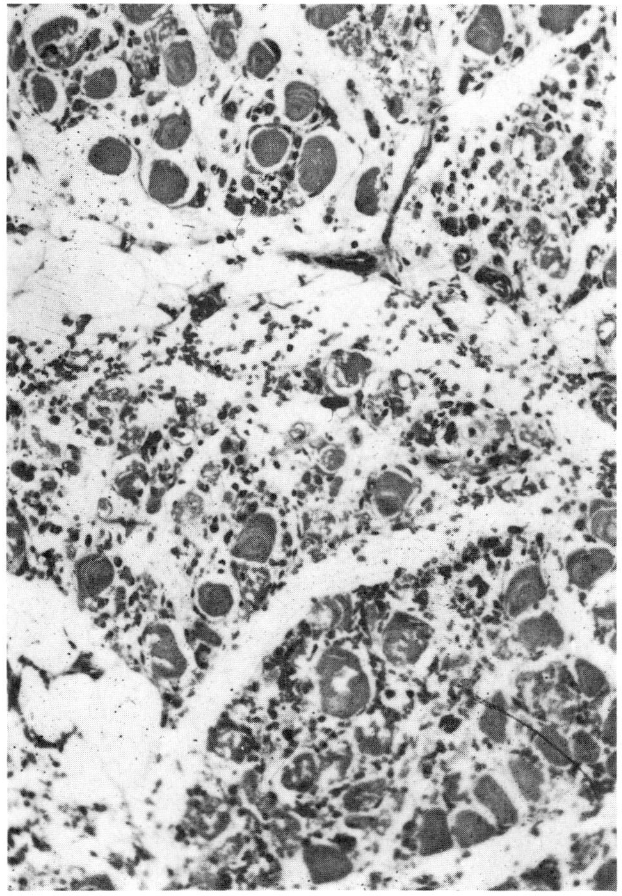

Figure 14-5: Muscle fibers showing evidence of degeneration and lysis associated with interstitial inflammatory reaction (× 130). (From Haimovici H: Arterial embolism, myoglobinuria, and renal tubular necrosis. *Arch Surg* 100:639, 1970.[107])

Evidence and extent of acute tubular necrotic lesions depend on tubular clogging by myoglobin and possibly to some degree hemoglobin. The above pathological picture is commonly referred to as myoglobinuric nephrosis or nephropathy. Sometimes the

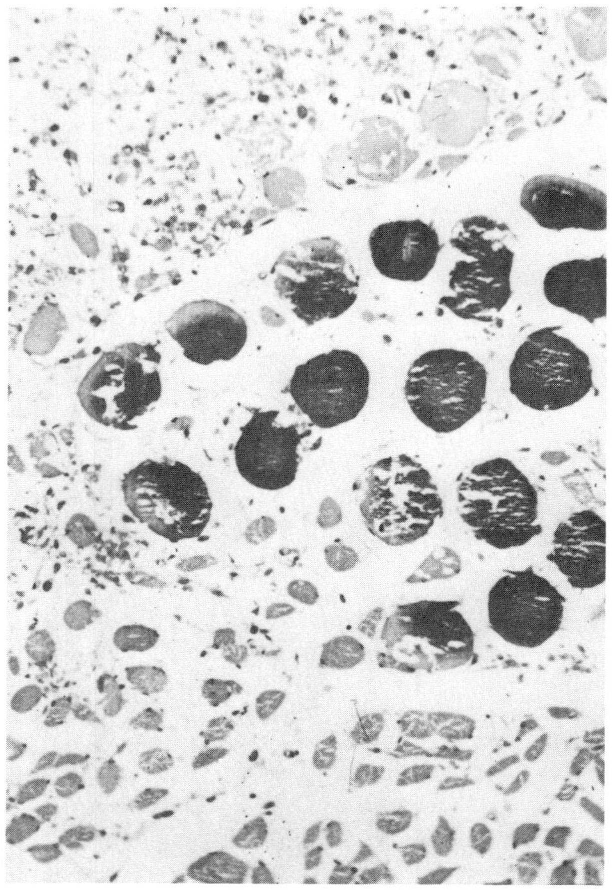

FIGURE 14-6: Muscle fibers showing areas of degenerative changes with many foci of necrosis (dark areas), interstitial edema, and inflammatory reaction. (H&E ×130) (In Haimovici H: *Vascular Emergencies,* Appleton-Century Crofts, p. 273, 1984.)

latter findings are mixed with preexisting nephrosclerotic lesions which are apt to aggravate the prognosis.

The pathogenesis of the acute renal failure associated with this syndrome of myoglobinuria has brought to light unsolved problems. However, on the basis of the histologic data reported

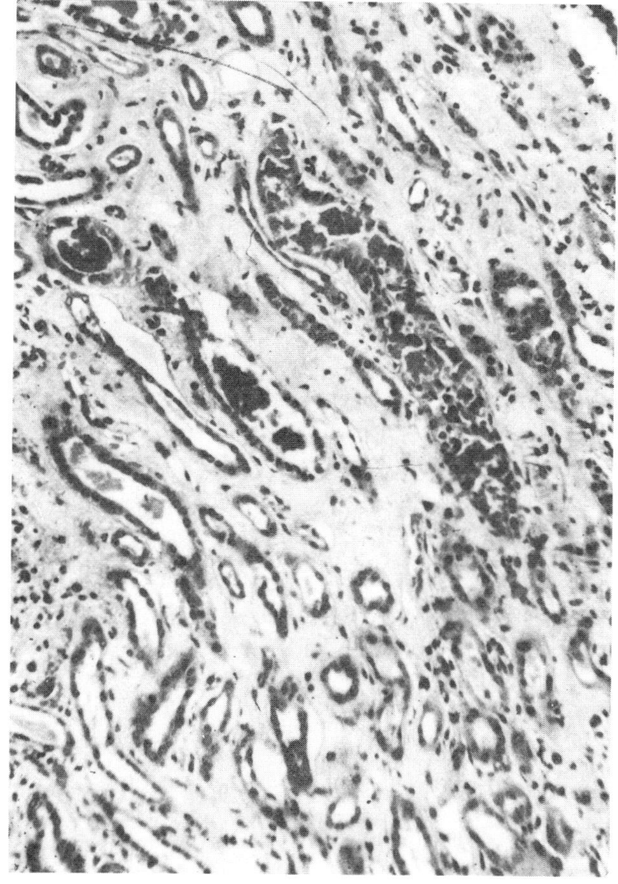

FIGURE 14-7: Renal tubules containing casts with evidence of discontinuity of epithelium showing necrosis and reactive epithelial cells indicating regeneration ($\times$ 130), (From Haimovici H: Arterial embolism, myoglobinuria and renal tubular necrosis. *Arch Surg* 100:639, 1970.)

above, obtained from both human autopsy material and experimental animal models, the presence of myoglobin casts in the renal tubules seems to strongly suggest a causal relationship between the tubular mechanical blockage by the myoglobin casts and the acute renal shutdown. In addition, there is some sugges-

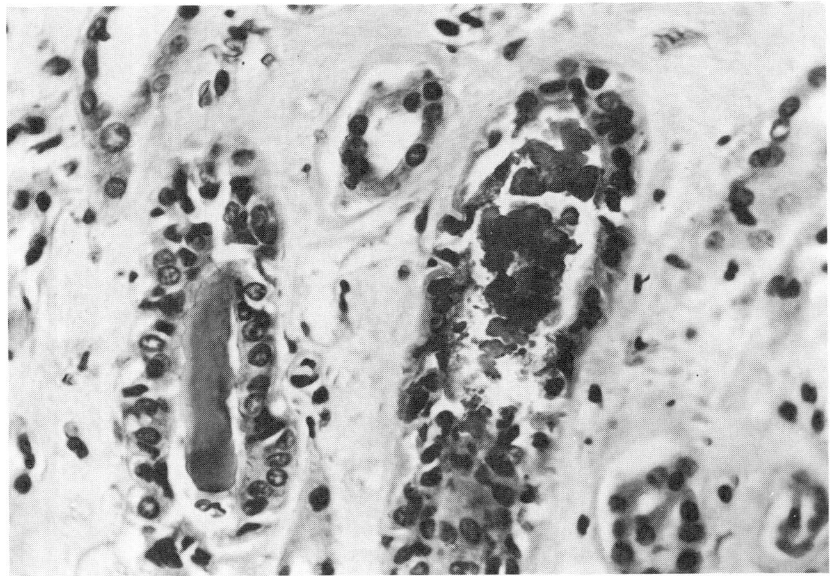

Figure 14-8: Renal tubules containing casts of myoglobin and showing reactive epithelium cells indicating regeneration ($\times 440$). (From Haimovici H: Arterial embolism, myoglobinuria and renal tubular necrosis. *Arch Surg* 100:639, 1970.)

tive evidence that myoglobin *per se* has a direct toxic effect on the tubules. Acute renal failure has indeed been induced experimentally by the infusion of myoglobin, but not by the use of hemoglobin.[293]

Clinical Course: Prognosis

The clinical course of this syndrome varies with the severity and duration of the metabolic complications, which in turn depend on the extent and degree of tissue damage. In mild or moderate cases of ischemia, the metabolic alterations—including hyperkalemia, myoglobinuria, and elevation of CPK—may last only a short period of time and are completely reversible. In severe cases of ischemia, the metabolic and structural repercussions are often largely irreversible. Although some of these metabolic changes can be easily corrected, the hyperkalemia and myoglobinuria may reach dangerous levels due to massive muscle necrosis.

The clinical course may be affected by several factors, of which the most important are: (1) the number, extent, and level of arterial occlusions; (2) the duration of the occlusions; (3) the extent of involvement of intramuscular arterioles and venules; (4) the awareness and early recognition of this syndrome; and (5) the immediate aggressive treatment of the ischemia and its early metabolic manifestations.

The overall limb loss due to gangrene is quite high, ranging between 30% and 50%. In our own experience, gangrene was present in 25% of the survivors and in 36% of the fatal cases. The more proximal the acute occlusion is (e.g., in the aortoiliac), the more massive the rhabdomyolysis. This leads to higher amputation rates and lower survival rates than are found in patients with femoropopliteal occlusions. Although late or delayed thromboembolectomy may represent a negative prognostic factor, it is primarily the degree of ischemia and not the chronology that is the determining factor in these cases.

The reported mortality rates range from 30% to 80%. Sarrazin[254] and Cassar,[37] both studying a group of 23 cases, reported a mortality rate of only 30%, while Gutierrez-Carreño[97] noted a mortality rate of 44.4% in a group of nine patients. In our series, seven of 15 patients (47%) died. On the other hand, Cormier and Devin[44] reported a mortality rate of 80% in 25 cases. The high rate of fatality is usually attributed to hyperkalemia, uncontrolled acidosis, and acute renal shutdown, with its inherent complications.

Skeletal Muscle Reperfusion Injury

While the initiating ischemia of the skeletal muscle results in rhabdomyolysis, the reperfusion phase is further complicated by free radicals-induced ischemia leading to additional superimposed necrosis.[27,28,52,55,123,182]

In the past few years, a large body of evidence has been accumulated mostly in connection with ischemic-induced myocardium, due either to primary occlusion of the coronary arteries or secondarily during coronary bypass surgery. It has become increasingly clear that during reflow or reperfusion into a region of a hypoxic or ischemic myocardium or skeletal muscle, one may observe paradoxical results consisting of marked increase of ischemic damage.[56,85,142,274] A number of experimental studies have shown that the blood flow to skeletal muscle obstructed for one-half to several hours may result in edema formation after release of the occlusion. The longer the period of ischemia, the more pronounced edema formation is noted, primarily due to changes in *vascular permeability*.

Recent studies in ischemic-reperfusion injury in skeletal muscle have shown that the role of oxygen-derived free radicals in the genesis of increased vascular permeability and the production of active oxygen species can be prevented by pretreatment with specific oxygen radical scavengers,[85,140a,155] as will be discussed in connection with treatment of this phase (see Chapter 26).

Clinical Cases

Table II illustrates 15 patients with metabolic syndrome associated with acute arterial occlusions. This table summarizes some of the essential clinical data on 15 patients seen between 1959 and 1977 from a group of over 200 patients with acute arterial occlusions who presented with the metabolic syndrome. There were 10 patients with arterial embolism (cases 1, 2, 4, 5, 7, 10, 11, 12, 13, and 15) and five with acute thrombosis complicating previously implanted grafts (cases, 3, 6, 8, 9, and 14).

In the 10 patients with arterial embolism, there were 16 extremities involved, of which 14 displayed severe ischemic manifestations, whereas the five patients with acute thrombosis had seven involved limbs and all were severely ischemic.

Eleven of these patients were men. The average age in the embolism group was 64 years (range 35 to 83 years) and in the thrombosis group 58.5 years (range 48 to 66 years).

The clinical manifestations of these cases were quite severe and of course in many ways very different from the common forms of acute arterial occlusions. Their distinctive features included (1) a metabolic syndrome due to ischemic rhabdomyolysis, and (2) a high incidence of limb loss as well as high mortality rates, as indicated in the table.

To provide a more detailed report on these patients, the

following three cases will illustrate most of the important features included in this table.

Case Reports

Case #1 (Patient #15)

A 54-year old man was admitted to Montefiore Hospital on February 13, 1977, for evaluation and management of an incapacitating left hip claudication. Except for mild arterial hypertension, he was free of diabetes or any cardiac disorder. A right transfemoral aortogram revealed a marked stenosis of the left iliac arteries (common and external), occlusion of the hypogastric at its origin, and stenosis of the origin of the superficial femoral. On February 16, a left iliac thromboendarterectomy involving all three segments was carried out uneventfully. Three days later, the reamed-out artery became thrombosed, requiring a 10 mm Dacron velour tube for a bypass between the proximal iliac and the common femoral arteries. Following this procedure, all pulses were restored. About 12 hours later, although the pulsation of the graft in the groin was bounding, the left leg up to mid-calf was found to be cold, mottled, very painful, and rigid. Motion of toes and ankle was absent, and calf muscles were hard, tense, and swollen, especially in the anterior compartment. At exploration, the superficial femoral, the profunda, and the popliteal arteries were all found to be occluded by thromboemboli. Patency of these vessels was restored by thromboembolectomy and a bypass graft with a 6 mm expanded polytetrafluoroethylene (PTFE Gore-Tex) tube from the Dacron graft in the groin to the mid-popliteal artery. In addition, fasciotomies of the anterior and posterior compartments also were performed. Appropriate muscle biopsies were secured for histologic identification of the lesions.

Hospital Course

Before the operation, in addition to the compartment syndromes, the urine was concentrated and dark brown, indicating the possibility of myoglobinuria. The patient was given in-

Table II
Patients with Metabolic Syndrome Associated with Acute Arterial Occlusions

Case No.*	Age (yr)	Sex	Site and nature of occlusion	Procedure	Results: Limb	Results: Patient
1	64	M	Right iliac embolism	Iliofemoral embolectomy	Gangrene	Died; renal shutdown
2	35	M	Left iliac embolism	Iliofemoral embolectomy	Gangrene; above-knee amputation	Recovered
3	65	F	Right iliofemoral thrombosis	Thrombectomy (concurrent with aortoiliac bypass graft)	Gangrene; above-knee amputation	Recovered
4	57	M	Aortic saddle embolism	Aortic embolectomy	Bilateral gangrene; bilateral above-knee amputation	Died; renal shutdown
5	42	M	Bilateral femoral embolism	Bilateral embolectomy	Bilateral gangrene; bilateral above-knee amputation	Recovered
6	66	M	Thrombosis of 6-yr-old aortoiliac graft	Right axillofemoral bypass; fasciotomies	Recovered	Died; renal shutdown
7	71	F	Left iliac embolism	Left iliofemoral bypass; fasciotomy	Gangrene	Died; heart failure & myoglobinuria
8	56	M	Thrombosis of 7½-yr-old aortobifemoral graft with lower extremity thrombosis	Replacement of aortobifemoral graft into profunda aortic artery; fasciotomies	Recovered	Died 4 days after operation

9	42	M	Thrombosis of 15-mo.-old right femoropopliteal graft	Thrombectomy of graft; fasciotomy of calf	Recovered (necrosis of soleus)	Recovered
10	83	F	Bilateral femoral embolism	Bilateral femoral embolectomy; right leg fasciotomy	Recovered	Died; heart failure
11	63	M	Right femoral and left iliofemoral embolism	Bilateral transfemoral embolectomy; right leg fasciotomy	Recovered	Recovered
12	83	F	Bilateral femoral embolism	Bilateral femoral embolectomy; right leg fasciotomy	Left recovered; right remained ischemic	Died 24 hr after operation; heart failure
13	79	M	Bilateral femoral embolism (after aortic graft)	Bilateral femoral embolectomy; fasciotomies	Recovered	Recovered
14	66	M	Thrombosis of left popliteal graft	Thrombectomy & popliteal-dorsalis pedis bypass graft; fasciotomy	Recovered	Recovered
15	54	M	Left femoral (superficial & profunda embolism)	Embolectomy; femoropopliteal bypass; fasciotomy	Recovered	Recovered

*Cases 1 through 4 have been reported fully previously.[14]

travenous sodium bicarbonate before and after surgery. Following the procedure, the foot became warm and the pulses returned. The calf remained swollen for about 4 to 5 days after operation and then progressively decreased in size. The urine cleared up progressively, with the output remaining excellent throughout. Of interest were the facts that the blood urea nitrogen and potassium levels had remained within normal limits throughout the postoperative course. Besides the presence of myoglobin in the urine for 48 hours, the only other chemical changes were those seen in the serum enzymes. The serum glutamic oxaloacetic transaminase, the serum glutamic pyruvic transaminase, and the lactic dehydrogenase levels all went up on the fourth day after operation and returned to control levels on the twelfth day after operation. The greatest changes were seen in the creatine phosphokinase, increasing progressively up to 1,725 units on the sixth day after operation and then decreasing to 102 units on the twelfth day after operation. Histologic examination of the gastrocnemius disclosed focal rhabdomyolysis. The patient improved progressively and was discharged in good condition.

Comments

In brief, the case of acute embolic occlusion of the deep and superficial femoral arteries illustrates early ischemic rhabdomyolysis with mild myoglobinuria. The immediate recognition of the syndrome prior to the revascularization and treatment of the condition during the post-revascularization phase were successful in preventing any serious complications. In this case, the muscular mass involved was much smaller, a fact that may account for a less severe metabolic syndrome, in contrast to the next two cases.

Case #2 (Patient #4)

A 57-year-old white man was admitted to the hospital approximately 10 hours following sudden onset of pain and paralysis of both lower extremities.

Except for chronic alcoholism, his past history failed to reveal any significant medical condition. On admission, the diagnosis of aortic embolism was made. The source of the embolus was not apparent until the next day when the electrocardiographic tracings disclosed changes consistent with coronary insufficiency.

A transperitoneal aortic embolectomy was carried out about 16 to 17 hours after the clinical onset. At the conclusion of the procedure, it was noted that the patient was putting out urine and that the femoral pulses had become readily palpable. Shortly after his admission to the recovery room, however, the clinical picture was that of persisting severe ischemia of both feet and legs associated with marked oliguria.

Approximately 16 hours postoperatively, the patient presented pre-gangrenous changes of both feet and legs, extreme rigidity of both ankles and calf muscles, absent pedal and popliteal pulses but palpable femorals, and urinary output of 5 to 6 cc per hour, the urine being of a dark red color.

The impression, in the presence of these findings, was that the patient had massive ischemia of both legs associated with renal shutdown secondary to possible myoglobinuria, which was confirmed shortly thereafter. Despite alkalinization, use of mannitol, and other measures in the management of his renal failure, the patient's condition deteriorated rapidly. The serum potassium level was 7.2 mg/100 cc. It was felt that early amputation would stop the toxemia and possibly slow down the renal failure. Consequently, a bilateral mid-thigh amputation was performed about 48 hours after the embolectomy.

At the site of amputation, there was no subcutaneous edema, although the thighs appeared swollen. Significant changes, however, were found in the muscles, which appeared edematous, pale gray, and tense. At the end of the procedure, the muscles had reddened considerably and assumed normal color, although remaining still somewhat edematous. Minimal stenosing atheromatous changes were present in the femoral and popliteal arteries, while the accompanying veins appeared occluded by old organized thrombi.

The patient's subsequent clinical condition deteriorated, with the daily urinary output being 147 cc and increasing slowly up to 381 cc about 2 weeks later, the day before he died. The BUN level on the last day rose to 186 mg/100 ml and his serum creatinine level was 16.6/100 ml. The electrolytes were maintained at normal levels. The potassium level was below 4. Four days before his death, a hemoptysis was noted and the diagnosis of pulmonary infarction was entertained. Chest x-rays were consistent with congestive heart failure with varying degrees of pneumonitis. His clinical picture followed a progressive downhill course and 17 days postoperatively, the patient died.

Comments

This case of aortic saddle embolus illustrates a most severe case of ischemic myopathy leading to myoglobinuria, renal shutdown due to renal tubular necrosis, and fatal outcome. Histologic studies of the muscles and of the kidneys disclosed severe changes in the muscles of the limb and myoglobin crystals in the tubules, with severe changes in the tubular epithelium.

Case #3 (Patient #6)

A 66-year old man was admitted to Montefiore Hospital on January 22, 1972, 5 ½ hours after sudden severe pain of both lower extremities. His past history showed that on June 6, 1966, the patient had an aortoiliac Dacron bifurcation bypass graft and bilateral lumbar synpathectomy for occlusive disease. On admission, the femoral pulse in the groin was absent bilaterally. The left lower extremity appeared to be moderately viable, while the right was mottled, cyanotic, associated with a swollen, hard, and tender calf. The electrocardiogram revealed premature ventricular contractions with no evidence of myocardial infarction. Operative findings 8 hours after onset revealed thrombosis of the graft and infrarenal aorta and disruption of the anastomosis. An attempt to sew in a new graft was futile because of friability of the infrarenal aorta due to extreme atheromatous changes. The infrarenal aorta then was ligated, and a right axillofemoral graft and fasciotomies of the leg compartments were carried out.

Following the axillofemoral bypass, a good femoral pulse returned, the limb became warm, but the swelling of the thigh, leg, and foot increased.

Laboratory Findings

The patient remained oliguric, and his urine was concentrated and contained myoglobin for the first 3 days, as determined spectroscopically. Table III summarizes the major biochemical findings.

On the first day, the arterial pH was 7.330, PCO_2 was 36, and PO_2 was 220. The next day the pH was 7.268, the PCO_2 was 59, the PO_2 was 200. After he was extubated, the pH still remained at 7.305, the PCO_2 at 44, and the PO_2 at 80. These arterial blood findings remained the same for 5 days after admission, in spite of use of sodium bicarbonate which had been started prior to and during the first surgical procedure. On the fourth day, his potassium went up to 6.8 mg/100 ml.

Because of oliguria since admission and due to the progressively rising blood urea nitrogen and creatinine clearance levels, he was put on renal dialysis, in addition to exchange resins (Kayexalate). A few days later he developed seizures due to hypocalcemia. In spite of intensive care and constant supervision of his metabolic disorders, he died on February 4, 1972, 15 days after the acute aortic occlusion.

Post-Mortem Examination

At the post-morten examination, except for focal infarction of the right kidney and of the bladder, all of the organs failed to disclose any serious disorders. The coronary arteries displayed only a moderate degree of atherosclerosis without occlusion, and there was no evidence of previous or recent infarction. Histologically the kidneys displayed acute tubular necrosis. Muscle biopsies taken during the fasciotomies of the anterior tibial and gas-

Table III
Laboratory Findings in a Patient with a Failed Aortoiliac Graft (6 Years after Implantation)

	Day 1	*Day 9*	*Day 14*
BUN (mg%)	20.0	171.0	264.0
Creatine (mg%)	1.3	10.5	17.1
Uric Acid (mg%)	8.2	19.8	30.6
Calcium (mg%)	10.3	6.4	5.3
Phosphate (mg%)	1.9	6.9	8.7
LDH (IU/L)	210.0	2,745.0	1,485.0
SGOT (IU/L)	50.0	1,980.0	1,593.0
CPK (IU/L)	210.0	10,800.0	17,910.0

trocnemius displayed swelling and hyalinization of the individual fibers characteristic of ischemic changes.

In brief, the acute thrombosis of the aortoiliac bypass graft implanted 6 years previously resulted in a dramatic clinical and metabolic syndrome which led to the death of the patient in spite of all measures taken to overcome the effects of the rhabdomyolysis, the acute tubular necrosis, and the electrolytic imbalance.

Discussion: Views on Pathogenesis

It is quite apparent from the preceding data that the cases of arterial embolism that result in the above-reported metabolic complications exhibit different features from those of the common clinical form. Among the several underlying factors, differentiating these severe forms from the latter, appear to be the following: (1) a massive obliterating process that leads to an "absolute" ischemia not necessarily related to its duration, since the clinical-metabolic syndrome often assumes an "explosive" onset; (2) a poor or ineffective collateral network, as a corollary of the massive occlusion of the main arterial tree; (3) widespread irreversible ischemic lesions of the skeletal muscles; and (4) combined severe hemodynamic and metabolic phenomena.

In attempting to analyze the underlying mechanism of the various changes due to an acute ischemia, as emphasized by Malan[175] and others, one should bear in mind that the responses of the various tissues to anoxia are not identical. First, the most vulnerable to massive ischemia are the peripheral nerves. Second to be involved in this "asphyxia metabolism" are the striated muscles. Because of the large mass of tissue represented by the muscles in the extremities, their involvement dominates the metabolic complications in these arterial occlusions. The level of plasma CPK is direct biochemical evidence of the degree of muscle damage.

The pathogenesis of this complex clinical, pathological, and metabolic syndrome is currently the subject of diverse investigations (see Chapter 13) (Table IV). A few laboratory experimental studies have attempted to clarify the mechanism of the metabolic effects, especially that of the liberation of myoglobin, by using tightly applied tourniquets across the thighs of dogs.[193] It was

Table IV
Pathogenesis of Myonephropathic-Metabolic Syndrome in Acute Arterial Occlusions

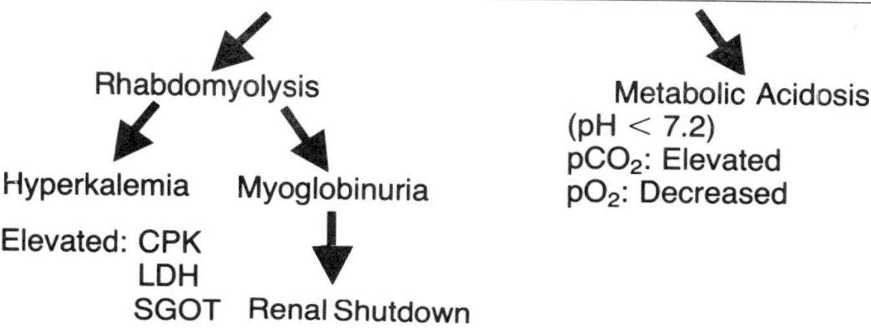

found that 4 to 7 hours after release of the tourniquets, myoglobin was liberated from striated muscles into both blood and lymph and was excreted in the urine. The peak concentration of myoglobin appeared in blood and lymph within 2 to 4 hours after release of the tourniquets, while its peak urinary excretion occurred during the second hour. Using a somewhat different experimental set-up (tourniquets and cross-circulation), Snyder and Campbell[267] have shown that reestablishment of blood flow to previously ischemic limbs is associated with myoglobinuria, hyperkalemia, and aciduria followed quite often by renal insufficiency. These experimental models were set up for reproducing a "crush syndrome" due to direct massive injury of all the traumatized tissues. Similar observations have been made during experimental and clinical replantation of limbs.

Clinical and biochemical observations on the relationship of acute arterial obstruction to muscle damage were carried out on the effect of transient femoral artery occlusion in patients undergoing cardiopulmonary bypass with retrograde femoral artery perfusion, and in patients before and after arterial embolectomy.[77] In the first group, severe venous hypoxia and moderate hypercapnia were noted in the limb with perfusion through the femoral artery. In the group with arterial emboli, restoration of flow after embolectomy was associated with transient but severe hypoxia, marked hypercapnia, fall in venous pH, and increased CPK. The biochemical findings in this study, on the whole, were of a mild nature, and no sequelae were noted. In these cases, the metabolic changes bore no resemblance to the severity of the syndrome reported in the preceding cases, but their significance as metabolic complications indicate that they may remain limited if recognized and treated without delay.

Contrasting with the above report of rather mild and transient hemodynamic and metabolic effects, the severe *myonephropathic-metabolic syndrome* associated with massive acute arterial occlusions appeared to be less frequent. However, the reports presented at the Symposium of the European Cardiovascular Surgery in 1972 (Brussels) and a more recent one of the Japanese Society of Cardiovascular Surgery (May 1987) are a clear reflection of the world-wide growing awareness and interest in this syndrome and suggest that it is less infrequent than the literature seemed to imply up to now.

The pathogenetic mechanism of the metabolic events, based on the preceding data, may be described as a successive series of biochemical alterations. The common denominator of most of the changes is the initiating severe ischemia of the skeletal muscles. The onset of these alterations is sometimes difficult to assess clinically. If muscle tenderness and rigidity are considered as an index, then muscle involvement must be present at a very early stage and is probably the first sign in the chain of events leading to the biochemical and metabolic changes. Among these, CPK and myoglobin are most important chemical indicators of ischemia. In some of my cases operated upon within 4 to 6 hours, the muscles appeared edematous and pale ("fish-flesh"). It is of interest to note that Carlström described an equine paroxysmal myoglobinuria syndrome in which the iliopsoas and the quadriceps femoris appeared edematous and pale, a condition apparently caused by thrombosis of the abdominal aorta.[36]

Microscopically, there is a great variety of morphological changes of the muscular fibers, ranging from slight to moderate degenerative changes to actual necrosis. As noted previously, these consist of loss of striations and of sarcolemmal nuclei of muscular fibers seen in most cases, especially in the early stages, while in more advanced cases, necrotic foci together with regeneration of fibers may be seen. As a result of these morphological alterations, chemical changes occur at the cellular level where myoglobin, potassium, CPK, etc., are released into the blood and lymph streams. The basic morphological derangement resides in permeability alteration of the membrane of the muscle fibers, due to decreased ATP as a result of ischemia (see Chapter 4, *Membranes: Their Role in Biochemical Interchanges*.

The amount of myoglobin released from the muscles, the duration of the myoglobinemia, and the resulting myoglobinuria appear to vary from case to case. The renal damage observed in these cases is due in large part to the precipitation of myoglobin and possibly due also to hemoglobin in the renal tubules. It is generally accepted that the renal lesion is primarily a function of the amount of myoglobin retained in the tubules. The precipitation of this pigment in the kidney depends on its degree of excretion and the urinary pH. Since most of those patients display metabolic acidosis, the latter will predispose to precipitation of this pigment in the tubules. The therapeutic implication is clear and indicates the need for alkalinization of the patient to prevent and counteract the acidosis, as already emphasized.

As already mentioned, the CPK level, which varies with the degree of muscle damage, is an important biochemical marker of the degree of muscle necrosis.

Hyperkalemia, seen in most of these patients, is likewise the result of release of potassium from the muscle fibers due to cellular membrane alteration. Awareness of this and the other biochemical complications, resulting from muscle ischemia, especially in prolonged occlusions, should evoke appropriate therapeutic measures for the prevention of a serious outcome.

Therapeutic Orientation

The basic principles and the specific modalities of management will be found in Chapter 27.

Postscript

This chapter dealing with arterial embolism was conceived to be more detailed than the subsequent clinical entities included in this section. As such, this chapter on arterial embolism represents the prototype of an acute arterial occlusion in which rhabdomyolysis and severe metabolic complications exemplify the hallmarks conveyed by this monograph. It is understood that not all the clinical entities in this section are characterized by the identical manifestations described here in this chapter, although the basic rhabdomyolytic and metabolic complications are to be found in every one of these entities.

15

Temporary Ischemia of the Lower Extremity Secondary to Clamping of Major Arteries

Introduction

With the advent of reconstructive surgery of the abdominal aortic segment, a number of hemodynamic and metabolic complications were encountered. These problems appeared to be primarily associated with resection of abdominal aortic aneurysms. These complications were noted in connection with operations of a major artery, mostly the aorta, [29,57,58,62a,141,176] and to a lesser extent the iliac or femoral arteries, as a result of temporary occlusion during the surgical procedure. The resulting mild or severe hypotension, often associated with variable degrees of metabolic changes, has led to a large amount of investigative work to explain these phenomena which were unexpected at that time. The sudden decrease in blood pressure, known as the "declamping phenomenon" or "declamping shock," has been extensively studied both in laboratory animals and to a lesser extent in conjunction with human reconstructive arterial surgery.

The results of declamping after experimentally induced occlusion of the abdominal aorta were dependent essentially on the method and extent of the associated arterial exclusions.

Experimental Data

Isolated Aortic Clamping

Mongrel dogs were used in most of these studies. The animals were anesthetized with pentobarbitol sodium in most experiments using concomitant ventilation through an endotracheal tube by a respirator.

In the temporary aortic cross-clamping, the hemodynamic and metabolic changes were usually mild and transient. They varied with the duration of the occlusion of the aorta. Strandness,[279] occluding the infrarenal aorta induced for 1 hour, found at declamping a 23% decrease in the average mean aortic pressure and a 21% decrease in the average cardiac output. Associated with these findings was a decreased hind leg volume after clamping and an increased volume within 60 seconds after declamping which later returned to normal. According to Strandness, the acute drop in blood pressure which occurred at the end of temporary abdominal aortic occlusion, was a result of translocation of blood into the vascular bed distal to the clamp and was independent of the duration of clamping if blood volume is unchanged. As pointed out by the author, the gradient of pressure across the clamp at the time of release of occlusion appeared to be the most important factor determining the magnitude of blood volume shift and resultant drop in pressure. To prevent this pressure change, this investigator felt that the rapid injection of a vasopressor distal to the clamp immediately prior to its removal could be effective in minimizing the drop of blood pressure.

Baue and McClerkin,[10] also using 1-hour cross-clamping, found no evidence for a change in myocardial function as measured by ventricular contractile force. After release of the clamp, both arterial and venous pH fell from 7.38 to 7.28 and from 7.31 to 7.16, respectively. This acidosis lasted 5 to 15 minutes. The acute drop in blood pressure was also attributed to a translocation of transient pooling of blood into a temporarily hypovolemic vascular bed. The magnitude of pressure drop was unrelated to the length of time of clamping, and its duration ranged from a few seconds to 2 or 3 minutes. Like the previous investigators, Baue and McClerkin found that the declamping phenomenon could be prevented or completely eliminated by the use of a vasopressor distal to the clamp immediately prior to its removal.

Combined Aortic Clamping with Multiple Ligations of Major Branches

To obtain an experimental setting approaching clinical situations, experiments were designed to exclude not only the aorta but also multiple branches between the renal arteries, the aortic bifurcation, and its distal branches. In contrast to the previous simple experiments of clamping only of the aorta, the results in this series were quite different. Thus, Engler et al.,[72] using a combined cross-clamping with multiple-branch ligation technique, obtained sustained hypotension associated with hypoxia and acidosis. These changes were prevented by using a small shunt from the aorta above the point of occlusion to the aorta below. It appeared that these experiments by Engler would suggest that the changes observed were due to inadequate arterial pressure perfusion of the muscles distal to the clamped aorta.

Other investigators, using more complex combinations of ligation of major branches, have obtained somewhat similar results to Engler and his group but definitely more involved than in single ligation or clamping of the aorta experiments. Lim et al.,[169] in addition to the cross-clamping of the aorta below the renal arteries, also carried out the ligation of lumbar arteries and all the collaterals of the aorta including the inferior mesenteric artery. Furthermore, marginal vessels of the sigmoid colon, both inferior epigastric arteries, and the spermatic or ovarian arteries were all interrupted to insure that all collateral channels were excluded from the hind limbs and pelvic area. Systemic blood pressure was stable at a mean of 135 mmHg throughout the period of aortic occlusion. At the time of aortic declamping, there was an average fall of 58 mmHg from the prerelease level in the aorta. The mean arterial pH was unchanged during the period of occlusion and was 7.418 after 3 hours of cross-clamping. One hour after declamping, it dropped to 7.399 and then returned to its preclamping level. In brief, severe regional acidosis developed which was not manifested in the systemic circulation when the aorta was occluded. With aortic declamping, there was a liberation of acid metabolites into the systemic circulation and a transient hypotension. Muscle blood flow was zero in the hind legs during the period of occlusion. There was a transient, marked increase in flow following restoration of the distal circulation. However, an important difference from the previous experimental method was the pretreatment with low molecular weight dextran. Although it did not alter the acidotic state, it did prevent the transient declamping hypotension.

Perry,[219] using somewhat similar experimental methods, found that the basic mechanism producing the declamping phenomenon is sequestration of large amounts of the functioning blood volume in the previously ischemic extremities. There was no strong evidence in these experiments to indicate that moderate alterations in pH or excess lactate exert significant depressant effects upon myocardial contractility and cardiac output. The blood volume deficit resulting from the cross-clamping was easily overcome by blood volume replacement.

According to Provan et al.,[230] the major factor contributing to the fall in arterial pressure using cross-clamping of the aorta and multiple ligations of branches appears to be the decreased peripheral resistance in the lower half of the body resulting in greatly increased aortic flow after the clamps were released. Provan et al. used 30 minutes of abdominal aortic occlusion in these experiments for the study of the metabolic and hemodynamic effects of the clamping phenomenon As in the previous experiments, the clamping was followed by a fall in pH in the inferior vena cava in all animals, a rise in caval CO_2 tension, and a fall in caval oxygen tension in two-thirds of the observations. In about a third of their experiments, there was a sustained hypotension after the clamping when the arterial oxygen tension was below 135 mmHg or the arterial pH was below 7.35, or the mean aortic pressure was below 100 mmHg before release of the clamp.

It is obvious that in this setting of experimental combined ligations and clamping, hemodynamic and metabolic phenomena were obviously present but were transient and the situation became normal within a short period after the release of this occlusion of the aorta and the ligated branches.

However, since the preceding experiments induced only temporary and transient changes, a more profound degree of ischemia appeared necessary to achieve results which would parallel those in humans. Thus, a greater number of branches have to be excluded from the vascular system. By excluding all collaterals in addition to all major branches below the femoral, Winninger[299] was able to reproduce hemodynamic and metabolic changes similar to those observed in acute occlusions in humans. The declamping hypotension reached the level of 35–41% of the preclamping level and the arterial pH was markedly decreased, together with a severe systemic acidosis. Stipa et al.,[276] using an even more extensive arterial exclusion technique, reported that during the declamping of the femoral arteries after a 10-hour ischemia, there was progressive acidosis and at least a 50% increase in limb volume associated with shock and rapid death.

In summary, to reproduce experimentally the hemodynamic and metabolic changes found in clinical situations, it is necessary to obtain a wider interruption of the arterial supply than a simple cross-clamping of a major artery. The preceding experiments have demonstrated unequivocally that a progressive increase in exclusion of not only the major arteries but also of the branches beyond the abdominal area, has definitely shown that what happens in the clinical setting with acute arterial occlusions needs to be an extensive arterial interruption process of a substantial degree. Then the hemodynamic and metabolic complications appear to be progessively severe depending not only on the number of occluded arteries but also, and more particularly, on the duration of the occlusion. The following report will illustrate the real role of the duration factor.

Such a set-up was carried out by Esato et al.[73] in 19 dogs in which cross-clamping of the infrarenal abdominal aorta was applied for 48 hours. The experimental animals were divided into three groups according to the treatment applied.

Untreated group. Simple occlusion released after 48 hours without any therapeutic measures. This group served as a control.

The THAM group. The THAM group was administered intravenously 1 hour after the occlusion at a dosage calculated for pH correction. Then, just prior to release of the occlusion, twice the previously injected amount of THAM was administered.

The perfusion group. The perfusion of the peripheral arterial tree performed immediately before release of the clamping using 30 ml/kg of lactated Ringer's solution.

The results were quite different in the three groups. In the untreated group, the SGOT levels increased significantly, reaching the highest levels of 239.9% in 12 hours after the release of the occlusion. They decreased thereafter but remained higher than the preocclusion level. In the THAM group, the SGOT levels in perfusion groups remained near the control values even after the release of the occlusion. Significant differences were seen at 1 and 3 hours only between the untreated and perfusion groups. Also of significance were the high levels of CPK in the untreated group, with the highest level at 3 and 12 hours after the release of the occlusion which remained high for the following 48 hours.

The same results showing marked differences between control and treated groups were noted with all the other biochemical parameters. It appeared from these data that metabolic derangements were effectively controlled by intravenous injections of THAM and by peripheral washout of the ischemic site with lactic Ringer's solution. (For more details see Chapter 13.)

Human Data

The human data obtained with arterial clamping in vascular surgery reflect to some extent the experimental findings summarized above rather briefly. While metabolic alterations may be noted after the declamping of most major arteries, serious hemodynamic changes usually occur mostly after declamping or grafting following excision of an aortic aneurysm.

Reconstructive Arterial Surgery for Occlusive Arterial Disease

In contrast to the experimental procedures designed to interrupt by clamping or ligation of major arteries, in the clinical setting the patient has already preexisting ischemic changes before the clamping of the major arteries required during the operation. Thus, the surgical procedure is a superimposed acute ischemia upon an extremity already suffering from a chronic occlusive arterial disease. Furthermore, at the declamping phase, arterial flow to the vascular bed which is suddenly restored with a larger flow and higher perfusion pressure than before clamping, one may therefore anticipate metabolic consequences of these events in addition to hemodynamic changes.

Metabolic Effects

1. In chronic occlusive disease in patients with only claudication of the extremities, it is usually associated with some degree of muscle hypoxia in which a decreased pH and increased blood lactate and pyruvate are present. Therefore, during reconstructive vascular surgery in such patients, arterial clamping necessary for the procedure has been shown to accentuate the oxygen deficit of the tissues distal to the clamp. The extent to which such cross-clamping of the aortoiliac and femoropopliteal segment produces significant metabolic changes during reconstructive arterial surgery is not widely known, since it has seldom been reported.

2. O'Donnell et al.[206] published a study on metabolic evaluation in 35 patients with chronic occlusive arterial disease, primarily on the basis of muscle *surface measurements of pH,* using the medial belly of the gastrocnemius. Their observations on pH appeared to correlate fairly well with the clinical degree of ischemia. Thus, there was no difference in tissue metabolism of lactate, glucose, and oxygen between control cases and the claudication group. By contrast, a lower pH and a significant increase in lactate release, glucose, and oxygen extraction were observed in the groups with rest pain and ischemic gangrene. After aortofemoral or femoropopliteal arterial reconstruction, muscle surface pH values were comparable with those of the control group (7.42 ± 0.05). Although these pH determinations are indirect measurements of tissue perfusion, O'Donnell et al. considered them to be a sensitive index and a useful clinical approach to metabolic evaluation in muscle ischemia.

Clamping of Femoral Artery

Sorlie et al.,[269] in a study on metabolic changes during *prolonged clamping of the common femoral artery* for femoropopliteal reconstruction, also reported significant changes. Regardless of the degree of preexisting chronic occlusive disease, the femoral cross-clamping for 80 to 180 minutes represents an important superimposed acute ischemia. A battery of biochemical determinations was carried out before, during, and after the release of the femoral clamp. The pH, the PCO_2, PO_2, O_2 saturation, lactate, LDH, and CPK were studied in the popliteal venous effluent and the systemic blood of eight patients. Marked acidosis and a rise in lactate, phosphate, and creatinine were found in all patients. The pH decreased to a mean value of 7.18 and the PCO_2 increased from 45 mmHg to 62 mmHg. There was no statistically significant correlation between the occlusion time and the degree of hypoxia. Of the electrolytes, the potassium concentration increased by 20% in the venous effluent over the preocclusion level. Of the muscle enzymes, only the CPK activity increased, gradually reaching its peak after 8 to 15 hours (mean value 700 units per liter) and returned to normal values in 5 days. As a rule, the maximum CPK level correlated well with the femoral occlusion time. The significance of these metabolic changes, as judged by the CPK activity in the eight patients, was moderate and without any apparent clinical lasting repercussions.

It is of interest to note that in such a simple procedure consisting of cross-clamping of the femoral artery for reconstructive surgery of the vessels below it, several metabolic changes had taken place. This study has demonstrated that there is a definite effect of the arterial occlusion on the local metabolism which was affected by the changes in blood gases, electrolytes, the energy metabolites and muscle enzymes, and the venous effluent from the ischemic lesion. There were systemic consequences from this occlusion of the femoral as reflected in the systemic circulation and, finally, the muscle damage induced by the ischemia of the superimposed clamping was evidenced by the CPK activity for 4 to 5 days postoperatively. Depending on the degree of the occlusive process prior to surgery, more serious metabolic consequences may be observed than in this particular instance.

Abdominal Aortic Clamping

Cross-clamping of the infrarenal abdominal aorta, which induces ischemia of a larger muscular mass than does cross-clamping of the common femoral, was reported by Anderson, Eklof, and their associates.[4] As in the case of the femoral artery clamping, during the reconstructive aortic surgery, the necessary cross-clamping of the aorta will temporarily lower still further the distal blood flow. The hemodynamic and metabolic changes thus induced decrease further and more severely in those patients having aortic aneurysm repair than in those operated on for occlusive aortic disease. Their studies carried out over a period of several years have been performed to determine disturbances in the energy-rich phosphagen metabolites in skeletal muscle of the ischemic limb and in the efferent venous blood. Their hemodynamic and metabolic changes were reported on aortic reconstructive surgery in 14 patients, 12 having occlusive aortic disease and two undergoing surgery for aortic aneurysm repair. Occlusion time of the investigated leg lasted for 69 to 150 minutes (mean 107).

Prior to cross-clamping, before and 30 minutes after aortic declamping, muscle biopsies were obtained from the lateral vastus muscle of the ischemic leg. Glycogen, lactate, phosphocreatine (PCr), creatine (Cr), ATP, ADP, and AMP were measured using enzymatic fluorometric techniques. The results of the cross-clamping and declamping have shown that lactate content increased four-fold and glycogen decreased. Although the PCr content fell, the muscle ATP could not be maintained. However, the muscle creatine did not significantly decline.

Thirty minutes after aortic declamping, the metabolic changes were more dramatic. However, in spite of recirculation of the limb, the lactate level was still high. Both ATP and ADP levels decreased significantly, together with the PCr and Cr contents. Except for one patient with an abdominal aneurysm, no declamping hypotension was noted in these cases. There was a significant post-clamping increase in mean lactate as already mentioned and pyruvate concentration in the iliac venous blood over the values noted before aortic clamping. The values for lactate and pyruvate ranged from 1.49 to 2.80 and from 0.08 to 0.19, respectively, 60 minutes after declamping. The metabolite concentration and the muscle samples 20 minutes after aortic declamping disclosed several significant alterations. The glucose, lactate, pyruvate, and lactate/pyruvate ratio had all increased, while phosphocreatine, ATP, ADP, and AMP showed significant declines to 80% of the preclamping values. These investigators postulated that these findings "might indicate damage in the mitochondria and the cellular membranes in skeletal muscle after temporary arterial occlusion," which is in accordance with the conclusions of other investigators.

The plasma concentration of PCr, Cr, and hypoxanthine in efferent venous blood from the investigated limb showed that while hypoxanthine arteriovenous differences are low, the plasma creatine content was found to increase all through the procedure. On the other hand, the PCr level did not change significantly. The hypoxanthine concentration rose during ischemia and the initial reperfusion, but returned to basal level after 10 minutes of recirculation. The hypoxanthine arteriovenous differences indicate a sharp outflow of this substance on the release of the clamp and during the first 5 to 10 minutes of reoxygenation.

In brief, in patients undergoing aortic repair, the mean muscle blood flow is decreased by 50–90% during cross-clamping depending on the size of persistent blood flow through the developed collaterals. Thus, a limited supply of oxygen and exogenous substrate is still possible. As mentioned, there are several changes in the phosphagen components but all metabolites return to basal level within 5 minutes of recirculation except for the lactate content. As shown by these investigators and others, the cellular transmembrane potential seems to lag behind in restoration and was not normalized until an hour later. The cross-clamping in the latest study induces only minor changes. One of the important conclusions from their latest studies indicates that there is a significant rise in creatine in efferent venous blood accentuated upon reperfusion which, in their opinion, strongly supports the concept of leakage through disrupted muscle cellular membranes. This point has already been made in previous chapters of this monograph.

Based on the current observations, they confirm the possibility of injury to the muscles in the presence of an oxygen-dependent autolytic degradation of the tissue enabled by the low remaining perfusion. The formation of oxy-radicals appears to be a contributing factor as pointed out elsewhere in this monograph.

In accordance with recent concepts of free-radicals, these authors have adapted their own thinking in this new understanding of the reperfusion syndrome. It appears, therefore, that it is not sufficient to simply restore an effective perfusion of previously ischemic tissue but also to protect membrane function at the time of reperfusion. Without mentioning the antidotes to these oxyradicals, they indicate, however, that the multipharmacological approach seems to be necessary. Probably severely ischemic limbs should be specifically treated before and during revascularization to abolish the adverse results of reoxygenation (see Chapter 26).

Abdominal Aortic Aneurysm: Ruptured Lesions and Metabolic Complications

The hemodynamic and metabolic responses to clamping and declamping of the aorta for aortic aneurysms appear to be far more complex than the responses to such clamping in aortoiliac occlusive disease. The preceding studies of Anderson, Eklof, and their associates[4,68] have dealt with cross-clamping of the aorta for abdominal aneurysms, and especially with the metabolic consequences of changes occurring in skeletal muscle as well as in the blood. These changes dealt primarily with the phosphagens and the reperfusion syndrome, in cases of ruptured aneurysms and their severe metabolic complications.

Ever since the early days of this type of surgery, cross-clamping of the infrarenal aorta has received the most attention because of potential metabolic and renal complications. A great variety of opinions have been expressed concerning the mechanism of "declamping shock," for example, the redistribution of blood volume below the clamp, fall in cardiac output, and liberation of a vasodilator substance from the hypoxic tissues during aortic occlusion, etc. It is likely that more than one of these factors and perhaps others are responsible for these complications, the most recently incriminated, among others, being prostaglandin E.

Mansberger et al.,[176] studying the metabolic responses in 15 patients undergoing elective resection of abdominal aortic aneurysms, consistently found a "washout acidosis" following aortic declamping. This was evidenced by a significant fall in pH, elevation of the absolute values of lactate and pyruvate, and excess lactate during occlusion. The venous PO_2 and its saturation were profoundly decreased.

In *ruptured* aortic aneurysms, metabolic and renal repercussions are increased manifold, especially in patients with severe shock, prolonged cross-clamping, and massive transfusions. Of these complications, a renal shutdown represents the single most important cause of mortality ranging from 50–90%. Several mechanisms have been postulated to account for renal complications—e.g., aortorenal reflexes with renovascular spasm, renal atheromatous embolization, and hypovolemic shock associated with multisystem failures. Why some of the postulated mechanisms, such as the aortorenal vasoconstrictor stimuli, have not been corroborated, is the fact that hypovolemic shock is recognized as playing a very important role in the etiology of the prerenal failure. The sudden decreased renal perfusion coupled with the presence of myoglobinuria secondary to prolonged muscular ischemia, related to cross-clamping, provide the intrinsic tubular factor ultimately responsible for the acute renal shutdown. The incidence of the latter factor rarely mentioned in the current literature is difficult to ascertain. Admittedly, a large number of other factors contribute to renal complications, of which rhabdomyolysis and myoglobinuria may play a most significant role in a number of cases as yet undetermined.

McCombs and Roberts[181] reported 17 cases of acute renal failure in a series of 398 cases of abdominal aortic aneurysm, of which nine were resected electively and eight were resected after rupture. The overall incidence was 2.5% following elective operations and 21% after rupture. Nine of the 17 patients had peripheral embolization and four of the nine had showed myonecrosis. However, other factors (e.g., prolonged cross-clamping and preoperative-interoperative hypotension in 11 other patients) were likely to have contributed to the renal problem.

While the surgeon's ability to deal with the multiple factors leading to renal complications is often limited, renal protective measures during aortic cross-clamping must be vigorously applied, along with measures designed to protect against acidosis, myoglobinuria, hyperkalemia, etc. In some cases, extracorporeal shunting during aneurysm repair may be considered, as has been recently advocated. Acute renal failure, although reported elsewhere in this monograph, is mentioned here only in relation to aortic cross-clamping associated with severe aortic disease, which represents, actually, the major factor of the kidney catastrophe. The anatomopathological and physiological factors are discussed elsewhere. Appropriate and urgent treatment may reduce considerably the usually poor prognosis attached to this condition (see Chapter 19).

16

Acute Abdominal Aortic Occlusions

Acute Abdominal Aortic Occlusions

Acute occlusion of the terminal abdominal aorta and its bifurcation displays clinical manifestations most often of a catastrophic nature. Two major etiologic factors are generally responsible for this condition.

Saddle Embolus of the Aortic Bifurcation

Its sudden and complete occlusion results usually in bilateral absence of femoral pulses, complete paralysis of the lower extremities, coldness, and mottled cyanosis with pallor, extending sometimes above the hip regions and reaching the umbilicus. In incomplete occlusion of the aortic bifurcation, there is a disparity in degree of manifestations between the two sides, with one side displaying a weak femoral pulsation and minimal neurovascular manifestations in contrast to the opposite side which shows maximum ischemic changes. An aortic embolus usually reflects a most severe co-existing heart disease (myocardial infarction, chronic decompensated cardiac failure).

The incidence of aortic embolism, based on the statistics of our own studies, was 11% out of a total of 300 cases involving the lower extremities. The natural course in the untreated aortic cases resulted in 28.5% of early death and gangrene of both limbs, while in the survivors gangrene and amputation occurred in 39%. Partial recovery occurred in 32.5%, especially in younger patients with incomplete aortic occlusion.[100]

Acute Arterial Thrombosis

Acute arterial thrombosis, the second major etiologic factor, as distinct from arterial embolism, may occur as a result of a great number of local arterial factors or as the consequence of associated systemic diseases. The relative incidence of acute thrombosis and arterial embolism is not always easy to establish, especially in elderly patients with combined cardiopathy and peripheral arteriosclerosis. As a result, all episodes of acute arterial obstructions, regardless of origin or etiology, have often been wrongly classified together as "acute arterial occlusion." Indeed, the classification into two separate groups is not merely a matter of semantics. Prognostically and therapeutically, it is important to distinguish embolism from acute thrombosis.

In a previously published compiled review of a total of 1,576 cases of acute arterial occlusions of the lower extremities, 892 or 56.6% were due to embolism and 684 or 43.4% were due to acute thrombosis.[101] Of these, the relative incidence of acute occlusion of the aorta due to embolism and acute thrombosis were also different. The former occurred in 14.9% while the latter occurred in 7.5%. It appears, therefore, that the nature of the acute aortic occlusion is predominantly embolic. This fact, besides other features, is of great therapeutic significance. The same holds true from a pathophysiological point of view, since the latter is somewhat different in the two conditions. In embolism, the degree of occlusion depends essentially on the size of the embolus and the local arterial response to its sudden impact. In acute thrombosis, the level of occlusion depends on (1) preexisting arterial lesions, and (2) their preponderance in certain areas, such as the abdominal aorta that displays a relatively great susceptibility to atherosclerosis.

Acute infrarenal aortic thrombosis is, however, less frequent than embolic occlusions and is also infrequent in contrast to the common entity of chronic aortoiliac occlusive disease (Leriche syndrome). Its sudden occurrence has the earmarks of a catastrophic event, not unlike a massive saddle embolism, which it mimics in all its clinical manifestations. The pathophysiology and hemodynamics are quite different in the chronic thrombotic occlusions from those in acute thrombosis. In the former, the increments of the atherosclerotic lesions of the aortic wall proceed slowly, over many years, until the reduction of the lumen reaches a critical stenosis (80% of the cross-sectional area). If acute thrombosis occurs at this stage, it may be well tolerated due to collaterals. However, when the terminal aortic thrombosis occurs in a lumen still below the critical stenosis or in a nearly normal lumen, the ischemic effects are sudden and severe, with pain in both legs followed by paresis or paraplegia.

The physical findings are similar to those encountered in aortic saddle embolism: absent pulses below the umbilicus, coldness, mottled cyanosis of the skin distal to the midabdomen and buttocks, and numbness and loss of motion in both lower extremities.

The medical background of this group of patients shows frequent associated disease due to generalized arteriosclerosis, involving the legs, the kidneys, the cerebral circulation, the heart, etc. Although these patients may display cardiac decompensation, they usually do not have an emboligenic cardiopathy.

While prior intermittent claudication may be present in some of these patients due to aortoiliac stenosis, the acute aortic thrombosis usually appears suddenly, without a previous history of arterial insufficiency. As a rule, the occlusive process involves not only the terminal aorta but also both common iliacs. The distribution of the thrombosis in nine cases reported by Danto et al.[51] was variable but extensive: (1) in four cases, the thrombosis extended up to the level of the renal arteries; (2) in five cases, the thrombosis extended up to or below the inferior mesenteric artery; (3) in three cases, the thrombosis was confined to the aortoiliac area, while in the other six there was considerable distal propagation of prior occlusion; and (4) in one case, the thrombosis occurred in an abdominal aortic aneurysm. Similar patterns have also been noted by others. In a recent article by Littooy and Baker,[171] out of 18 cases of acute aortic occlusion, 10 were embolic and eight were due to acute thrombosis. Of these, six had thrombosis of preexisting aortoiliac occlusive disease. One of these was induced by blunt trauma. The other two patients had totally occluded previously patent aortobifemoral bypass grafts, and one of these was induced by blunt trauma in a biking accident.

Differential Diagnosis

The differential diagnosis of embolism and thrombosis from other conditions must first ascertain the presence of an emboligenic cardiopathy or absence of a prior history of intermittent claudication. The differentiation between these two entities, however, is not always easy. A dissecting aneurysm, if it involves the abdominal aorta and iliac arteries, may mimic an acute occlusion. Chest and abdominal pain, together with an enlarged mediastinum and a double lumen on the aortogram, will help to establish the correct differential diagnosis.

Management

While the exact nature of the acute aortic occlusion can be difficult at times, as mentioned above, the diagnosis of the occlusion *per se*, in contrast, is relatively straightforward by the symptomatology described. The clinical presentation is dependent on the extent of the obstruction, presence of propagated clot, distal emboli, and the patient's collateral circulation.

The suspected diagnosis of either embolic or thrombotic occlusion of the abdominal aorta mandates immediate use of IV heparin as well as fluids including Ringer's lactate solution, and sodium bicarbonate given in large amounts in the attempt to overcome the potential metabolic acidosis which is quite frequently encountered and very rarely mentioned in the papers dealing with this subject. This has a double advantage: first it provides the necessary fluids for patients who are very often hypovolemic and, most importantly, it provides the necessary antidote to the metabolic acidosis and prevents the myoglobin from precipitation in the tubules, thus preventing renal shutdown. Although myoglobin is one of the important metabolites released by the ischemic muscle, other biochemical factors released by the same muscle through the damaged myofibrillar membranes are rarely mentioned. CPK, potassium, calcium, LDH, SGOT, etc. are significant from diagnostic and prognostic points of view. All of these biochemical factors will determine the prognosis not only of the viability of the limb, but also of the survival of the patient.

The problem that arises often in these cases is the necessity of preoperative angiography. This is somewhat controversial because of the potential hazards involved. Standard angiography without digital subtraction techniques is often difficult. The patient should always be well hydrated regardless of whether angiography is being contemplated because of renal failure, which could either be caused or worsened by the contrast material.

Time Interval to Revascularization

Early or immediate recognition of the acute condition is essential for the successful management of these acute embolic or thrombotic occlusions of the abdominal aorta. Recognition of the diagnosis in acute thrombosis appears to be somewhat delayed by comparison with the acute embolic occlusion. Thus, the time from the onset of symptoms until the revascularization of the extremity averaged 10.3 hours in embolic cases in contrast to 26.1 hours in cases of acute thrombosis.[171] The delay between the onset of the symptoms and the revascularization of the extremities may result in metabolic complications secondary to acute rhabdomyolysis. Thus, renal failure and mortality are much higher in cases of acute thrombosis if recognized late by comparison with those seen much earlier in acute embolic occlusions. Renal failure occurred in 11 patients reported by Littooy and Baker.[171] Mortality occurred in eight out of 11 patients, problably due to acute myoglobinuria with acute tubular necrosis. Although these findings were not mentioned specifically in this article, it is inferred "that as a result of muscle cell ischemia and cell death, these would lead to the release of myoglobin, potassium, and lactic acid." Myoglobin develops and peaks about 3 hours after reperfusion, which may lead to its precipitation in the renal tubules if the urine is concentrated and acidic. Another complication that occurs in these late recognized cases is pulmonary insufficiency resulting from the revascularization syndrome.

If preliminary findings suggest embolism, one may attempt a thromboembolectomy through a transfemoral approach. With few exceptions, however, in acute thrombotic lesions, this will fail to achieve a forceful and sustained arterial flow. This would then indicate the nonembolic nature of the occlusion. Nonoperative treatment of acute aortic embolic or thrombotic occlusion leads to a fatal outcome of approximately 75%. Thromboendarterectomy is not recommended as a safe procedure, since re-thrombosis occurs often, if not as a rule. Deterling et al.,[62a] by direct transaortic thromboembolectomy, had a 33% mortality rate, while Busuttil et al.[30] reported a 23% rate by the transfemoral aortic technique. With the same procedure, Kornmesser et al.[154] noted a mortality rate of 41%. Aortofemoral bypass and axillo-bifemoral bypass are other alternatives. The latter is a preferable means of correcting this condition, if direct aortic approach is not feasible. Since the natural course of these cases is ominous, aggressive efforts are justified as they may be rewarded by survival of some of these gravely at-risk patients.

Prognosis is extremely serious because of the potential of metabolic complications and risks involved, not only for the salvage of the lower extremities, but also for the survival of the patient. This is in contrast to the prognosis of the arterial occlusions of similar etiologies below the inguinal ligament. This fact is consistent with the well-documented prognostic rule of the size of the occluded vessel: the larger the acutely occluded artery, the greater the loss of limb and the greater the mortality.

Postoperatively, the patients should be anticoagulated for prophylaxis of recurrent thromboemboli. Elliott et al.[70] have thus reported benefits both for salvage of limbs and patient survival.

The latest reports confirm clearly that acute occlusion of the abdominal aorta still carries a severe prognosis if unrecognized or treated without delay.

17

Acute Thrombosis of Abdominal Aortic Aneurysms

Introduction

Aneurysms of the abdominal aorta are well known to have a tendency to enlarge at varying rates, and as a result, a substantial number is prone to eventual rupture. The latter, which is the major and potentially catastrophic complication, is in contrast to a sudden complete thrombosis of the aneurysmal sac, an event which is much less frequent, but no less dangerous. A few recent publications have disclosed that such a complication is associated with severe clinical and metabolic manifestations and high mortality rates.

That sudden thrombotic events occur is not surprising in these cases, since most abdominal aortic aneurysms contain in their sac laminated thrombi which, in the majority of instances, do not completely occlude the lumen. The latter may be reduced to a stenosis of a high degree, in which case collaterals are formed and may account for the relative tolerance of total sudden occlusion of the abdominal aortic aneurysm. This event may occur even in the presence of 80% stenosis of the lumen, due to the preexisting collateral circulation formed progressively during the thrombotic process. The ultimate slow occluding terminal thrombosis may still be tolerated in such cases. However, if the noncritical stenosis of the lumen becomes suddenly occluded either by a cardiogenic embolism or by a massive extension of the *in situ* thrombosis, the sudden occlusion will lead to a severe clinical syndrome. This event poses, then, enormous diagnostic and therapeutic challenges.

These cases seem to have drawn little attention in the past. Shumacker[275a] mentioned briefly one such instance in 1959 in a series of 134 cases of surgically treated aortic aneurysms, but it was Janetta and Roberts[137] who reported the first well-documented case in 1961. In 1974, Johnson and associates[140] collected 10 cases from the literature and added seven of their own. Since then more cases appeared in the literature, especially between 1981 and 1982.[2,6,12,14,17,21] It is somewhat surprising that with the recently increasing incidence of aortic aneurysms, acute thrombosis of the terminal abdominal aorta is not being reported more frequently. It is likely that their significance and diagnosis are mistaken for routine cases of abdominal aortic aneurysms complicated by thrombosis or by simple cases of acute thrombosis of the terminal abdominal aorta.

Clinical Manifestations

Clinical manifestations are those of a sudden occlusion of the terminal abdominal aorta which is usually associated with severe arteriosclerotic disease distal to the aneurysm. The clinical characteristic is mottling noted to the level of the iliac crest, or even to the umbilicus. The symptoms and findings are those of severe ischemia, including severe pain, paresthesia, pallor, absence of pulses, and paraplegia, the latter noted in six of the 17 cases reported by Johnson et al. The paraplegia may be due to the anterior spinal artery syndrome associated with lumbar artery occlusion and low flow state. Significantly, a high mortality is also noted in these cases ranging from 46% to 53% occurring within 48 hours of onset. Associated conditions responsible for the immediate cause of death were irreversible shock, myocardial infarction, and cerebral vascular accidents. Renal failure, as already mentioned in the form of anuria or severe oliguria, was seen in most patients who died. Myoglobinuria, secondary to severe ischemia of the muscles, most likely played an important part in renal tubular dysfunction, as noted by Johnson and a few others.

Diagnosis

While the clinical manifestations are usually dramatic and relatively easy to identify, it is difficult to determine the nature of the aortic occlusion. Absence of femoral pulses and the severity of the ischemia of the lower extremities may lead initially to the diagnosis of an acute Leriche syndrome, but the exact nature of the aortic lesion may often be difficult to determine by palpation alone of the abdomen. Translumbar aortograms may ascertain the location of the occlusion without revealing the nature of the aortic lesion. Use of Doppler ultrasound, rarely used in the reported cases, is at present instrumental in revealing the nature of the occlusion. In addition, it is quite helpful in delineating the presence and size of the aortic aneurysm and it is a simple and expeditious noninvasive and accurate method. According to Criado,[46] who applied this noninvasive method which is used routinely under other circumstances, he found it quite helpful as a diagnostic tool in his case. In addition to the absence of visualization, it is of crucial diagnostic significance to focus on the possibility of renal artery involvement by extension of the thrombotic process. In this regard, the assessment of urinary output by an indwelling bladder catheter and its response to parenteral fluid administration are of decisive importance. The presence of oliguria otherwise constitutes the only clear-cut indication for emergency aortography.

Most of the aneurysms appear to be rather small, i.e., around 4 to 5 cm. In my own experience with three cases of acute thrombosis of abdominal aortic aneurysms, two occurred as large aneurysms of 8 cm and the third was 4 cm. In these three cases, the thrombosis occurred rather slowly over a period of a few days or possibly longer due to the preexistence of laminated thrombi in the sac and obviously with preexisting collateral circulation. No acute clinical manifestations occurred in such instances. This type of thrombosis of abdominal aortic aneurysm is rarely mentioned in the literature due to its lack of dramatic onset. Two other possible mechanisms that can precipitate acute, complete thrombosis of abdominal aortic aneurysms, are: (1) superimposed aortic emboli originating in the heart, and (2) possibility of the shift in position of the intrasacular mural thrombus leading to complete obstruction of the aneurysm by the latter. These two phenomena occur suddenly and result in complete occlusion of the lumen. The syndrome is quite different from that of the small aneurysms which progress slowly and occlude the lumen after some time when collateral circulation had developed and prevents the sudden severe ischemia of the lower extremities.

Diagnosis of acute aortic thrombosis is based on clinical findings consisting of the possible palpation of an abdominal mass with the clinical manifestation of acute ischemia of the lower extremities. The precipitating factors are not always clear. Abdominal injury may initiate the sudden thrombosis. Criado reported in 1982 one case of a 77-year-old women who, several minutes after sustaining a fall at home, experienced acute lower back pain and increasing painful numbness of the lower extremities, which gradually progressed to total anesthesia and motor paralysis. Mottling cyanosis from the umbilicus distally associated with absence of lower extremity pulses bilaterally together with presence of flaccid paraplegia and absent reflexes helped make the diagnosis of the presence of an acute thrombosis of an abdominal aortic aneurysm. This, of course, was confirmed by ultrasound which indicated the presence of infrarenal aortic aneurysm with no discernible lumen. This was subsequently confirmed by laparotomy which was performed within hours after intensive fluid therapy and correction of the existing metabolic acidosis with a pH of 7.29.

The differential diagnosis in such cases is with saddle embolus, acute atherosclerotic thrombosis of the terminal abdominal aorta, acute aortic dissection, and acute thrombosis of an abdominal aortic aneurysm.

Saddle embolus is the most frequent cause of acute aortic occlusion and is relatively simple to diagnose when the patient has no significant peripheral arterial disease, but presents a cardiac source of embolization, especially such as atrial fibrillation, mitral stenosis, or recent myocardial infarction. Sudden thrombosis of the terminal abdominal aorta occurring in the absence of obvious aneurysm appears to manifest itself clinically almost in a similar fashion displaying symptomatology, prognosis, and management similar to the acute abdominal aortic aneurysm. In either instance, more often than not, the diagnosis has been mistaken for embolism of the terminal abdominal aorta, due to the similarity of the clinical manifestations.

Acute aortic dissection can frequently be distinguished by the presence of severe chest or back pain, signs of major distal artery occlusion, and an abnormal chest roentgenogram in a hypertensive patient. The most difficult differentiation lies between simple atherosclerotic thrombosis of the aorta and aortic aneurysm thrombosis, particularly the thrombosed aneurysm which is small and impalpable on physical examination. As already mentioned above, delineating the presence and size of aortic aneurysms is helped by use of ultrasound which is expeditious, noninvasive, and quite accurate. This statement is based primarily on the use of ultrasound and the diagnosis of aneurysms in general. In doubtful cases it should be routinely employed in all patients presenting with a syndrome of acute aortic occlusion regardless of the presumed nature.

One critical diagnostic aspect should be focused on the possibility of associated renal artery involvement by the thrombotic process. This may be overlooked due to lack of awareness of the potential presence of myoglobinuria, a fact that carries a serious prognosis and represents a vital complication. The latter's significance stems from the role of myoglobin which may precipitate in the tubules in patients with associated metabolic acidosis.

Prognosis of acute thrombosis of an abdominal aortic aneurysm appears, therefore, to be a catastrophic event and presents a major surgical emergency. The surgical procedure may depend on the nature of the lesions and the condition of the patient.

Management

Aneurysmectomy with graft replacement and distal reconstruction of arterial lesions of the lower extremity, when applicable, is the routine procedure. The metabolic complications are among the serious complications and, therefore, should be anticipated. The patient should be managed with hydration and intravenous bicarbonate to combat the existing acidosis and prevent possible precipitation of myoglobin in the renal tubules. Use of intravenous heparin as an initial gesture is obviously mandatory. In the event that an axillary bifemoral bypass is considered instead of aneurysmectomy, especially if there is evidence of acute myocardial infarction, it is obviously more desirable. The adequacy of blood flow to the kidneys must be ascertained in each case. In the event that renal artery thrombosis has been diagnosed, its disobstruction is life-saving when the thrombotic process extends to a critical level, involving the origin of the renal vessels. Presence of oliguria, unresponsive to fluid challenge, signifies renal involvement and should prompt the performance of preoperative aortography. In general, transaortic renal thrombectomy or thromboendarterectomy done before constructing the proximal aortoprosthetic anastomosis will restore blood flow to the kidneys.[20]

The question of which procedure is best suitable in the management of acute thrombosis of abdominal aneurysm will depend on whether the renal arteries are free of thrombosis as determined by preoperative testing. In the absence of renal artery involvement, the current opinion in the presence of the severity of clinical manifestations favors *axillary bifemoral bypass* as the most suitable procedure. One of the chief advantages of the procedure is that it can be carried out under local or light general anesthesia instead of an intra-abdominal aortic reconstruction which may be too great a risk in patients with severe renal or other visceral involvement.

Summary

In conclusion, acute complete thrombosis of abdominal aortic aneurysms is a rare but catastrophic event, its presentation being frequently dramatic as it assumes that of an acute Leriche syndrome. Ultrasound should be used to delineate the existence and size of the aneurysm and the management should be an emergent procedure consisting of systemic heparinization, rapid restoration of fluids, correction of metabolic acidosis, and assessment of the renal response to intravascular fluid replenishment. Axillobifemoral grafting instead of aneurysm replacement should be considered in most instances where an operative risk is too great to enter the abdomen.

18

Vascular Trauma

Introduction

Arterial injuries, penetrating or blunt, may often induce a syndrome of acute arterial occlusion. As in cases of acute thromboembolism, traumatic arterial interruption may still be amenable to surgical correction many hours after the event, provided adequate collateral supply is still available for maintaining viability. Unfortunately, often an arterial injury may become aggravated by a number of associated features induced by the same original trauma.

It is not within the scope of this chapter to delve into these associated lesions. Suffice it only to mention that in the present context, their concomitant evaluation is essential, since they may contribute significantly to the myonecrosis-renal-metabolic syndrome. The main subject of this chapter will therefore deal only with events relevant to the syndrome of complications mentioned above.

The clinical picture of an arterial trauma varies greatly due to a wide number of factors. Rhabdomyolysis and its biochemical complications seem to occur infrequently in simple arterial injuries in contrast to those combined with other lesions. Indeed, development of the metabolic-renal syndrome secondary to arterial trauma is usually the result of: (1) delayed repair; (2) multiple traumatic lesions; (3) fractures and dislocations; (4) soft tissue trauma; (5) venous injuries; (6) nerve lesions; and (7) traumatic shock. These factors, alone or combined, lead quite often within hours to severe ischemia of the various tissues. The two most significant determinants of the outcome are extensive soft tissue trauma and delayed vascular repair. Supporting these two criteria, among others, are a series of experiments carried out on dogs, by Miller and Welch.[187] They have shown that survival rates of extremities subjected to varying periods of acute ischemia under standard conditions lead to gangrene in 10% of the cases within 6 hours, and that the salvage rates decreased 50% between 12 and 18 hours, and remained as low as 20% after 24 hours. These findings were further confirmed by Nolan and McQuillan[204] who found that permanent muscular damage may be present after 6 hours of complete ischemia.

Fractures and dislocations are usually associated with extensive muscle damage making arterial repair more complex and worsening the prognosis. When muscle necrosis persists for any length of time, severe edema usually develops that further adds to the compression of the adjacent tissues, thus creating a vicious circle of increasing ischemia.

The arterial lesions in civilian practice encompass a great variety of patterns varying from a simple blunt traumatic arterial compression or arterial wound to the disruption of a major artery combined with multiple injuries.

Manifestations of Critical Ischemia

Blunt Arterial Lesions

The local manifestations consist of: (1) pronounced ischemia of the limb characterized by coldness, waxy pallor, cyanotic mottling, and sensory anesthesia; (2) rigor of the limb, a most striking sign due to contracture of the muscles; and (3) edema of the extremity reflecting essentially the enlargement of the fascial compartments and, to a lesser extent, that of the subcutaneous tissue.

In conjunction with the muscular rigor (rigidity) is the presence of myoglobinemia and myoglobinuria. In cases of vascular trauma, one should always be alert to these two biochemical accompaniments. The simplest way to determine this is by routine urine examination for presence of myoglobin which should be mandatory. Lack of awareness of this fact may result in acute renal tubular blockade by this muscular pigment leading to acute renal failure. Metabolic acidosis nearly always present or preceding myoglobinuria should evoke the danger of myoglobin's precipitation in the tubules in the presence of an acidotic pH.

In addition to myoglobinuria, among other biochemical abnormalities, one should look for creatine phosphokinase (CPK), which is an excellent indicator of the degree of myonecrosis.

Penetrating Arterial Lesions

In this category, the potential for myonecrosis-renal-metabolic complications is greatly increased. Arterial reconstruction in this vascular-skeletal complex is more difficult to achieve. Even after reestablishing main arterial patency, reperfusion of ischemic tissues, especially of skeletal muscle, remains often inadequate (see below, paradoxical reperfusion phenomenon).

The clinical manifestations in penetrating arterial lesions are more extensive and complex than in those seen in blunt trauma. The muscles are often lacerated and crushed. As already noted previously, fractures and dislocations may further add to the complexity of vascular repair and increase the potential for myonecrosis-metabolic complications.

Arterial Repair

It is noteworthy that before the 1950s, the incidence of metabolic complications secondary to arterial trauma of the extremities was rarely reported. The high rate of primary amputations carried out during that pre-reconstructive arterial era most likely prevented the full-blown clinical development of such events. By contrast, after the 1950s following nearly routine repair of arterial injuries, both in civilians and in those during the Korean and

Vietnam conflicts, the revascularization syndrome and its aftereffects have become increasingly noted.

Indeed, shortly after the beginning of the new era of reconstruction of arterial lesions, it became evident that not infrequently reperfusion of ischemic tissues would result in extension of myonecrosis and metabolic complications (see Chapter 26, *Role of Free-Radicals in Post-Ischemic Skeletal Muscle Reperfusion Injury*). While early arterial repair carries a better prognosis due in part to persistence of some degree of arterial inflow through the injured artery, and collateral flow, in contrast to late cases of repair, the poor results are ascribed primarily to associated crush injuries of skeletal muscles and to the extensive debridement of these damaged tissues.

Clinicopathological Course

The relative incidence of post-traumatic rhabdomyolysis associated with myoglobinuria and secondary renal shutdown is difficult to estimate for two major reasons: (1) vascular trauma is usually only part of a wider picture of multiple severe injuries; and (2) the priorities for salvaging the patient's musculoskeletal, visceral, and shock problems overshadow the limb ischemia, if present.

Resuscitation of the patient and control of bleeding with control of open wounds are the immediate preoccupations of the trauma surgeon. Vascular damage often takes second place which may account also for the usual late revascularization in the presence of critical ischemia. It is in these latter cases that myonecrosis, myoglobinuria, and renal problems appear to take precedence over other critical aspects of the total trauma picture. Keen awareness of potential metabolic complications arising from ischemic muscles is probably the greatest prerequisite for the diagnosis and its immediate treatment.

Despite an increasing number of large series of case reports on vascular injuries, it is quite surprising that little or no information has been reported on myoglobinuria or acute renal failure. Thus, in a rare recent publication on major arterial trauma dealing with 267 injuries, Robbs and Baker[239] described only 14 cases out of a total of 114 lower limbs involved with signs of critical ischemia of the lower extremities meeting the criteria of rhabdomyolysis and metabolic complications. Arterial reconstruction in these 14 cases resulted in eight salvage and six major amputations. Of these, only two developed acute renal failure which was successfully treated by hemodialysis. In addition to the 14 cases in which reconstructive surgery was done, the authors also report 12 major amputations after "arterial repair," the exact nature of which is not specified. It is not clear from their description what was meant by the distinction between the two groups of patients and their methods of management.

A few rare publications have pointed out the significance of the metabolic complications and acute renal failure.[181] It is of interest to note that a number of European papers dealing with such cases have provided detailed information on this post-traumatic vascular syndrome.[208]

A typical example is the following summary of a case report recently published, which illustrates this complex problem:

"A case is presented with severe muscular trauma to the lower leg and ischemia of 9 hours' duration secondary to a totally disrupted popliteal artery and vein. Following successful revascularization and fasciotomies, the patient developed an extreme local muscular edema, pigmenturia, and impaired renal function. It was concluded that the pigmenturia was a mixture of both myoglobinuria and hematuria, dependent on an acute toxic nephrosis, due in part to rhabdomyolysis and in part to the effect of delayed revascularization. Extensive fasciotomies completed at the time of revascularization almost certainly attenuated the metabolic toxic process to a large degree and contributed to the fair functional outcome. The patient's oliguria responded to mannitol infusion, and on the second postoperative day, the urine was already much lighter in color."[269]

This case is illustrative of the major clinicopathological and management aspects of rhabdomyolysis, myoglobinuria, and acute renal failure, which will be described in more detail below.

Before doing so, a few brief examples may further illustrate this problem. The arterial lesions observed in civilian practice encompass a great variety of patterns. They may range from a simple traumatic arterial compression or arterial wound to that of disruption of a major artery combined with multiple injuries. The following examples may best illustrate these features:

A case reported by Glen[88] of temporary compression of external iliac vessels caused by a central dislocation of the hip with rupture of the pubic rami resulted in a fatal metablic renal syndrome. As the vascular decompression was carried out, sudden and profound collapse occurred comparable to a sudden release of a tourniquet.

Moloney et al.[192] reported a case of ischemic muscle necrosis as a result of superficial femoral artery contusion associated with compound fracture of the femur. The patient developed metabolic acidosis and myoglobinuria. In spite of fasciotomies, an above-knee amputation was carried out, but the patient recovered his kidney function.

Another case reported by Letac et al.[167] involves a wound of the common femoral artery in a 17-year-old butcher apprentice caused by an inadvertent thrust of a knife. Although the artery was repaired within 1 hour, the patient developed metabolic complications (metabolic acidosis, hyperkalemia, and incipient tubular necrosis) resulting in death.

As an example of late repair, Natali[200] stressed the poor prognosis of delayed repair in several cases. One case with severe wound of a superficial femoral artery was operated on successfully within 12 hours. A second case with total division of the popliteal was repaired successfully in spite of revascularization syndrome with shock-like complications. In the third case, the patient was operated on 32 hours after the trauma, and in spite of successful repair, the patient had an above-knee amputation and developed acute renal shutdown for which peritoneal dialysis failed to save the patient.

Similar complications were reported by Breger et al.[22] in a 26-year-old man who, following repair of an axillary artery, developed shock-like symptoms at declamping of the vessel. The patient developed myoglobinuria on the same day and 2 days later became anuric, but was treated successfully with peritoneal dialysis.

Morton et al.,[197] in a series of 30 patients with acute problems of arterial injuries of the lower extremities, reported one patient who in spite of successful arterial reconstruction developed renal shutdown and died of a "crush syndrome."

From the brief summaries of these few cases, it is apparent that the clinical setting of patients presenting with arterial injuries is obviously different from that encountered with other entities involving acute arterial occlusion. Although similar diagnostic criteria for identification and treatment of the metabolic manifestations are applicable, the multiplicity of other injuries usually complicates management.

Based on the preceding few examples, it would appear that greater awareness is essential for diagnosis and treatment of these post-traumatic complications of rhabdomyolysis leading to myoglobinuria and renal shutdown.

Management

General Considerations

Management of these cases deals with an emergency of limb- or life-threatening condition. Upon arrival, after vital signs assessment, the patient should be transferred either to vascular radiology, or directly to the operating room for evaluation of the extent of the vascular injuries and associated visceral involvement (abdomen, chest, neck, etc.). There should be, immediately upon arrival, aggressive fluid and blood volume replacement, and an evaluation of the status of muscle consistency (rigor, laceration). The use of semi-rigid dressings or orthopedic devices for external support before repair of vessels is an important consideration. Urine testing for myoglobin, pH, and urine output, and prophylactic control of infection due to wound contamination, are mandatory from the outset.

Special Factors

Most of these factors are related to muscle ischemia (rhabdomyolysis), the earliest and most important being: myoglobin, hyperkalemia, lactic acidemia, creatine phosphokinase (CPK), blood pH (below 7.2), etc.

Myoglobinuria

Within a few hours of the trauma (less than 6), the urinary output is usually decreased and the urine displays a dark cherry-red or burgundy-red color, due to myoglobin. Not infrequently, myoglobin may escape detection due either to a laboratory mishap or to delay in testing the urine. However, its presence can be determined as a guaiac- or benzidine-positive pigment in the urine containing *no* red cells, especially if the serum is clear. The most common mistaken diagnosis is hemoglobinuria. Of course, specific methods available for detecting these pigments are chemical, spectrophotometric, or immunologic. For emergency purposes, the simplest method should be used first as a screening test and later confirmed by a quantitative method.

From a practical point of view, if there is myoglobinuria or if it is anticipated, alkalinization of the patient should be initiated as soon as it is suspected. Sodium bicarbonate or THAM are to be used, and should be continued throughout the first 2 days until the blood pH, especially from the blood of the involved limb, has been restored to a normal level.

Hyperkalemia

In severe cases of rhabdomyolysis, increased serum potassium is noted after revascularization. It usually represents a poor prognostic factor translating into an advanced degree of muscle cytolysis. Its sudden release after removal of a tourniquet or arterial clamp may lead to cardiac arrest.

Should hyperkalemia and BUN fail to yield to appropriate fluid and electrolyte replacement, hemodialysis may have to be considered.

Rhabdomyolysis

The degree of ischemic damage to the skeletal muscle is of central significance, since it determines the viability of the limb and to a great extent the severity of the metabolic syndrome. The muscular lesions range from diffuse cell injury of variable extent to frank massive necrosis (myonecrosis). It is important to reemphasize that the muscle cell changes are translated into biochemical alterations and metabolic complications.

Focal lesions can be excised and there can still be an attempt to salvage the limb. Wide debridement is often necessary, unless amputation is unavoidable.

Acute Renal Failure

Hypovolemia associated with vascular injuries due to gunshot, stabbings, vehicular accidents, or crushing injuries, alone or combined, may lead to acute renal failure. Prolonged period of hypotension and extensive muscle damage with resultant myoglobinuria are the two determinants of renal failure. Under these conditions, fluid volume replacement, besides the use of sodium bicarbonate, are essential for combating the effects of hypovolemia and myoglobinuria.

Mannitol

Hypertonic mannitol, advocated in the 1960s by Barry[9] and others for its use in the prevention of renal shutdown during aortic surgery, is again being strongly recommended in vascular reconstructive surgery, this time for additional biological reasons. Experimental and clinical data suggest that its administration may play the role of a scavenging agent of oxygen-derived free radicals. The current clinical data indicate that mannitol, like superoxide dismutase, catalase, and allopurinol, can significantly reduce the extent of lesions during reperfusion of ischemic tissues (McCord[182]). The mechanism of action of mannitol and the other allied substances is not entirely clear. The clinical results of their use in myocardial, brain, and intestinal ischemic injuries have been most encouraging. Similarly, administration of mannitol in cases of skeletal muscle ischemia, especially in the prevention of the revascularization syndrome after acute arterial ischemia, seems to respond to the same mechanism of action. Thus, in a report by Buchbinder et al.,[26] hypertonic mannitol administered prior to revascularization prevented the signs and symptoms of the reperfusion syndrome. Consequently, the authors feel that the survival rate and rate of limb salvage have improved significantly. Thus, 14 patients out of 15 survived, with no evidence of rethrombosis or compartment syndrome.

Hypertonic mannitol (20%) should first be given as an intravenous bolus of 10 cc, to be followed by an infusion of 10 g/hr, the latter schedule to be continued for 6 to 24 hours. The duration of this treatment is determined by the severity of the ischemia and the overall condition of the patient. Its administration, to be thoroughly effective, should start before any reconstructive procedure is initiated.

Fasciotomy, preferably of all four compartments in severe cases, is often limb-saving. It should be carried out before myonecrosis is suspected.

Indications for Revascularization

The foregoing therapeutic measures, administered almost concomitantly, are designed to control the metabolic acidosis by alkalinization of the patient as well as to prevent myoglobin precipitation in the renal tubules. In addition, aggressive fluid and blood volume replacement are essential for the same prophylactic purpose.

Revascularization indications of the limb will depend on (1) the extent of the arterial lesions, and (2) the viability of the extremity and absence of advanced rigor of muscles. An enlarged, swollen limb is most often due to compartment syndrome requiring wide fasciotomies.

In the presence of rigor, revascularization of the limb should be undertaken without delay. However, in the presence of frank myonecrosis involving a large muscular mass, primary amputation may be unavoidable. In the presence of focal myonecrosis, excision of the latter may not represent a major contraindication to revascularization.

As stated earlier, to prevent the reperfusion side-effects, it is essential that mannitol be administered prior to the vascular repair concurrently with all the other procedures designed to combat the biochemical-induced metabolic complications.

19

Acute Renal Complications Secondary to Myoglobinuria

Introduction

Acute renal failure secondary to myoglobinuria consists usually of blockage of the renal tubules by myoglobin. This condition has been found in patients after a variety of types of rhabdomyolysis. These complications may be found mostly in five major arterial conditions:

1. Acute arterial occlusions,
2. Aortic aneurysms,
3. Following open-heart surgery,
4. Post-traumatic acute renal failure, and
5. Nontraumatic rhabdomyolytic entities.

Acute Arterial Occlusions

Myoglobinuria may occur in a variety of arterial occlusions, the most common being arterial embolism, acute thrombosis, cross-clamping of major arteries, arterial cannulation during cardiopulmonary bypass, and arterial trauma.

While the acute renal failure occurring in any of these conditions may vary in intensity or duration and prognosis, most of them, however, do exhibit similar symptoms and signs throughout their evolution. The most typical entity which may serve as a prototype for the other conditions is acute arterial embolism.

Within a few hours after onset of an embolic occlusion of a major artery, oliguria is present, the urinary output usually becomes decreased, and the urine displays a dark cherry-red or burgundy-red color, due to myoglobin. Myoglobin, before reaching the urine, is or should always be detectable in the plasma. Furthermore, some of the problems in detecting the myoglobin in the urine include lack of awareness of its presence or the fact that only small amounts of myoglobin may be cleared through the kidney thus causing difficulty in identification. The test for myoglobin in the plasma has not been used often in these cases and, therefore, its identification in the urine had been overlooked.

Myoglobinuria may reach a peak within 48 hours after the onset of acute arterial occlusion and may last several days depending on the extent and severity of the rhabdomyolysis. Occasionally, myoglobinuria may escape detection due either to laboratory mishap or to delay in testing the urine. Its presence can be determined as a guaiac- or benzidine-positive pigment in the urine containing no red cells, especially if the serum is clear. The most common mistaken diagnosis in myoglobinuria is that of hemoglobinuria. Berman[13] suggested that a naked-eye look at the plasma may suffice as a screening test to suspect myoglobin by applying this rule: "red plasma plus red urine equals hemoglobin; clear plasma plus red urine equals myoglobin." Of course, the specific chemical tests available described elsewhere for detecting these pigments in the urine provide the final accurate diagnosis. The methods available for estimating myoglobin are chemical, spectrophotometric, immunological, or radioimmunological. Most of these tests are primarily qualitative in nature. Recent methods have been described for quantitative investigation of myoglobin in the urine, thus making possible earlier detection of this pigment in the serum or plasma.

Acute renal impairment usually varies with the degree of muscle ischemia, acidosis, and the degree of myoglobinuria. In the mild or moderately severe cases, renal function is temporarily impaired and completely reversible. Urinary output may be decreased during the devascularization phase and may be further impaired after the revascularization. Most patients display either oliguria or anuria. Their BUN and creatinine rise to very high levels quite rapidly after the renal impairment is detected clinically. In cases with severe complications, prolonged myoglobinuria in the presence of acidosis, if not treated promptly, leads to irreversible shutdown and usually to the death of the patient unless rigorous peritoneal or hemodialysis is undertaken and continued for quite a number of weeks until the situation appears to stabilize.

Post-mortem examination usually shows the kidneys to be of normal shape and consistency. The capsule can be stripped with ease. One may find focal infarctions even though the renal tissue does not appear to be entirely within normal limits. Histologically, however, the renal tubules contain casts of myoglobin, with reactive epithelial cells occasionally indicating their regeneration. Evidence and extent of acute tubular necrotic lesions depend on tubular clogging by myoglobin and possibly hemoglobin to some degree. The above pathological picture is commonly referred to as myoglobinuric nephrosis or nephropathy. Sometimes preexisting nephrosclerotic lesions are present which are apt to aggravate the prognosis.

The pathogenesis of the acute renal failure associated with this syndrome of myoglobinuria has brought to light unsolved problems. However, on the basis of the histologic data reported above, obtained from both human autopsy material and experimental animal models, the presence of myoglobin casts in the renal tubules seems to strongly suggest a causal relationship between the tubular mechanical blockage by the myoglobin casts and the acute renal shutdown. In addition, there is some suggestive evidence that myoglobin *per se* has a direct toxic effect on the tubules. A number of experimental data is available to support this contention.[293]

In summary, myoglobinuria, which is one of the consequences of rhabdomyolysis, may lead to renal shutdown which represents a major factor in the prognosis of such cases. Its early identification and vigorous aggressive treatment of renal shutdown with hemodialysis is absolutely indispensible.

Abdominal Aortic Aneurysms

Although renal complications may occur in elective excisions of abdominal aortic aneurysms (AAAs), they are more commonly encountered in ruptured cases. In elective cases, one may note occasionally the so-called declamping phenomenon of the aorta. This syndrome is due to accumulation of a significant amount of acid metabolites, as evidenced by a significant fall in venous pH, a profound fall in venous PO_2, and an increase in venous CO_2 saturation. This metabolic syndrome, at the time of release of the aortic clamp, may induce severe hypotension, which in the presence of decreasing blood volume may have potentially serious consequences.

In patients with ruptured AAAs, preoperative oliguria may lead to a complete renal shutdown lasting several days to several weeks postoperatively. Mortality due to renal shutdown is quite significant. Thus, Chawla et al.,[38] in a collective review of 756 patients from 19 centers, found that the operative mortality of ruptured abdominal aneurysms ranged from 34–85%, with a mean of 56%. They further stated that when a ruptured aortic aneurysm is complicated by acute renal failure, mortality approximates 91% with otherwise seemingly successful operations. Similar results have been reported by others in cases of combined ruptured aortic aneurysms with renal complications.

Clinically, the patient who is going to develop renal complications as a result of the ruptured AAA arrives at the hospital in profound shock, oliguric or anuric, and the operative findings indicate a large retroperitoneal extravasation of blood extending from the diaphragm to the pelvic area, with a hypotensive episode of several hours. During or after resection of the aneurysm, the patient may already appear oliguric, putting out only a few milliliters of urine, which is highly concentrated and contains hemoglobin or possibly myoglobin. The incidence of the latter factor is rarely mentioned in the current literature. Admittedly, a large number of other factors contribute to the renal complications, of which rhabdomyolysis and myoglobinuria may be more significant than realized.

McCombs and Roberts[181] have reported 17 cases of acute renal failure in 398 cases of AAAs, of which nine (2.5%) were resected electively and eight (21.0%) after rupture. The renal failure is usually irreversible in a large percentage of patients. However, hemodialysis should be started immediately with the hope that within a few days or weeks the renal tubular necrosis will resolve itself to a certain extent and allow the function of this organ to restart. Occasionally, after 3 to 5 days in the milder instances, the renal function will recover almost spontaneously without the use of hemodialysis, using only the measures designed to improve the blood volume, blood pressure, and restoration of acid-base balance.

Unfortunately, based on clinical events and necropsy findings, multiple organ-system failure is added to the renal complications. While the treatment of established massive tubular necrosis is dismal, it behooves the surgeon and the team of the intensive care unit to treat prophylactically the potential factors that may lead to these complications. Decreasing the aortic clamp time, operating time, and blood loss seems to be essential as demonstrated in a recent small series of 61 consecutive cases.

Moderate hypothermia, if indicated, during surgery and prophylactic diuretics together with adequate therapy may help to protect the renal tubules and thus prevent this often fatal complication.

Luft et al.[172] have reported on 38 patients with acute renal failure following surgery for aortic aneurysms who were analyzed retrospectively in search of predictors of survival. Of 14 potential predictor variables considered, none taken singly were significant; however, the combination of age, operative interruption of renal blood flow, and prior renal dysfunction served as significant predictors. Low survival rates occurred if the patient was over 70 years of age, if renal blood flow required interruption, or if preoperative renal impairment was present. High survival rates occurred in patients less than 70 years of age, who had no interruption of renal blood flow, and who had normal preoperative renal function. Although the total mortality rate of these patients with acute renal failure was 71%, only one of 12 patients with favorable prognostic indicators died. Acute renal failure following aortic aneurysm repair has no worse prognosis than that stated in the literature for acute renal failure following other surgical procedures. A vigorous therapeutic approach should be maintained despite the presence of complications.

In spite of the general dismal outlook of these abdominal aortic aneurysms complicated by acute renal failure, a more encouraging finding emerged from a study by Whelton.[293] His experience with acute renal failure complicating abdominal aneurysm rupture is based on recent clinical experience with 11 consecutive patients; he saw eight survivors with recovery of renal function. That is a mortality rate of only 27% in contrast to the pooling of such data where he found 12 of 89 patients survive, with a mortality rate of 83%. Whelton emphasized that this improved prognosis in his cases simply reflected maximum-effort, intensive-care management, together with prompt and vigorous dialysis. As a result of these measures, the outlook for this subset of acute renal failure was clearly improved.

Following Open-Heart Surgery

Acute renal failure following open-heart surgery represents a significant complication contributing substantially to morbidity and mortality of patients in this group. Abel et al.[1] have determined the incidence of renal dysfunction in a clinical study based on the records of 507 adult surviving patients following open-heart surgery. Of these, 309 patients (61%) were considered to have maintained normal renal function throughout the postoperative period compared to 198 patients (39%) who developed renal dysfunction consisting of BUN more than 50 mg per 100 ml and a serum creatinine level greater than 2.0 mg per 100 ml. The mortality rate in the former group was only 1.6% compared to 30.3% in the patients having abnormal renal function.

A retrospective analysis of the incidence and degree of renal dysfunction in the postoperative period following open-heart surgery was carried out during a single calendar year. In evaluating potential risk factors for the development of renal dysfunction in the postoperative period, the authors singled out the age of the patient and the type of cardiac procedure considered. The mean age of all patients was 53.1 ± 11.5 years. Of the normal group, the mean age was 51 ± 11.4 compared to 56.4 ± 10.8 years for the so-called abnormal group. The mean difference of 5.42 years is surely not a significant reason for the "abnormality" of this group. The others point out, however, that the unresolved feature observed postoperatively is the one that arises during the latter period. There is certainly a group of patients in whom hypotensive episodes either preoperatively, intraoperatively, during cardiopulmonary bypass, or in the immediate postoperative period, can be incriminated as having led to a period of prolonged renal ischemia which resulted in a state recognized as acute tubular necrosis. They point out that this state was characterized by high urinary sodium excretion, and was associated with a progressive rise of urea nitrogen and serum creatinine levels with a concomitant decrease in creatinine and inulin clearance. Other alterations observed postoperatively are less definable than acute tubular necrosis. The explanation given by Abel et al.[1] may be due to "possible multiple renal emboli from an atrial thrombus or valvular calcification, that may cause a decrease in renal function. Other factors such as renal artery or venous occlusions, subclinical aortic dissection following retrograde aortic perfusion, nephrotoxic damage on the basis of administered drugs, and low cardiac output states may lead to decreased renal perfusion and may result in a severe state of prerenal azotemia without frank tubular damage."[1]

It appears, therefore, that all these changes enumerated by the authors do not consider at all any possibility of rhabdomyolysis occurring during the procedure as a result of the cardiopulmonary bypass. A possibility that has not been considered is the rhabdomyolysis with myoglobinuria which might have contributed to the renal dysfunction discussed in this chapter. However, no evidence is given in this anaylsis in order to be able to state with finality that this kind of an etiology was the basis for the renal dysfunction. Other similar instances in the literature, however, indicate that rhabdomyolysis with myoglobinuria represent such cases where the patient ends up having acute renal tubular necrosis and renal failure.

Earlier metabolic acidosis emerging from the ischemically cannulated limb was noted, but without affecting the systemic blood adversely because of the mild type of arterial insufficiency and the short duration of the cardiac bypass. However, Rowland et al.[243] described a case of fatal myoglobinuria in a 25-year-old man who underwent open-heart surgery for aortic valve replacement in whom the right external iliac artery was used for the perfusion. The patient developed an acute renal failure postoperatively and died within 2 days of his surgery. Details of this clinical case are to be found in Chapter 23, *Arterial Cannulation During Cardiopulmonary Bypass*.

Likewise, similar examples were provided by a group of Japanese cardiac surgeons who presented a series of 420 patients in whom massive ischemic myopathy with myoglobinuria occurred in eight patients or in 1.9% of the entire group. They were typical cases of acute renal failure associated with open-heart surgery. Details of these cases are also to be found in Chapter 23.

If the rhabdomyolytic process is not very severe, the myoglobin release from the ischemic muscle is minimal and the kidney damage is likewise not too severe. Kagen[144] thus reported six cases with myoglobinuria in a group of 16 patients after open-heart surgery for valvular replacement. The patients who did not develop a renal problem had considerably shorter procedures than those with myoglobinuria. Only one of the six patients with myoglobinuria died in the immediate postsurgical period of renal failure and progressive jaundice. The incidence of myoglobinuria in this group of patients is closely related to the total surgical time, including that of the period of the pump for cardiac bypass. The source of myoglobin in these patients is likely to originate partly from the myocardium as a result of surgical trauma but mostly from the lower extremity skeletal muscle ischemia due to prolonged pump perfusion.

Similar observations were made by Kugimiya and associates[159] published in a presentation entitled *Myopathic Nephrotic Metabolic Syndrome as a Complication of Cardiopulmonary Bypass*.

As shown by Bywaters,[31] it is known that the renal lesions are directly related to myoglobinuria. This was demonstrated by injecting solutions experimentally containing myoglobin. In the absence of rhabdomyolysis, it appeared therefore that the renal damage and eventual shutdown was induced by myoglobin alone.

Post-Traumatic Acute Renal Failure (PTARF)

Post-traumatic, ischemic rhabdomyolysis followed by anuria has been known since the early part of this century beginning with the reports of von Colmers (1909)[42] and Minami (1923).[191]

Later Husfeldt and Bjering (1937),[134] McClelland (1941),[180] and Glenn (1941)[88] emphasized that anuria and uremia can be sequels to traumatic shock. This clinical syndrome of post-traumatic acute renal failure has been well recognized after both the civilian and military experiences during WWII, especially after the Battle of Britain due to the crush injury syndrome. It is fundamental for the clinician to remember, regardless of the location and degree of trauma sustained, that it is necessary, as emphasized by Whelton, to consider three etiologic categories of acute renal failure:

1. *Prerenal* due to decreased renal perfusion;
2. *Renal* (intrinsic anatomic and vascular defects) characterized by acute tubular necrosis secondary to prolonged decreased renal perfusion and myoglobinuria; and,
3. *Postrenal* due to outflow obstruction.

Although frequently observed in the past, this condition is clinically seen less frequently except in catastrophic situations such as falling debris from earthquake damage to buildings, etc. The decrease in this complication reflects a better understanding of the syndrome's pathophysiology and rapid management of trauma victims.

Due to the complexity of the metabolic complications in this group of patients, renal failure requires aggressive management because invariably one cannot predict their clinical outcome. In the presence of oliguria or anuria, prompt and rapid dialysis is essential. The exact pathophysiology of the post-traumatic renal problem requires a close analysis of the glomerular and tubular functions in order to understand the sequence of events which led to the shutdown of the kidney.

The incidence of this complication due to trauma has been decreasing dramatically in the past few years. Thus, during the early 1940s, PTARF was seen in one out of every three seriously injured soldier; by the early 1950s, the incidence was one in 200, whereas by the end of the 1960s, the incidence in military casualties was one in 600 or lower.

Management must be carried out without delay. The patient's physical examination must be evaluated with emphasis on the fluid-volume status, the serum electrolytes with particular attention to potassium and bicarbonate levels, and blood chemistry determinations with particular attention to blood urea nitrogen and serum creatinine. Urinalysis must be determined for the presence of protein, glucose, and other chemical abnormalities with microscopic evaluation of the presence of cellular elements or cast formation and particularly the presence of myoglobin and its amount.

The principles of management are directed toward the following:

1. Fluid replacement and restoration of electrolyte balance;
2. Extracorporeal hemodialysis and/or peritoneal dialysis;
3. Control of infection;
4. Nutritional care;
5. Management of hyperkalemia which is included in point #2.

It is always difficult under those circumstances when the patient arrives at the emergency room to answer the question of when is optimum time to start hemodialysis. If there is any doubt about the time to begin, it is always wiser to err on the side of early dialysis (Whelton). Although urea is not the key factor in induction of the uremic syndrome, blood urea nitrogen provides only a yardstick measure to the accumulation of other end-products of nitrogen metabolism that should have been excreted by the kidneys. One of the important chemicals that must be taken into account is hyperkalemia, which may have disastrous effects on the myocardium and the CPK, which is an index of the degree of rhabdomyolysis. The latter may offer a guide as to what to anticipate in terms of biochemical changes resulting from the destruction of the muscular fiber membranes.

Nontraumatic Rhabdomyolytic Entities

Rhabdomyolysis and myoglobinuria may occur in the absence of acute arterial occlusions or crush injuries of the skeletal muscle. This group of entities may occur as a result of a variety of etiologic factors such as exertional states in otherwise normal individuals, convulsive disorders from chronic alcoholic myopathy, defects in carbohydrate metabolism such as McArdle's disease, syndrome of abnormal glycolysis, hypokalemia and potassium depletion states, toxic factors due to heroin use or any of a great variety of drug abuse which may lead to myoglobinuria and indirectly to muscular lesions due to compression of an arm or any part of the body. Finally, myositis syndromes occupy an important portion of this group of nontraumatic cases: of these, dermatomyositis, polymyositis, systemic lupus erythematosus, etc., are the most noteworthy.

Ischemic pressure necrosis may occur as a result of patients being in coma due to a number of different factors (alcoholism, drug addiction, carbon monoxide poisoning). In many of these cases, the ischemic pressure necrosis is the dominant pathogenetic factor of myoglobinuria and muscle necrosis.

Exertion in otherwise normal individuals has been already mentioned previously in Chapter 6. Exercise may induce myopathic disorders in patients who have predisposing lesions of the muscular system which appear to be in the category of apparent healthy normal individuals. Other accounts leading to overexertion occur in athletes and in military recruits subjected to strenuous training programs. This is classically associated with the anterior tibial compartment syndrome more than with any other musculature. For instance, a study of 586 Army officer candidates in training disclosed that 23 men, approximately 4%, had chemically detectible myoglobinuria. When the exertion occurred in a gradual fashion, such changes of muscle leading to myoglobinuria was not observed. The suggestion is that prior conditioning may lessen such a complication.

Metabolic Factors

Among these factors, alcoholic myopathy has received some attention because of increasing numbers of this group of patients. The lesions observed in the skeletal muscle were classified by Perkoff as subclinical, acute, and chronic alcoholic myopathies.[217]

The subclinical form is characterized chiefly by elevation of serum levels of enzymes, considered to be of muscle origin after excessive alcohol intake, and probably represents a mild form of the acute illness. Acute alcoholic myopathy on the other hand appears after heavy consumption of alcohol and is marked by muscle cramps, weakness, and myoglobinuria. Affected muscles are painful, swollen, and tender. Myoglobinuria, which may be complicated by renal failure, is a striking feature of this illness. Myonecrosis and evidence of muscle regeneration are seen in the tissue. The relationship of the reversible abnormality in carbohydrate metabolism induced by alcohol was pointed out by Perkoff et al.[217] in 1966 who called attention to decreased lactate release from muscle after ischemic exercise in affected patients.

In chronic myopathy occurring in association with alcoholism, the major clinical finding is slowly progressive weakness without muscle pain or tenderness. Muscle biopsy may show focal degeneration, increase in fibrous tissue, or focal infiltration with fat.

The pathogenic mechanism of alcoholic myopathies is not entirely understood. Current theories, however, suggest that ethanol, or a metabolite, may be directly injurious to muscle. As an example, administration of ethanol to three nonalcoholic men for 4 weeks increased serum creatine phosphokinase activity and produced ultrastructural changes in skeletal muscle.

The list of factors responsible for this group of rhabdomyolysis and myoglobinuria is a long one and, because of new entities, appears to increase since the publication years ago of Rowland's and Kagen's tables.

Myositis Syndromes

Among the many factors responsible for this category of rhabdomyolysis, the myositis group appears to be more significant in certain respects from a clinical point of view. The number of known causes as mentioned above of acute renal failure secondary to myoglobinuria is increasing rapidly due to a variety of syndromes affecting the skeletal muscle. The well-recognized causes of rapid muscle necrosis with release of myoglobin include a great variety of polymyositis. In dermatomyositis and polymyositis, it is well known that trace myoglobin is present in the serum and in the urine, yet there were only five cases in the literature of myoglobinuric renal failure associated with these disorders reported by Kreitzer in 1978.[156] Since then, a large number has been published increasing considerably the experience with polymyositis and this syndrome.

Kagen described myoglobinemia in inflammatory myopathies found in the sera of patients with dermatomyositis, polymyositis, scleroderma, and systemic lupus erythematosus, as already mentioned earlier, with active myopathy. In addition to myoglobin found in the sera of these patients, the muscle-originating enzymes are also to be found, such as creatine phosphokinase (CPK), lactic dehydrogenase (LDH), and SGOT. These biochemical factors show activity much higher in samples containing myoglobin but there was considerable overlap between those with and without myoglobinemia.

Kagen determined myoglobin by immunoassay in the serum samples obtained from 62 patients over a 5-year period. Of the 62 patients, 21 had dermatomyositis, 21 had polymyositis, and there were 20 additional patients with myopathy associated with other connective tissue disorders. Most patients in each group were women, particularly in the category of "other connective tissue disorders." This group contained seven patients with systemic lupus erythematosus (LE), six with scleroderma, three with juvenile rheumatoid arthritis, one with rheumatoid arthritis, two with arthritis, and one patient with an unclassified connective tissue disease who had joint, cardiac, dermal, muscular, and renal involvement.

The etiologic factors of myoglobinuria seem to have increased considerably in the past 10 years since a number of unsuspected conditions have been associated with muscular ischemia. Rhabdomyolysis and myoglobinuria have become more common, although their nature is not entirely elucidated in relation to infectious disease and other conditions.

For further details, see the chapter on non-traumatic rhabdomyolysis (Chapter 21).

20

Ischemic Muscle Contracture: Volkmann's Syndrome and Anterior Tibial Compartment Syndrome

Volkmann's Syndrome

Historical Data

The theories of the pathogenesis of muscular contracture have been a subject of debate ever since Volkmann described an entity which bears his name. Volkmann, in 1869 and later in 1875, described a deformity of the hand and wrist resulting from an interference of some nature of the blood supply of the muscles of the forearm. This condition was usually preceded by the application of splints or bandages for fracture of the humerus in the region of the elbow joint which resulted in a "stoppage of the arterial blood." In his classic article published in 1881,

Volkmann[287a] said that he believed that "the contraction was due to ischemia caused by the muscular tissue being deprived of arterial blood, in consequence of which the muscle perished from want of oxygen." He called attention to the fact that the contracture comes on some time after the initial paralysis, and that it becomes more marked as more repair tissue is laid down; and from the onset of the condition, there is considerable rigidity which is increased as more scar tissue is formed. He reported one case in 1875 of a 16-year-old child. Mention of this case had already been made in his book published in 1869.

Early Clinical and Pathological Data

The credit for calling attention to the condition and establishing it as a real entity belongs to Leser.[166] In 1884, he reported seven cases. A little later he investigated the condition experimentally, using dogs in his research work. Leser's description of the clinical manifestations of Volkmann's ischemic paralysis and contracture was as follows:

> Shortly after the constricting bandage is applied to the forearm, the hand begins to swell and there is severe pain. The patient may complain of numbness or paresthesia of the fingers. The pain and swelling may develop so rapidly that the bandage is removed in an hour. If the bandage is removed only after 24 hours, then the fingers show marked contracture and the muscles of the forearm feel hard and stiff. Not the slightest active movement is possible and attempts at passive movement of the fingers cause great pain. Soon after the removal of the bandage, often within an hour, a marked swelling in the muscles of the forearm begins. This acute inflammatory reaction in the muscles reaches a maximum in about 24 hours and then gradually subsides and a marked contracture of the muscles follows.

Leser's explanation for these changes following the constriction of the forearm was attributed entirely to an ischemic origin and was independent of pressure on the nerves. Leser stressed the fact that these manifestations were solely dependent on a deprivation of arterial blood to the extremity. However, an accompanying venostasis, which is also present, merely hastens the development of the pathological condition. The oxygen deprivation of the muscle results in a degeneration of the muscle fibers and later their absorption, and the ultimate contracture is to be considered simply as a rigor mortis.

Of further interest is Leser's detailed description of the endothelium of small vessels. It appeared to be thick and he interpreted this as being due to the fact that endothelial cells were elastic and, hence, when the blood pressure in small vessels was decreased, the endothelium became much thicker. He states that the changes seen in the muscle indicate two processes at work: (1) degeneration of the muscle tissue; and (2) a marked inflammatory process in the muscle.

Views other than those expressed by Volkmann and Leser were held by several surgeons and investigators who failed to demonstrate the actual ischemia and the cause of the contracture. Powers described the muscles as they appeared in a patient operated upon 16 months after the onset of the disease.

> The muscles were pale, red and very tough and fibrous. Microscopic examination revealed a great hyperplasia of connective tissue around and between the bundles of muscle fiber. The fibrosis was so complete that in many areas no muscle tissue could be identified. Muscle tissue appeared atrophic and fragmented. Many fibers had lost their nuclei and transverse striations, having the appearance of broad ribbons of delicate fibrillar tissue. Their appearance and reactions strongly suggested hyaline degeneration. Moderate amounts of fatty infiltration of the connective tissue was present but no actual fatty degeneration of the muscle fibers was found.

Experimental Data

Several other investigators have subsequently tackled this problem but it was Jepson[139] who carried out the first experimental study of this phenomenon and attempted to correlate these findings with the clinical entity. Jepson's experimental work carried out in 1924 was designed to determine the mechanism of the ischemic contracture as seen in man. For this purpose he attempted to reproduce this condition in animal experimentations for the purpose of finding means of preventing the deformity of the paralysis and contracture of the skeletal muscles.

After a number of experimental models, Jepson concluded that in a typical case of Volkmann's contracture, the deprivation of oxygen is not complete.

Jepson used dogs for his experiments and applied splints, casts, and bandages as a means of constricting the extremity. He used several models of experiments, and in one he applied simple ligation of the femoral vein. He obtained deformity in these animals, resembling that in a human, which was maintained from 6 to 9 days. The dogs with simple ligation of the vein maintained deformity slightly longer than those with the partially encircling incision which was the control series. While Jepson recognizes that muscles completely deprived of their oxygen supply finally disintegrate, he did not find from his experiments in a typical case of contracture that the deprivation of oxygen is complete. In addition, in the models bruised by the trauma where he used splints, bandages, and casts, there is extravasation of blood and serum in the subfascial tissues. As a result, the tension may be so great as to cause cyanosis of the entire forearm. The intrinsic pressure causes local myositis and then a pressure on the nerves, usually the median and ulnar, and the blood vessels. If the intrinsic pressure is relieved within a short time after the formation of the hematoma, the patient will usually recover.

Clinical Conditions Exclusive of Fractures

Since the original description which referred mostly to fractures of the upper extremity in children, Volkmann's ischemic contracture has been observed following a variety of clinical conditions, exclusive of fractures of the arm or leg, such as: injury to the soft tissues alone, acute arterial occlusions due to embolism or thrombosis, or vascular injuries. In more recent years, this syndrome has been seen to occur sometimes after arterial reconstruction despite apparently successful restoration of the circulation. In such cases, although gangrene is completely avoided, and in spite of restored arterial circulation, the hand and wrist or ankle and foot may become acutely flexed, usually in a severe claw. The forearm or calf muscles appear hard, painful, and tender, with passive dorsiflexion being quite impossible because of the resistant contracture of the flexor muscles.

Mechanism of Contracture

The mechanism of the ischemic contracture is not always apparent but, as already stated, the prerequisite for its development is the localized severe circulatory insufficiency to a group of muscles without affecting the rest of the limb. As a result, these muscles become first ischemic and later fibrous, thus leading to the contracture. The early gross changes are like the ones found in the anterior tibial compartment syndrome. They are localized usually to the tissues distal to the arterial occlusion or injury.

Microscopic changes consist of small areas of white-cell and round-cell infiltration, and various degrees of dilatation of venules and arterioles. There is considerable reduction in the nuclei of the muscle fibers over certain areas, representing the "islands of necrosis." By the time the chronic stage is reached, the loss of nuclei is complete. One sees then masses of ischemic muscle in which individual fibers are recognizable, but there is hardly a live nucleus even in the interfibrilar fibrous tissue. These masses resemble nothing more closely than a muscle sequestrum, upon the surface of which is a sheath of dense fibrous tissue.

Pathogenesis: Clinical Data

Several important theories of the pathogenesis and treatment of Volkmann's ischemic contracture were contributed following the early part of this century. Thus, Griffiths[93] in 1940 based his observations on 32 cases of which 29 were concerned with post-traumatic lesions and three with arterial embolism. Analysis of these 32 cases provided evidence in support of the theory that Volkmann's ischemic contracture was due to arterial injury and the accompanying spasm of the collateral circulation. This view was supported by clinical signs of arterial occlusion in acute and chronic cases. The histology has shown that there was muscle infarction. Jepson's theory that the contracture results from venous occlusion was rejected in view of the absence of any venous compression by hematoma in acute cases. By contrast, arterial lesions were found during operations at all stages.

The venous obstruction theory had originally received almost universal acceptance particularly after the experimental work of Brooks in 1922 and that of Jepson in 1926. Although venous occlusion as a clinical entity is well-known and separate from the muscle contracture of Volkmann's syndrome, the interpretation of the previous investigators was at great variance with the known facts of venous thrombosis which may lead to gangrene as demonstrated abundantly in other areas of vascular pathology.

Lesions found in chronic cases may be due to trauma of the vessels, particularly of the arteries which may have been contused severely at the time of the fracture and produced the upsetting of the mechanism leading to the muscular contracture of the Volkmann's type. Typical cases of this nature had been presented by several surgeons, particularly by Rich[237] and many others who have found old ruptures, lacerations, and thromboses of the brachial artery.

As already mentioned earlier, Volkmann's contracture after arterial injury and embolism provide pathological conditions illustrating the effects of pure arterial occlusion which may lead to ischemia of a group of muscles which in turn leads to contracture. Three patients reported by Griffiths, despite apparently successful restoration of circulation, developed typical Volkmann's contracture after embolectomy. This author illustrates the point by mentioning a case of a 42-year-old man with an embolism of the brachial artery at its bifurcation, after the embolectomy restored the circulation 2½ hours after it had lodged in the arterial tree. Although the radial and ulnar arteries were freed of the thromboembolic material and the operation restored the circulation and radial pulse, the patient rapidly developed a contracture of moderate severity in the forearm flexors with a typical Volkmann claw and firm resistance to correction. The explanation for this phenomenon was due to the fact that collateral circulation was not restored in this case.

Based on his clinical experience and on experimental work on rabbits in whom arterial ligature was used in production of skeletal muscle contracture, Griffiths was at variance with the experiments reported by Jepson as already mentioned earlier. Based on the above data, the arterial origin of the ischemia leading to muscular contracture has gained wide acceptance.

Seddon[262] pointed out in 1963 that the lesions of Volkmann's ischemia are usually a circumscribed deep-seated affection of voluntary muscles and to a lesser degree of other tissues in the ischemic zone. In its grossest form, it differs from gangrene only in that the necrotic area is encased in a fibrous envelope with more or less normal superficial tissues. The general shape of infarct—for that is what it is—is an ellipsoid shape with its main axis in the length of the limb.

Degree of Lesions: Evolution

The level of the infarct is variable, though it most often occurs in the distal two-thirds of the forearm or leg. This usually depends on the level of the vascular damage. Accordingly, there are several degrees of damage, including reversible damage in cases of mild ischemia, and mild fibrosis, usually represented by a fairly diffuse change which precludes spontaneous recovery of the muscle. Severe fibrosis due to profound ischemic changes of the muscle results virtually in its destruction. For all practical purposes, the muscles become converted into a shortened fibrous mass. Finally, necrosis of the muscle occurs with metabolic and renal complications. When contracture develops in such cases, it is not in the necrotic part but in the less ischemic fibrotic muscle that envelops it.

Seddon, in concluding, states that the arterial damage is the chief cause of Volkmann's ischemia, the initiating damage being anything from complete severance of an artery to minimal injury that sends the vessel into spasm. It is indeed the latter that is so peculiarly noxious. Seddon states that classification of the ultimate damage in these cases is quite difficult because the ischemia can vary spatially as well as in intensity.

Of course it is of great significance to focus attention on the reversible damage where therapy can be of help, but this requires immediate attention and diagnosis of the condition. One has to keep in mind that the overwhelming majority of cases which lead to muscle contracture present originally striking changes of the skeletal muscle of the forearm or leg which overshadow those in other tissues. In the statistical study of Seddon, many cases of Volkmann's ischemia of the forearm muscles fell between two extremes: mild–17, localized lesions–5, and severe–28.

Comment

Considering the vulnerability of skeletal muscle to acute ischemia, it is surprising that clinically significant metabolic and renal complications have not been more frequently reported. Indeed, in contradistinction to the severe entities where the ischemic changes involve large masses of skeletal muscle, those in the forearm or leg muscles result in complications which seem to be moderate and are not recognized. This is only an apparent absence of any degree of metabolic ill effects in these cases. This is likely due primarily to a lack of awareness rather than to a negative identification of the metabolic-renal elements. Indeed, as shown by abundant data throughout this monograph, biochemical reponses in the so-called "uncomplicated" acute arterial occlusions induced by cross-clamping seem to be most often transient and therefore may be overlooked. In cases of intermediate severity, however, the most conspicuous findings may be the clinicopathological features, which remain confined to a limited area, often without obvious systemic manifestations. Of these, two classical examples are most often encountered: the anterior tibial compartment syndrome and Volkmann's ischemic contracture affecting the forearm or the leg muscles. While these entities are likely to occur for the most part as an integral part of a more complex clinical picture, their specific mention in this discussion is of particular interest in the context of the rhabdomyolytic process in general.

Management

Treatment of these cases is based on accurate diagnosis which is a matter of urgent importance. It may be reversible as already mentioned if the blood supply is restored within a reasonably short period of time. Fasciotomies with long adequate incision in the skin and fascia should be performed promptly. Otherwise, continued edema of the muscle within the closed fascial compartment may lead to necrosis. Fortunately, Volkmann's contracture has become rare because of a better understanding of the etiology and pathogenesis of the condition.

Volkmann's contracture is often exhibited as a result of chronic vascular injury. It may be reversible if the blood supply is restored within a reasonably short period of time as mentioned. If circulation returns, the muscles swell and fasciotomy should be considered without delay.

Rich and Spencer,[237] in their book *Vascular Trauma*, state on several occasions throughout the book that spotting necrosis and replacement by fibrous tissue will lead inevitably to Volkmann's contracture and will need without fail the appropriate and immediate management. They also emphasize the necessity for adequate fasciotomy and point out that it must not be "too little and too late." Among other measures besides the surgical procedures, such as fasciotomy and restoration of the arterial flow depending on what arterial lesions have been detected, the use of dextran and heparin must be instituted as a prophylactic measure.

Injuries to the ulnar and radial arteries may lead to Volkmann's contracture if an expanding hematoma is present in addition to the ischemia of the muscles of the forearm. Its evacuation through a wide fasciotomy is indicated promptly to avoid permanent neuromuscular deficits in the hand. Little and Ferguson[170] reported 11 such cases with blocked ulnar arteries.

Volkmann's ischemic contracture of the leg is encountered more frequently than in the past following procedures on the arterial tree whether it is on the popliteal or on arteries proximal to it. It is imperative after any reparative procedure of the arterial tree from the aorta distally to keep in mind the possibility of severe ischemia of the leg muscles which may lead to a compartment syndrome that needs immediate attention. Fasciotomies and evacuation of hematomas, if present, are indicated among other measures. Occasionally, prophylactic fasciotomies may forestall disastrous consequences of an overlooked ischemic complication of the skeletal muscles of the leg.

Anterior Tibial Compartment Syndrome

Like Volkmann's ischemic contracture, compartment syndromes are confined to limited muscular areas. These two entities are occasionally mistaken for one another when Volkmann's ischemic contracture affects the leg muscles. It is, therefore, appropriate to deal with these two entities in the same chapter although they are distinct syndromes.

Localized rhabdomyolysis to a group of leg muscles in acute arterial occlusions occurs either isolated or for the most part as an integral part of a more complex clinical picture. It is generally surprising that clinically significant metabolic and renal complications have not been more frequently reported. In contradistinction to the usual severe entities, only a small number of compartment syndromes have been mentioned in the literature.[21]

The most common compartment affected is the anterior tibial group of muscles, usually due to an acute arterial occlusion, rarely the result of an isolated interruption of the anterior tibial artery. More often than not it is secondary to the occlusion of the more proximal arterial tree (i.e., the iliac, femoral, or popliteal).

Recently, several etiologic factors were noted to be associated with the occurrence of an anterior tibial compartment. Bogaerts et al.[19] reported an acute rhabdomyolysis secondary to a nephrologic condition. Likewise, Lang[160] noted several cases of this complication associated with intra-arterial perfusion of streptokinase. Other etiologic factors reported were following use of heroin addiction,[75] during the course of cardiopulmonary bypass,[125] following acute embolic occlusion,[174] and in burn patients.[143]

The main clinical features of these cases range from superficial edema to actual necrosis of the muscles of the anterior tibial compartment. In milder forms, such lesions may end up in fibrosis of connective tissue, or, if uncorrected, they may result in complete necrosis of these muscles or even result in loss of the leg. Due to the relatively small area of rhabdomyolysis, systemic complications are usually mild and rarely lead to renal complications.[79,132,160,174] While such cases of compartment syndrome rarely occur isolated, their diagnosis in the context of the entire clinical picture may sometimes be overlooked.

Awareness of potential occurrence of the compartment syndrome as a complication seemingly as an independent event shoud be kept in mind so that appropriate treatment can be applied without delay, especially in the presence of severe rhabdomyolysis and renal complications.

21

Nontraumatic and Nonocclusive Arterial Rhabdomyolysis with Acute Renal Failure

Introduction

Inspired by the earlier description of the crush syndrome, associated with myoglobinemia and myoglobinuria resulting from rhabdomyolysis, a clinical awareness developed in relation to a great variety of medical nontraumatic and nonsurgical conditions. Originally, these cases were observed in nephrology, neurology, biochemistry, and other medical subspecialties. Patients in these various subspecialty areas were seen because of skeletal muscle complaints with urinary changes in whom myoglobin had been detected. Shortly thereafter, in medical subspecialties, an increasing number of cases were noted displaying the above syndrome of myoglobinemia and myoglobinuria associated with rhabdomyolytic processes. It appears at the present time that such instances are more frequently encountered than originally suspected.

Grossman et al.[94] reported in 1974 from the Renal-Electrolyte Section of the Department of Medicine and Department of Neurology from the University of Pennsylvania School of Medicine a paper entitled "Nontraumatic Rhabdomyolysis and Acute Renal Failure." The identification of these patients in a group of individuals during a 3-year period was invariably accompanied by a triad of orthotolidin-positive urine, pigmented granular casts in the sediment, and marked elevation of serum creatine phosphokinase (CPK) levels.

Several years later, Chugh et al.[40] from the Department of Nephrology and Biochemistry, reported in 1979 from Chandigard, India, acute renal failure due to nontraumatic rhabdomyolysis with a mortality rate among the myoglobinuric patients of over 29% while the overall mortality due to acute renal failure ranged from 40% to 60%. Following these reports, especially the one by Grossman, a great number of case reports dealing with similar clinicopathological manifestations made increasing appearance.

Due to a great variety of etiological factors involved in this form of rhabdomyolysis with and without myoglobinuria, the present discussion of this type of rhabdomyolysis may be divided into two separate sections: (1) reports of the two mentioned authors, and (2) a review of a great variety of groups of cases due to a wide spectrum of causes. An assessment of the pathogenesis of the rhabdomyolysis of these cases may lead to a more comprehensive classification of these nontraumatic and nonacute arterial occlusive processes.

Grossman and his associates, in a 3-year period, have observed 15 cases of acute renal failure in which muscle necrosis with myoglobinuria in the absence of overt trauma or surgery was the sole identifiable explanation for the acute renal failure. They have concluded from their experience that myoglobinuric acute renal failure from causes other than trauma or surgery is a frequently encountered process and probably misdiagnosed most of the time. Grossman pointed out that the lack of awareness of these entities led to cases of myoglobinuria often overlooked by those usually found in other abnormalities in acute renal failure of other causes. This is true in acute arterial occlusions as well as in traumatic cases. One of the distinguishing features, however, is hypercalcemia during diuresis and hypocalcemia in the early phase when diuresis is decreased, both of which are a unique feature of this type of acute renal failure.

These authors have identified three groups of patients with this type of myoglobinuria: (1) patients having myoglobinuria without acute renal failure; (2) patients with prior surgery or trauma as a probable cause of myoglobinuria and finally (3) patients who in the absence of surgery or overt trauma had myoglobinuria and went through a clinical course of acute renal failure for which no cause of rhabdomyolysis could be found. This last group of patients was the one representing the subject of this study. It is important to have a clear definition of rhabdomyolysis and acute renal failure in order to identify this entity as described by Grossman and Chugh.

Rhabdomyolysis is indicated by the presence of diffuse muscle cell injury, as based on biopsy specimens or autopsy material.

Acute renal failure is defined by acute tubular necrosis and is an acute loss or marked reduction of renal function associated with a rise in blood urea nitrogen and serum creatinine levels that persist despite the absence or correction of hemodynamic or mechanical causes of reduced renal function. Ruled out from this group of acute renal failure were cases of usual acute glomerulonephritis, acute renal infections, obstructive uropathy, and other specific acute and chronic renal diseases.

During the period of 1969–1972, Grossman and his associates observed 44 patients with myoglobinuria;[94] of these, acute renal failure developed in 19. Excluded from this group were four of the 19 with myoglobinuria from lower limb ischemia after reconstruction of arterial surgical problems. The remaining 15 patients had myoglobinuria and acute renal failure without either surgical or accidental trauma; this group constituted at least 5% of all cases of acute renal failure seen in their consultation service of renal lesions. This is an interesting statistical fact since it indicates the relative incidence of this type of myoglobinuria in relation to the total statistical study of this group of patients.

Chugh, on the other hand, studied 27 patients with established acute renal failure of whom 17 on preliminary screening revealed positive evidence of myoglobinuria and 10 were nonmyoglobinuric and served as controls.[40] In all these instances of the two groups, the diagnosis of acute renal failure was established on the basis of a history of oliguria/anuria of more than 2 to 3 days in most patients, all of whom were previously healthy, but developed progressive elevation of blood urea and serum creatinine, a urinary sodium concentration of more than 40 mmol/L of sodium, and low urinary osmolality.

The specific studies demonstrating the presence of myoglobinuria and rhabdomyolysis consisted of evidence of myoglobin in the urine, estimation of the serum creatine phosphokinase (CPK), serum aldolase, and serum levels of potassium, uric acid, and calcium. On the basis of the positive or negative evidence of urinary myoglobin, the patients were divided into two groups: myoglobinuric and nonmyoglobinuric.

With regard to the presence of CPK and absence of myoglobin, there is a difference of opinion between some investigators with regard to the method used for identifying myoglobin either in the blood or in the urine. Kaiser et al.,[147] in a letter to JAMA of March 26, 1982, took issue with those authors who report on the positive presence of CPK and absence of myoglobin. According to their experience with 23 cases of atraumatic rhabdomyolysis, this positive CPK-absent myoglobin condition seems to be impossible to these authors. In their opinion, muscle damage causing enzyme leakage invariably leads to concomitant increases in serum myoglobin concentrations. Even in cases with minor degrees of rhabdomyolysis (as judged from serum creatine phosphokinase levels), serum myoglobin is regularly and notably elevated according to Kaiser and associates. Normal serum myoglobin levels seem to be improbable since in this situation renal elimination of myoglobin is impaired and serum myoglobin levels are elevated. In cases of myoglobinuric renal failure, serum creatine phosphokinase levels always return more rapidly to normal than do myoglobin levels. The reason for this discrepancy between their findings and those of other investigators is from their point of view due to the method or technique used for the assay of myoglobin. Even with relatively insensitive myoglobin assays such as gel immunodiffusion assay, complement fixation assay, or spectrophotometric methods, elevated myoglobin values should have been found in these patients. Nevertheless, they suggest that the highly specific, sensitive, and reliable radioimmunological method should be used in the measurement of serum myoglobin levels.

This serious difference of opinion is mentioned because of

the discrepancy in the two papers by Grossman and by Chugh covering renal failures with elevated CPK in the absence of myoglobin. It is possible that the technique of determining myoglobin was not sensitive enough to provide a positive finding. It is also possible that such cases may exist in the absence of myoglobin but may be due to other factors. Those involved in this area of nontraumatic rhabdomyolysis and renal failure should review their cases and see whether the difference between one method of assay of myoglobin and another would verify the assertion by Kaiser and associates.

Etiology of Rhabdomyolysis

As already mentioned above, the great variety of medical conditions responsible for the nontraumatic rhabdomyolysis includes a large number of myopathies, grand-mal seizures, and prolonged coma, the latter probably related to drug abuse associated with toxic effects or muscle injury due to compression during immobility in the course of the comatose stage, infections, either bacterial or viral, burns, epilepsy, poisoning with various metals, etc.

Clinical Manifestations

The clinical picture in such cases consists of complaints of pain referable to musculoskeletal system, and muscular pain mild in nature which, in retrospect, was diagnosed as myoglobinuria when the urine had been tested. Absence of musculoskeletal complaints may be correlated retrospectively after the diagnosis of myoglobinuria is established. Physical examination is often misleading. In 12 patients of the 15 reported by Grossman who were able to cooperate for full muscular examination within 48 hours of admission, four had completely normal results without weakness, swelling, pain, or tenderness. Definite dehydration on initial examination appeared probable. However, another group of patients never gave any clinical evidence of dehydration. Laboratory tests in all 15 patients demonstrated evidence of myoglobinuria. However, visible myoglobinemia was not observed in any of these patients. Again, this may be related to the type of chemical assay for detecting the myoglobin, as mentioned above. Gross pigmenturia, a reddsh-brown discoloration of the urine, was seen in 12 of 15 cases. Exceptionally, some patients claimed never to have discoloration of the urine, although myoglobinuria was confirmed biochemically.

Associated Metabolic Changes

In all of these patients, hyperkalemia (potassium of more than 6 mEq per liter) developed within 3 days of the rhabdomyolytic insult (in five of the seven within 1 day). In 12 patients during the first 3 days after the insult, serum creatinine levels rose at unusually rapid rates, more than 2.5 mg per 100 ml per day. Three patients had increments in serum creatinine levels of more than 6 mg per 100 ml per day.

Serum calcium levels decreased during oliguria to less than or equal to 7 mg per 100 ml within 3 days of the insult. In five of six cases, hypocalcemia coexisted with hyperphosphatemia (a level of more than 8 mg per 100 ml). In three of these patients with hypocalcemia, hypercalcemia was displayed during the subsequent diuretic phase of the acute renal failure. These biochemical alterations occurred early after the beginning of the rhabdomyolytic process. Although hypercalcemia and hypocalcemia coexisted in a few patients, there were no definite cardiac arrhythmias. After the initial period, the patients behaved similarly to those with acute renal failure of other etiologies. Large and rapid increments in serum potassium, creatinine, and phosphate levels ceased. Dialysis was required in seven of the 15 patients for control of uremic symptoms.

In Chugh's cases of 17 patients, 15 were oliguric on admission and two were nonoliguric. The duration of oliguria varied from 2 to 30 days with a mean of 9 days.

Concerning the calcium level, it should be noted that 82% of Chugh's patients had hypocalcemia during the oliguric phase, while hypercalcemia was noted in 66.6% of these patients during the diuretic phase. These two findings during the evolution of the myoglobinuric syndrome are regarded by these authors as characteristic findings in the patients with acute renal failure following rhabdomyolysis. The mechanism underlying these findings is not entirely clear. Hypocalcemia has been attributed to the release of phosphate compounds from damaged muscles into the extracellular fluid leading to hyperphosphatemia which, in turn, facilitates deposition of calciophosphate in the damaged muscles. The latter has also been demonstrated radiologically, as well as in the muscle biopsy tissue.

According to Chugh, the exact mechanism by which myoglobinuria induces acute renal failure includes destruction of the tubular lumina by myoglobin casts, back diffusion of glomerular filtrate through breached tubular epithelium, and a diminished glomerular filtrate rate. Dehydration, as mentioned previously, is known to facilitate the induction of acute renal failure in animal experiments. It should be also noted, however, that myoglobin in the presence of acidosis precipitates readily in the tubules and produces an obstructive lesion of these tubules leading to the acute tubular necrosis. These authors seem to omit this possibility of the myoglobinuric nephrosis. The mortality reported by Chugh was five deaths in 17 patients, with the remaining 12 having recovered. Those who died were primarily patients with severe burns, extensive tissue necrosis, and septicemia.

Of the blood chemistries characteristic of myoglobinuric syndrome, it was already mentioned above that significant elevation of serum creatine phosphokinase (CPK) and aldolase were noted in all patients. Renal histology was significant and available in 10 of the 17 patients. It showed appearances consistent with acute tubular necrosis in all cases. It should be noted that of the 10 patients only five died and had autopsy material while the others had changes probably by biopsy.

As to the prognosis in the overall nontraumatic rhabdomyolytic cases, again these authors emphasized the significant contrast between their cases and those with the very severe metabolic renal syndrome secondary to acute arterial occlusions as described in Chapter 14 of this monograph.

Nonmyoglobinuric Renal Failure

Due to the controversy mentioned earlier concerning the detection of myoglobin in all of these renal failure cases, it is of interest to review briefly by comparison the two groups of patients. The fact that myoglobin was not detected in such instances may be the result of the method of assay rather than the actual presence of myoglobin either in the blood or in the urine. In cases reported by Grossman where myoglobinuria was definitely detected, no myoglobin was seen in the serum, which, again, is not consistent with what should actually happen. If myoglobinuria is detectable, myoglobinemia should also be present and the fact that it is not detectable may be due to a technical problem rather than to the presence or absence of the pigment.

Myoglobinuric versus nonmyoglobinuric renal failure showed no apparent difference between the two in relation to the duration of oliguria or severity of renal failure between the two groups of patients. Statistical evaluation in Chugh's series revealed significant differences in the peak levels of serum creatine phosphokinase (CPK), serum aldolase, and uric acid levels between the two groups. Although the mean serum potassium was higher in the myoglobinuric patients, the difference was not significant showing more than $p < 0.05$ which would appear nonsignificant. No significant difference was found between the mean levels of blood urea and creatine and creatinine in the two groups. Whereas the difference between the serum calcium levels of the oliguric and diuretic phases was statistically significant in the myoglobinuric patients, this difference was not significant in the nonmyoglobinuric group.

Chugh attributes the characteristic features of rhabdomyolysis, besides the pathological changes, to the presence of myoglobin in the urine and elevation of the serum creatine phosphokinase and aldolase in the blood. These criteria have enabled him and his group to identify the pathogenic role of muscle cell injury in many patients with acute renal failure in whom gross clinical evidence of muscle necrosis was absent. The rhabdomyolytic process responsible for this group of patients appears to range between 5% and 7% according to Grossman[94] and Coffler.[47a] It appears from the two studies of Grossman and Chugh that the condition may be more common than has been recognized thus far. Based on the comments by Kaiser regarding the detection of myoglobin, it would appear that a more sensitive test for detecting this pigment in either the blood or the urine would be necessary to evaluate more properly the incidence of this condition.

Myoglobinuria associated with copper or zinc or other metal intoxication has been reported as isolated instances. However, it would appear that muscle cell injury and rhabdomyolysis may have been due to the direct cytotoxic effect of these substances.

Prolonged coma and immobilization in one position have been incriminated as important factors, as already mentioned above. This is due to direct compression of the muscle or partial occlusion of the regional vascular supply because of weight of the body in an immobile position.

Although in these papers very few potassium deficiency cases have been reported, it is nevertheless pertinent to mention that animals with advanced potassium deficiency have been observed to have a subnormal muscle membrane potential, suggesting loss of integrity of the muscle cell membranes and thus leading to severe hypokalemia. This is considered to be a major contributory factor for massive muscle cell injury in one of the patients seen by Chugh.

In conclusion, it appears from these two major studies that myoglobinuric acute renal failure from nontraumatic causes is probably more frequent than is generally appreciated, although it is being recognized increasingly in the past 15 years since the first paper published by Grossman. Failure of diagnosis is a reflection of two factors as mentioned previously in other chapters, namely, lack of awareness of the common clinical settings in which nontraumatic muscle necrosis may occur and the absence of a widely available specific test for myoglobin in body fluids. The latter point mentioned by Grossman may be controversial or debatable in the context of the comment made by Kaiser and associates.

Case Reports

The recently increasing number of nontraumatic myoglobinuric conditions is due to a great variety of etiologic factors. However, it is not the intent of this section to include individually all of the reported cases. A classification of these conditions may provide a brief idea of their diversity.

Classification

Myopathies
Dermatomyositis
Polymyositis
Systemic lupus erythematosus
Grand mal seizures

Prolonged coma
Strenuous exercise
Infections
Viremias
Toxic factors

In spite of the multiple factors, a number of common features, both biochemical and management, link them together, albeit somewhat remotely, in some instances. Only the most common of these groups of cases will be mentioned here.

Paroxysmal Paralytic Myoglobinuria

Paroxysmal paralytic myoglobinuria was reported by Elek et al.[69] early in 1953, shortly after this condition became related to the crush syndrome following the Battle of Britain. It is a rare disease of unknown etiology affecting the skeletal muscle and resulting in myoglobinuria. The two chief complaints are painful muscle spasms and brownish urine. It occurs as minor or major conditions, which differ only in extent of lesions. Minor forms are characterized by painful tonic spasms affecting the lower limbs, mainly the calf muscles, followed within a few hours by transient myoglobinuria. Major attacks consist of pseudo-paralysis of the whole body and are much rarer than the former. The disease has a tendency to recur but the prognosis is good. The pathological changes in the affected muscles consist of focal necrosis. Etiology has remained unknown.

Rhabdomyolysis and Myoglobinuria Due to Potassium Depletion

Several papers have appeared on this subject and provide somewhat different pathogenic mechanisms to account for them. Rhabdomyolysis and myoglobinuria occur commonly in men who sustain environmental heat injury during extensive physical training in hot climates. They also occur in patients with potassium depletion. Since physical training in hot climates may be accompanied by serious losses of body potassium, the possibility was considered that performance of strenuous exercise resulting in potassium deficiency might enhance susceptibility to rhabdomyolysis. It is known that potassium is released from contracting skeletal muscle fibers and its rising concentration in interstitial fluid is thought to dilate arterioles thereby mediating the normal rise of muscle blood flow during exercise.

Knochel[151] supports the hypothesis by comparing the effect of electrically stimulated exercise on muscle blood flow, potassium release, and histology of the intact gracilis muscle preparation in normal and in potassium-depleted dogs. In normal dogs, muscle blood flow and potassium release rose sharply during exercise. In contrast, muscle blood flow and potassium release were markedly subnormal in dogs despite brisk muscle contractions. Although minor histologic changes were sometimes observed in nonexercised potassium-depleted muscle, frank rhabdomyolysis occurred in each potassium-depleted animal after exercise. These findings by this author support the hypothesis that ischemia may be the mechanism of rhabdomyolysis with exercise and potassium depletion.

Nadel et al.[199] reported the case of a patient who developed hypokalemic rhabdomyolysis and acute renal failure following prolonged nasogastric suction and total parenteral nutrition. Severe rhabdomyolysis and acute renal failure ensued. A review of the literature failed to disclose a similar case, according to Nadel, of hypokalemic rhabdomyolysis and acute renal failure, although the syndrome has been associated with other causes of hypokalemia and its pathophysiology has been investigated in experimental models. The morbidity associated with extensive myonecrosis and severe, acute renal failure in the patient indicates that hypokalemia and other electrolyte abnormalities should be aggressively corrected in similar clinical settings.

Although hypokalemia had long been suspected as a cause of rhabdomyolysis, the basic mechanisms of potassium depletion resulting in muscle destruction have, until recently, been elusive. In 1950, Smith et al.[266] described experimental data of dogs showing that depletion of potassium led to degeneration of skeletal muscles. Previously reported causes of this syndrome were attributed to: (1) drug therapy (diuretics, carbenoxolone, and amphotericin B); (2) licorice ingestions; (3) alcoholism, probably multifactorial causes of the decreased potassium in most of these patients; (4) gastrointestinal potassium losses due to regional enteritis with stearate therapy, laxative abuse, and nutritional deficiency syndromes with diarrhea; (5) renal tubular acidosis; and (6) exercise in hot weather.

The pathophysiology of hypokalemic rhabdomyolysis has been extensively studied by several investigators. Paramount to the integrity of the skeletal muscle is maintenance of an adequate blood flow in response to metabolic demand. With exercise, there is a reactive hyperemia that occurs in all normal muscle vascular beds. The mediators of this vasodilatation and increase in muscle blood flow may include hypoxia, changes in adenosine nucleotides or pH, or increases in osmolality, phosphate, or potassium levels.

Another paper dealing with the subject of rhabdomyolysis and myoglobinuria in association with hypokalemia of renal tubular acidosis was reported by Campion et al.[34] The case was of a 44-year-old woman who had severe hyperchloremic acidosis and hypokalemia. She had paralysis, muscle tenderness, and myoglobinuria. There was no history of previous muscle abnormality. In this case, the rhabdomyolysis appeared to be the result of potassium deficiency without concurrent drug therapy. The relative rarity of rhabdomyolysis in potassium-deficient states may result from the generalized weakness and paralysis, both of which might prevent sufficient muscular activity to stress energy-producing enzyme systems to a point of breakdown of cellular integrity. Nevertheless, potassium-deficient muscle must be under some stress, as evidenced by high serum muscle enzyme levels seen in potassium-deficient states. Conceivably, the marked acidosis seen in this patient by Campion, together with potassium deficiency, played a role in the production of rhabdomyolysis.

Comment

From knowledge of the role of the sarcolemmal membrane in the leakage of various biochemical substrates of the skeletal muscle, it is difficult to conceive how a patient loses only potassium without losing any other substances. In this particular case, myoglobinuria was present as well as hypokalemia. The potassium is usually lost at the same time through the membrane and should end up in hyperkalemia. Instead, the syndrome is characterized by the opposite condition—hypokalemia. An explanation for this paradoxical finding has not yet been found.

Inflammatory Myopathies and Myoglobinurias

In recent years, several papers on inflammatory myopathies appeared in connection with myoglobinuria and renal problems. Of these, Kagen,[146] Kreitzer,[156] and Pirovino[223] published their experiences with this topic.

Kreitzer, in a paper published in 1978 on dermatomyositis and polymyositis, mentions the clinical and biochemical findings in these cases. Myoglobin was present in the serum and in the urine, but he could find only five cases in the literature of myoglobinuric renal failure associated with these disorders. He proved the presence of myoglobin by immunologic techniques. The pathogenesis of renal failure associated with myoglobinuric syndromes remains controversial in his opinion and in spite of many attempts, he feels that the problem was not elucidated. He states, however, that the differential renal cortical blood flow occurs secondary to myoglobin's toxic property. Nevertheless, he is not sure whether this disorder is rare or if it is just transiently mild and, therefore, is being easily overlooked.

Pirovino discusses the problem of myoglobinuria and acute renal failure associated with acute polymyositis. He also feels that this association between myositis and myoglobinuria is rather rare. The data obtained in this case of polymyositis and acute renal failure was based on renal biopsy and quantitative assessment of myoglobin. A renal biopsy performed while the patient had active myositis and proteinuria shortly after recovery from renal failure revealed primarily glomerular changes of increased mesangial matrix and cells. Tubular and interstitial changes that might be expected following acute tubular necrosis were almost completely absent.

Kagen, in a most comprehensive study on this subject, includes his clinical and laboratory data based on dermatomyositis, polymyositis, scleroderma, and systemic lupus erythematosus with active myopathy. His immunological techniques permitted specific and sensitive detection of his low-molecular-weight, oxygen-binding protein normally found in the striated muscle cell.

He points out that the myoglobin assay has been useful not only in assessing the presence of muscle disease, but in alerting the physician to the risk of renal failure, which may complicate myoglobinuric states. The myoglobinemia in these cases was detected in 74.1% of sera taken from the patients with active myositis before therapy, with a slightly greater frequency in the groups with dermatomyositis and polymyositis. After the use of steroid therapy, the incidence of finding positive myoglobinemia fell to 43.4% and 59.5% in patients in clinical remission not requiring therapy. In addition to myoglobinemia and myoglobinuria, serum enzymes such as creatine phosphokinase, lactic dehydrogenase, and SGOT activity were higher in samples containing myoglobin. The number of patients studied amounted to 62 and the cases were divided into the following categories: 15 dermatomyositis, 14 polymyositis, 17 other connective tissue diseases such as systemic lupus erythematosus, scleroderma, juvenile rheumatoid arthritis, two with arthritis, one with rheumatoid arthritis, and one with an unclassified connective tissue disorder. Due to this wide spectrum of cases, the results mentioned by Kagen are of great scientific significance in terms of the appearance of myoglobinemia and consequent myoglobinuria in these inflammatory processes of myopathies. Sequential serum determinations demonstrated in some patients some reduction in the levels of serum myoglobin with therapy, namely, steroid drugs, usually before enzyme values had returned to normal.

The method of myoglobin assay described by Kagen has been used by a number of investigators who have found it to be quite reliable. In view of a previously mentioned comment by Kaiser and associates about the radioimmunoassay, it is of interest to mention that the methods described by Kagen were performed both by immunodiffusion and by complement fixation. Both of these methods were specific for myoglobin and did not detect other components of human serum, urine, red blood cells, or muscle extracts. The sensitivity of the immunodiffusion method was approximately 10 micrograms/ml, while that of complement fixation was approximately 0.3 micrograms/ml of serum. Kagen recognizes that because of interference factors present in some human sera, very low concentrations were underestimated by the complement fixation method.

Steroid therapy seems to be helpful in these inflammatory

myopathies. Corticosteroid treatment, primarily prednisone, was used for management of these cases.

It is of interest to note that in the study of Kagen, he was able to find that myoglobin is more commonly determined in the serum than in the urine of patients with myositis, and that urinary findings did not always accurately reflect the rapid changes that the serum does.

Because myoglobinemia is usually regarded as difficult and unreliable to test, Kagen points out that the frequency of myoglobinemia has not been fully explored. This is in agreement with Kaiser's statement that myoglobinemia and myoglobinuria are more frequently missed because of poor technique or method used for their detection.

Myopathy Associated with Alcoholism

Skeletal muscle biopsies from patients with various forms of alcoholic myopathy have been studied by light and electron microscopy by Klinkerfuss.[150] The morphological features of the acute myopathy consisted of severe intracellular edema and destruction of mitochondria and myofilaments. Morphology of the chronic myopathy was characterized by evidence of earlier destruction, and active regeneration of others, presumably reflecting the results of multiple alcoholic bouts. Altered cell membrane permeability is probably the initial alteration leading to these morphological changes.

Miscellaneous Etiologies

Myoglobinuria and acute renal failure have been reported in connection with *septicemia*.[270] O'Connor reported myoglobinuria associated with parainfluenza type 2 infection and Rheingold et al.[235] have presented a similar case due to typhoid fever.

Acute myoglobinuria and heroin drug abuse has been the subject of several articles in recent years. Several of these papers have reported various types of heroin use, either by snorting or direct oral use or injection intravenously (D'Agostino[48] and Tuller[286]). The latter author has personally seen 17 patients with rhabdomyolysis and myoglobinuria in the New York area. The diffuse inflammation of muscle described by Richter in the microscopic abnormalities in the patients described in this paper were identical to those illustrated in their article. In no case could the muscle lesion be attributed to accidental compromise of its blood supply, which is of interest since the rhabdomyolysis was due primarily to muscle breakdown by compression of the muscle directly during immobility of the patient. The rhabdomyolysis was confirmed by muscle breakdown following myoglobinemia and myoglobinuria and is a relatively minor manifestation of a profound metabolic disturbance which drastically alters integrity of a number of biological membranes. The role of heroin is merely one of the many agents capable of precipitating the rhabdomyolysis syndrome.

Conclusion

This succinct description of a few myopathies, either inflammatory, traumatic, or due to bacterial or viral infection, indicates the wide spectrum of etiologic factors that may affect the skeletal muscle and result in myoglobinemia and myoglobinuria leading to renal complications ranging from transient effects to complete shutdown and death of the patient if not treated in time with hemodialysis.

As a result of the greater number of reports on this subject, the role of acute ischemia of the skeletal muscle leading to a profound metabolic compromise of the homeostatic mechanisms of the human body has or will become a well-accepted concept.

22

Myocardial Infarction

Introduction

While there are similarities between the two muscular tissues, myocardium and skeletal muscle, some specific differences do exist.

Since myoglobin is found in both myocardial infarction and rhabdomyolysis, it would be helpful, on this basis, to review briefly their structures. Indeed, review of the myocardial features appears relevant in this monograph, although it is specifically devoted to the acute ischemia of the skeletal muscle.

The cardiac muscle has distinct characteristics from those of skeletal muscle. Nonetheless, the morphological features of both possess a certain common number of basic elements. Similarly, a number of important biochemical substances are present in the fibers of both myocardial and skeletal muscle.

There are of course some fundamental differences between the two types of muscles. It would, therefore, be appropriate that, before discussing the problem of myocardial infarction, a brief review of the cardiac muscle precede its morphological and biochemical features.

Cardiac Muscle

The cells of fibers of adult cardiac muscle fit together so tightly that under the light microscope they give the false impression of comprising a syncytium. Electron micrographs show, however, that cardiac muscle is definitely composed of elongated branching cells with irregular contours at their junctions. The fibers are usually about 14 mm in diameter in a normal adult heart, but they vary during normal growth and under pathological conditions.

Each fiber is enclosed in a sarcolemma which is similar to that of skeletal muscle. The structure seen with a light microscope includes a cell membrane, as external lamina outside the plasmalemma, and associated reticular fibers.

The nuclei, unlike those of skeletal muscle, are generally located in the central portion of the fiber, and number one per cell, or occasionally two, in contrast with a multinucleated condition in skeletal muscle. They are oval in shape and somewhat larger, sometimes one-half the diameter of the fibers.

The fibers contain myofibrils with constituent actin and myosin, and the myofilaments are organized in sarcomeres similar to those in skeletal muscle.

The *sarcoplasmic reticulum* consists mainly of smooth-surfaced membranes, but small segments occasionally have polyribosomes attached.

Skeletal muscle usually contracts only after an external stimulus is provided under normal conditions by the motor nerve endings. By contrast, as is well known, cardiac muscle cells possess the ability to contract rhythmically at an intrinsic basic rate in the absence of the nerve supply or other external stimuli. The mechanism underlying this capability remains largely unexplained. Interestingly, when myocardial cells are growing *in vitro*, they display a rhythmic contraction individually until the colony is crowded enough that intercellular contacts are established. At this time, contraction is coordinated among the cells, apparently mediated by nexuses (gap junctions).

Blood Vessels and Nerves of Cardiac Muscles. The blood supply of cardiac muscle surpasses that of skeletal muscle. Branches of sympathic and parasympathetic nerves follow the connective tissue pathways and terminate in fine endings scattered among muscle fibers.*

Role in Myoglobin in the Diagnosis of Myocardial Infarction

In addition to the well-established and currently used analysis of enzyme changes in myocardial infarction, determination of myoglobin has also recently been found to be of diagnostic significance. Alone or combined with the enzyme studies, it may be of great help in borderline cases.

Serum Enzymes and Isoenzymes in Myocardial Infarction

The specificity of a number of enzymes designed to detect acute myocardial infarction or acute myocardial ischemia, although generally accepted for their diagnostic value, has led to extensive studies of isoenzymes that are of different molecular forms but catalyze the same chemical reaction. Thus, two of the most common enzymes, lactic dehydrogenase (LDH) and creatine phosphokinase (CPK), are known to have five isoenzymes and three for the respective enzymes. Thus, lactic dehydrogenase has five isoenzymes generally designated numerically as one through five, with one representing the fraction that migrates most quickly toward the anode. Creatine phosphokinase includes three isoenzymes designated as MM, MB, and BB which have been identified by either electrophoresis or column chromatography.

CPK-MM is found predominantly in skeletal and cardiac muscle, but lesser amounts are present in brain. CPK-BB is predominantly present in brain, although it is also present in lesser concentrations in various viscera. The myocardium contains predominantly CPK-MM, but 15% to 20% of the total CPK activity is contributed by the MB dimer. Consequently, myocardial necrosis

*The preceding data on cardiac muscle are based on the article by D.E. Kelly et al. in Bailey's *Textbook of Microscopic Anatomy*, 18th Edition, Williams & Wilkins, Baltimore, 1984, p 909.

results in the appearance of significant amounts of the MB isoenzymes in the serum. However, serum CPK-MB isoenzyme activity may be increased in conditions other than myocardial infarction, particularly when significant skeletal muscle destruction has occurred. The latter occurs primarily in rhabdomyolysis with myoglobinuria. Thus, a number of other muscular conditions and a great variety of pulmonary, hepatic, inflammatory conditions, etc., have also shown a similar, but to a lesser degree, presence of these isoenzymes. Although CPK-MB is most specific for myocardial infarction, CPK-MB is predominantly, as mentioned, seen in skeletal muscle necrosis.

Myoglobin Determination in Myocardial Infarction

In 1962, Luginbuhl[173] noted that cardiac muscle myoglobin appeared to be immunologically identical to that obtained from human skeletal muscle. Since that time, several investigators have demonstrated myoglobin in serum and urine in varying amounts after injury to heart muscle, particularly after acute myocardial infarction. These observations suggested that a rapid test system to detect myoglobin in the urine may be a reliable method for the measurement of the presence, duration, and severity of acute myocardial necrosis in man.

Immunologic Detection of Myoglobinuria After Cardiac Surgery

In 1967, Kagen[144a,b] reported detection of myoglobin by a variety of chemical and physical methods as well as by the use of antibody techniques. In general, he found that immunological methods allow detection of smaller amounts of myoglobin than do chemical techniques. He then prepared a specific precipitating antiserum to human myoglobin that did not form precipitates with normal human serum, urine, hemoglobin, liver extract, uterine muscle extract, or with components of striated muscle tissue extracts other than myoglobin. The antiserum that he prepared could identify as little as 0.005 mg/ml myoglobin and reproducibly quantify amounts in excess of 0.015 mg/ml. With the use of this antiserum, myoglobinuria was detected in six of 16 patients after cardiac surgery. Of these patients, six out of 16 demonstrated myoglobinuria on the first day after cardiac surgery. None of 20 patients recovering from other surgical procedures had this finding. Myoglobin was detected in the serum of seven patients after surgery. In six of these seven patients, only trace amounts were present, while one patient had a slightly larger amount of this pigment in the serum. Three of the seven patients with myoglobinemia had coincident myoglobinuria. All the myoglobinuric patients had open-heart surgery and antecedent valvular heart disease. Five of the six had antecedent congestive heart failure, while five of six had heart valve replacement operations. The prevalence of myoglobinuria was related both to the total time of surgery and to the time of use of pump cardiac bypass apparatus.

Kagen[144] was not sure of the origin of the myoglobin present in the serum and in the urine of these patients. He postulated, however, that it seemed likely that it was of cardiac origin, although it was possible that skeletal muscle may also have been a source. This is one of the first studies of the presence of myoglobin in serum and urine associated with cardiac surgery and explains to a great extent the uncertainty of the values quantitatively and otherwise of the myoglobin in the urine and serum, as well as the technique used for detecting myoglobin.

Following this study with immunological detection of myoglobinuria after cardiac surgery, Kagen used an immunofluorescent technique for demonstrating myoglobin in the kidney. He used this technique in 43 patients with a variety of conditions ranging from open-heart surgery to a severe burn involving a great number of cases; among others femoral artery ischemia due to thrombosis and embolism were also included.

The patient who was the subject of this case report in his article[145] involving the myoglobin and the kidney developed postoperative renal failure 6 days after the onset of myoglobinuria and died as a result of this condition. The myoglobinuria was secondary to ischemia of the lower extremities. The vascular condition for which he was operated upon and from which he developed myoglobinuria was a fusiform aneurysm of the abdominal aorta. In addition, he had occlusive arterial disease of both lower extremities for several years preceding this operation.

The mention of this procedure was specifically for the use of immunofluorescent demonstration of myoglobin in the kidney which appeared to be quite useful in a variety of other conditions in which myoglobinuria was detected.

Urinary Myoglobin: A Clinical Test for Myocardial Infarction?

Adams and Elliott,[2] in a clinical study, undertook to determine whether myoglobinuria was a helpful diagnostic test for myocardial infarction.

Myoglobin has been noted quite early to be present in certain ischemic conditions of cardiac muscle and it became obvious that its presence in urine and in the plasma in amounts above normal levels might be of diagnostic significance with regard to damage to the myocardium. Several studies have appeared in the literature confirming this opinion.

Adams and Elliott's investigation was designed as a test that might displace the serum enzyme study. The results of this investigation were obtained in 44 patients with myocardial infarction and in 36 patients without myocardial infarction. In those with myocardial infarction, myoglobin was detected in the urine in 35, was equivocal in four, and was not detected in five. The combined enzyme tests (LDH, SGOT) were positive in 37, equivocal in four, and negative in three. It appears that the urinary myoglobin tests and the serum enzyme tests together were more definitive than either were alone, correctly identifying 42 with two equivocal. Thus, myoglobin determinations with ECG identified 43 of the infarctions with only one equivocal.

False-positive myoglobin tests were obtained in 16 patients in whom no diagnosis of myocardial infarction was made; 10 of these were patients with other heart disease, such as angina, congestive heart failure, and arteriosclerotic heart disease.

These investigations pointed out that while myoglobinemia can be caused by myocardial infarction, there may be other causes for it as well. This also holds true for false-positive tests with the enzymes, as mentioned above.

The Detection of Myoglobinuria by Radioimmunodiffusion Assay: A New Diagnostic Test for Acute Myocardial Infarction

This technique consists of a gel impregnated with myoglobin antiserum, which was used on urine samples from 60 patients with acute myocardial infarction, from 20 patients with chest pain due to ischemic heart disease without infarction, and from 20 normal subjects. Saranchak and Bernstein,[253] using this technique, have shown that these patients had marked elevations of myoglobin in the urine. The level of urinary myoglobin determined by this technique exceeded 5 mg/100 ml for patients who have suffered infarcts. High levels were associated with more massive infarction. In one-third of the patients studied, myoglobinuria preceded cardiac serum enzyme elevation and serial electrocardiographic changes indicative of acute infarction. These investigators felt that detection of myoglobinuria by this technique or by a similar one would be quite helpful as a new diagnostic test for acute myocardial infarction.

They felt a need for a rapid, reliable diagnostic test to be used in conjunction with clinical and electrocardiographic findings in acute myocardial infarction. Two-thirds of patients who had the complaint of chest pain were subsequently found in their experience not to have an acute infarct. Most of these patients, by present-day techniques, are admitted to coronary care units and carefully observed with monitoring for several days before the diagnosis of infarct can be effectively ruled out. They also confirmed other investigators' findings that patients who do have acute infarction of the myocardium often do not demonstrate the classic electrocardiographic changes or abnormal elevation in levels of serum enzymes early in the course of their disease. Their studies showed that determination of serum CPK level appeared to be the most reliable serum enzyme test for assessment of acute myocardial infarction, as has been well known by others. In their opinion, the ability to detect myoglobin in the urine makes this test more suitable in the study of infarction than CPK which may not be absolutely specific for infarction of the myocardium. This point of view may be disputed by present-day knowledge and by the opinion of some other investigators.

This technique enabled these investigators to quantitate myoglobinuria so that levels above 5 mg/100 ml could be employed as a diagnostic test of acute infarction. It was used as a rapid latex fixation test at the bedside, in the emergency room, or in the coronary care unit without wasting too much time. Their data indicated that myoglobin in its initial outpouring from damaged cardiac muscle may be an earlier prognostic sign than enzyme determinations and may eventually be correlated with infarct size.

While the preceding methods for detecting myoglobin in the urine in patients with acute myocardial infarction appear to be satisfactory, other tests appear to be as reliable, according to other investigators. The following few tests will therefore be discussed further.

Radioimmunoassay for Human Myoglobin in Myocardial Infarction

A test using radioimmunoassay for human myoglobin was studied by Reichlin et al.[234] in 13 normal individuals and in 68 patients admitted to a coronary care unit because of chest pain.

Myoglobin (MB) as a potential marker of myocardial damage was first published, as mentioned above, by Kagen[144] in 1967. Following this report, during the early 1970s, several groups attempted to determine the frequency with which myoglobin appeared in the urine in the early stage of myocardial infarction. The results were variable, related in part to the sensitivity and specificity of the precipitin and hemagglutination inhibition procedures used to detect myoglobin, and perhaps also in part to an incomplete understanding of the renal handling of myoglobin. An early study in 1973, using a radioimmunoassay for quantitating myoglobin in the dog by Lwebuga-Mukasa and colleagues,[171a] presented a preliminary report of this method capable of quantitating myoglobin in the dog in the nanogram per milliliter range. Studies were performed in chronically instrumented animals, focusing on plasma rather than on urinary MB. The findings indicated that MB appears in canine plasma 1 to 2 hours following coronary occlusion, peaks at approximately 6 hours, and disappears at approximately 10 hours. (For the exact technique of radioimmunoassay, see the paper by Reichlin.[234])

The results of this study indicate that myoglobin could be detected in the serum from the normal individuals.

> Values range from 3 to 75 and averaged 25 ± 3 ng/ml (ng = nanogram). Peak values in 32 patients with acute infarction were uniformly elevated, ranging from 200 to 5,500 and averaging 1,368 ± 1,357 ng/ml. All infarct patients had been admitted to the CCU within 12 hours of the onset of chest pain and all had elevated MB levels within 12 hours of the onset of

> pain, and all had elevated myoglobin levels within 12–48 hours after admission. Peak total CPK levels ranged from 160 to 2,000 and averaged 818 IU/L (upper limits of normal were 103 IU/L in males and 60 in females). MB-CPK was confirmed in the serum patterns. In eight patients the admission myoglobin level was clearly elevated while the total CPK level was still normal. In this study, myoglobin levels rose faster than CPK levels and reached peak values several hours earlier (mean of 18 versus mean of 28 hours); in no case did the CPK peak before the myoglobin.

The findings in patients with myocardial infarction confirm that elevations in serum myoglobin are an early and an extremely sensitive index of acute necrosis. Of interest in this study was that the highest serum levels in the infarction patients occurred in individuals with diminished peripheral perfusion, and skeletal as well as cardiac muscle myoglobin may have contributed to the elevated values (Reichlin et al.[234]) Elevations originating from skeletal muscle present problems in interpretation in cardiac patients. Since the cardiac and skeletal muscle myoglobin are immunologically identical, there is no way to obviate this important limitation in specificity of serum myoglobin elevations.

The usefulness of measurements of the urinary myoglobin concentrations in the detection of acute infarction remains unsettled. Encouraging reports have been presented, but false-negative values occur rather frequently in typical cases. It appears from this study that myoglobinuria in patients with infarction having positive serum myoglobin elevation has been of little value since negative results have been obtained in a large number of patients.[234]

Additional information about the renal handling of myoglobin and potential urinary degradation of myoglobin would be helpful. Studies of plasma concentration curves following intravenous injection of tracer amounts of radiolabeled sperm whale myoglobin in four normal individuals illustrated this point. Only a small percentage of the injected myoglobin was recovered in the urine.

Eight of the 19 CCU patients presenting with chest pain thought clinically to be cardiac in origin but showing no subsequent evidence of acute infarction showed mild elevations of serum myoglobin. Peak values ranged from 102 to 180 and averaged 162 ± 52 ng/ml. These patients showed no subsequent enzymatic or electrocardiographic evidence of infarction, suggesting that a more detailed examination of this patient subset is warranted. It is certainly possible that these elevations represented a small amount of myocardial necrosis not apparent by the criteria employed (which did not include myocardial scans or MB-CPK by radioimmunoassay). There were no clinical events to suggest that the elevations were related to skeletal muscle damage, and none of the group had laboratory evidence of renal insufficiency. The conclusion of this group of investigators was that further experience with CCU patients with cardiac chest pain and normal conventional studies for myocardial necrosis seems needed before specific conclusions are drawn.

Comment

Kaiser et al.[147] in 1979 and later in a letter to JAMA of March 26, 1982, offer their experience with this technique and state that the radioimmunological methods should be used in the measurement of serum myoglobin levels. With these assays, in healthy subjects, even below normal levels of serum myoglobin may be detected. They further suppose that the negative results obtained by other investigators were due to the insensitivity of their method or to technical problems in their assay system.

It is obvious that there is a fundamental difference of opinion based on their personal experience with this technique of radioimmunoassay. Further experience by others is of course warranted in order to ascertain whether these methods for myoglobinuria and myoglobinemia offer any specific and helpful values in the diagnosis of myocardial infarction.

Myoglobinemia and Reperfusion in Myocardial Infarction

Drexel and Dinstl[60] have recently shown that a pattern of myoglobinemia suggestive of a stepwise release of myoglobin from ischemic myocardium exists in all cases. In a study of spontaneous reperfusion in myocardial infarction, Ong et al.[208,209]

found that early CPK-MB peak was present. On the other hand, Drexel and Dinstl have shown that if an early peak of CPK-MB indicates reperfusion, prolonged drops between the myoglobin peaks are equally suggestive of reperfusion. In their studies, these investigators have shown that the peaks in their myoglobin curves occur at times when creatine kinase MB curve increases evenly. Other workers have demonstrated multiple peaks of myoglobin with consecutive flat creatine kinase peaks about 10 hours later (Kagen et al., 1977[146] and Sylven, 1979[281a]). Analysis of the above data underlies the critical role of reperfusion in myocardial infarction. (*Note:* while they do not mention the free-radicals of the superoxide oxygen, it sounds quite appropriate to mention here that these investigators were dealing in the reperfusion phase with this type of superimposed lesion of the myocardium.)

Ong et al.[208,209] feel that myoglobin is more rapidly cleared from the serum than is creatine kinase MB. Therefore, the recurrent elevation of serum myoglobin would suggest either episodic release after a single initial insult, recurrent ischemic events, or a combination of both. (*Note:* interpretation by Ong seems to be in the direction of superoxide free-radicals causing these recurrent ischemic events.)

In a related study, Sederholm and Sylven[261] have analyzed serum time activity curves for myoglobin and changes in the ST and QRS vectors for 18 consecutive patients with acute myocardial infarction who were admitted within 4 hours of the onset of pain. They found that myoglobin release was completed within 16 hours average after onset of symptoms and that the QRS vector changes were completed after 14 hours, and the ST vector decline ceased after 11 hours. They found that stepwise release of myoglobin and changes in ST and QRS vectors were often related. Additional events are often simultaneously reflected in these independent markers of myocardial ischemia and necrosis.

Ischemic Contracture of the Left Ventricle

Under certain biometabolic conditions, not necessarily including myoglobin, the myocardium may respond in a similar fashion to the skeletal muscles. One of these responses is the ischemic contracture of the left ventricle. This condition has been reported in patients and also reproduced experimentally. The condition is called "stone heart" or "myocardial rigor mortis." Cooley and associates[47b] have reported this condition as a rare complication of cardiac surgery, occurring in only 13 (0.3%) of 732 patients who had undergone a variety of open-heart procedures. However, its significance resides with the fact that it accounted for over 25% of the operative deaths from acute myocardial failure.

The pathogenesis of myocardial rigor has been attributed to a derangement of the usual spatial relationship between the actin and myosin myofilaments because of low concentrations of ATP. Investigations by Cooley et al.[47b] and later by Lie and Sun[168] indicate that the ultrastructure of tissue in "stone heart" reflects a state of global anoxia.[168] Anaerobic glycolysis is grossly inadequate compared to oxidative phosphorylation. Added to this is the overload of hypertrophied hearts which are more susceptible to the development of the ischemic contracture because they have been functioning precariously with severely depleted sources of high energy phosphate compounds. Muscle tension develops when the concentration of magnesium-ATP falls below a critical level independent of the presence or absence of calcium ions.

The metabolic response of ischemia of any individual heart, normal or diseased, varied considerably. Clinically, "stone heart" has been observed to occur after 22 to 110 minutes of ischemia. Experimentally, myocardial rigor can be produced after 38 to 70 minutes of ischemia. It is possible that this condition might be causally related to the release of endogenous catecholamines. The therapeutic protection afforded by propranolol, a beta-adrenergic receptor blocker, in both clinical and experimental situations, lends support to the theory that catecholamines may play a rôle in the pathogenesis of "stone heart" (Cooley et al.,[47b] Lie and Sun[168]).

The "stone heart" or "rigor mortis heart" offers a number of analogies to the skeletal muscle ischemic contracture observed in the lower extremity, particularly that of the calf. The pathogenesis of the latter is not unlike the one invoked in the production of the "stone heart." After all, these muscles obey the same biochemical responses under ischemic conditions.

23

Arterial Cannulation During Cardiopulmonary Bypass

Introduction

Cannulation of a common femoral artery for extracorporeal circulation may result in metabolic acidosis usually due to prolonged ischemia of the lower extremity. Its development and biological significance have been noted by a number of researchers. Horsley and Nelson[129] reported in 19 patients the metabolic acidosis emerging from the ischemically cannulated limb as mild, which did not affect the systemic blood adversely. Extended periods of cannulation, however, have been shown to result in severe metabolic acidosis.

While awareness of these metabolic changes has been instrumental in preventing any lasting ill effects, by promptly instituting the necessary measures, the possibility of myoglobinemia and myoglobinuria after open-heart surgery has been largely unreported. Rowland et al.[243] described a case of fatal myoglobinuria in a 25-year-old man who underwent open-heart surgery for aortic valve replacement, in whom the right external iliac artery was used for the cardiopulmonary bypass.

This complication of open-heart surgery was due primarily to the prolonged femoral artery cannulation. Since 1974, the cannulation site for the bypass has used the aorta instead of the femoral site which has been largely abandoned. As will be mentioned later, there are a few problems regarding the site of the aorta for its cannulation, necessitating therefore occasional use of a peripheral site for the bypass. However, in 1964, when Rowland reported his case, femoral artery cannulation was being used.

Case Reports

Following is a summary of the case as reported in his paper:

> A 25-year-old man had evidence of aortic insufficiency, both clinically and by cardiac catheterization. This was thought to be due to rheumatic heart disease, although there was no history of acute rheumatic fever. At age 21, a serological test for syphilis was positive, and he had been treated sporadically with penicillin; in 1963 there was still serological evidence of syphilis, and a Treponema mobilization test was positive. Surgery was offered because of angina pectoris.
>
> On October 17, 1963, open-heart surgery was performed for aortic valve replacement. Attempts at percutaneous puncture of the right common femoral artery for monitoring arterial blood pressure were unsuccessful, but there was no evidence of local hematoma. The right external iliac artery was exposed and cannulated in the usual manner for arterial perfusion. Cardiopulmonary bypass lasted 3½ hours. Moderate hypothermia (27°C or 80.6°F) was induced for approximately 1¾ hours. Flow was maintained at 4–4.8 liters per minute. The lung perfusion was due to a slow return of adequate ventricular function necessitating continuous circula-

tory assistance. The operation was completed at 5:30 p.m., and the patient's condition was thought to be good. Blood electrolytes at that time were good. The tissue removed at operation showed histological evidence of chronic rheumatic valvulitis.

At 7:15 p.m., he was seen to move all extremities except the right leg. The urinary output from 5 to 10 p.m. was 677 ml, but during the next 2 hours the rate dropped to 30 ml per hour. At 11:30 p.m., the entire right leg was swollen, tense, and anesthetic. Urinary output had diminished further, and the urine appeared dark brown. The right femoral pulse was palpable, but no other pulses were felt in either leg. The skin temperature was not overly different on the two sides. He complained of pain in the right thigh. The circumference of the right thigh was 67 cm, the calf 41.5 cm. Corresponding measurements on the left were 61 cm. and 38.5 cm.

After midnight the urinary volume ranged from 5 to 15 ml per hour. On the next day, he complained of pain in the buttocks and numbness of the right leg. The electrocardiogram showed evidence of hyperkalemia, with atrial fibrillation. The serum potassium was 8.0 mEq per liter.

There was no volitional movement of the toes or foot which were rigid and only a flicker of motion was seen at the knee. There was weakness of the hip flexion, the same on the left side whereas distal motion on the left was good. Deep reflexes were not elicited on either side. Vibratory sensation was absent below the lower third of the tibia, some positions were impaired from the knee down, and cutaneous sensation was absent below the knee.

Oliguria and hyperkalemia continued, and the urine remained dark brown despite the administration of glucose, insulin, and polystyrene sulfonate exchange resin (Kayexalate). After 8:00 p.m., urinary excretion virtually ceased and he died at 3:00 a.m. on the second postoperative day. The total urinary output for the last 24 hours was 337 ml. Post-mortem

> examination was not permitted. The urinary pigment was identified as myoglobin by spectrophotometry and starch gel electrophoresis.

While such tragic cases, as a result of a major artery cannulation for cardiopulmonary bypass, are presumably uncommon or even very rare, the possibility of ischemia of the lower extremity resulting in myoglobinuria should be borne in mind. Systematic search for myoglobinuria after cardiac surgery, especially in prolonged procedures, may help detect more instances than is presently suspected.

Kagen reported six cases with myoglobinuria in a group of 16 patients after open-heart surgery for valvular replacement.[144] The patients who did not develop a renal problem had considerably shorter procedures than those with myoglbinuria. Only one of the six patients with myoglobinuria died in the immediate post-surgical period of renal failure and progressive jaundice. The incidence of myoglobinuria in this group of patients is closely related to the total surgical time including that of the period of the pump for cardiac bypass. The source of the myoglobin in these patients is likely to originate partly from the myocardium as a result of its surgical trauma and, mostly, from lower extremity skeletal muscle ischemia due to prolonged pump perfusion.

A few other cases of open-heart surgery in which cannulation of the femoral artery was used for the bypass were reported in two patients by Herman et al.[125] in 1966 and in 4 patients by Fisher et al.[77] in 1970. Herman's cases resulted in anterior tibial compartment syndrome, while those reported by Fisher developed metabolic complications of mild to moderate severity which were treated successfully by appropriate medical management.

While femoral cannulation for cardiopulmonary bypass is used less often or rarely, as mentioned above, the incidence of femoral occlusion has increased, however, with the use of intubation of this vessel for intra-aortic balloon pumping (IABP) (Alpert et al.,[3a] Lefemine et al.[164a])

The following report by a group of Japanese cardiac surgeons was presented by Kugimiya[159] in 1979 at the 14th World Congress of the International Cardiovascular Society, and since published in 1983. Cardiopulmonary bypass in this series in which femoral artery cannulation was used, was carried out in 420 patients. Massive ischemic myopathy with myoglobinuria occurred in eight patients, or in 1.9% of the cases.

A review of one case will illustrate this complication. This concerned a 15-year old male who underwent patch closure of the ventricular septum defect, and an infundibulectomy with cardiopulmonary bypass. The complete cardiopulmonary bypass time was 2 hours and 8 minutes and the left femoral artery occlusion time was 4 hours and 21 minutes, and was cannulated for arterial perfusion. Moderate hypothermia, in addition to the cannulation and cardiopulmonary bypass, was induced during the bypass. During the early postoperative period, the general condition of the patient was good. But as soon as he awoke from anesthesia, he complained of tenderness and pain in the left lower extremity. There was marked swelling and rigidity in the left thigh and leg. The urine appeared to be dark red, and urinary output decreased during 10 hours after the operation. Fasciotomies of the anterior and posterior compartments of the calf were performed 2 hours after operation and peritoneal dialysis was begun on the second postoperative day.

The urine remained dark red in the early postoperative period. Although the urine appeared almost clear within 7 days, urinary myoglobin was positive for more than 3 weeks. A sample of calf muscle in the fasciotomy wound indicated necrotic muscle removed from that area on the 30th postoperative day. A specimen of muscle biopsy obtained about 20 hours after the operation showed severe interstitial edema, but the normal structure of the muscle cell was preserved (Figure 23-1). Another specimen obtained by a calf muscle biopsy performed on the 30th postoperative day showed thrombosed vessels in the left part which was typical of the findings of coagulation necrosis of muscle due to ischemia. The other laboratory data indicated, as already mentioned, myoglobinuria which appeared immediately after operation and continued for more than 3 weeks. Peritoneal dialysis begun on the second postoperative day was continued for 20 days. Marked oliguria improved within 2 weeks, but increase of blood urea nitrogen (BUN) lasted for more than 30 days. Serum potassium level rapidly elevated with progress of oliguria, but it soon returned to normal value following the use of peritoneal dialysis.

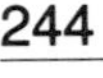

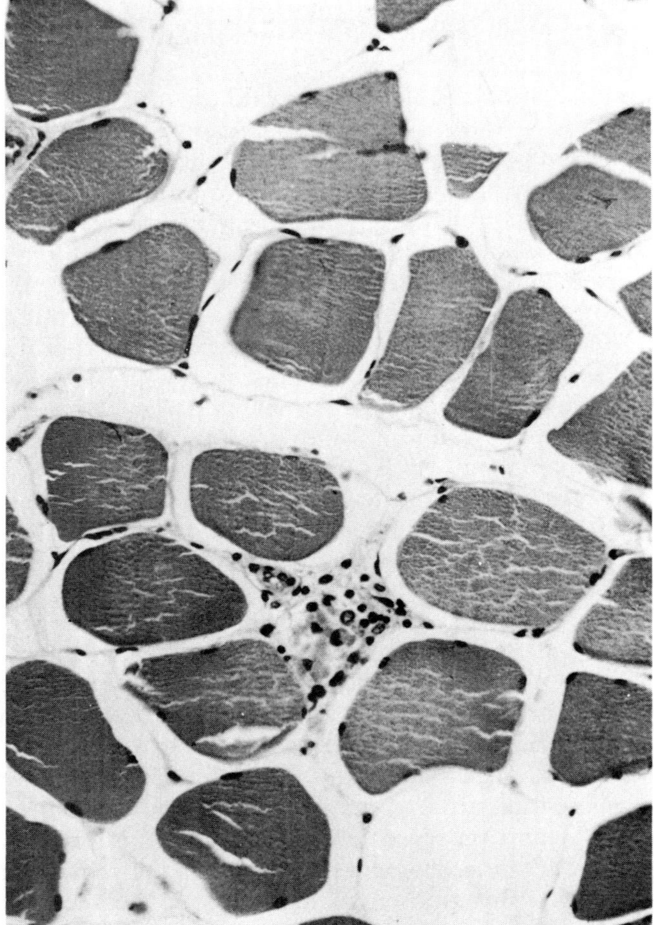

Figure 23-1: This specimen was obtained by muscle biopsy from the fasciotomy wound about 20 hours after operation. The section of muscle stained by hematoxylin-eosin reveals a severe interstitial edema, but the normal structure of muscle cells is preserved. (From Kujimiya,[159] with permission.)

SGOT and LDH serum level decreased but persisted a little longer than the former. With intensive general and local management, the patient improved gradually and was discharged without sequelae 4 months after the operation.

Conclusion

Experience with these eight cases has shown several important features. Seven out of eight cases were male, with an average age of 10 years ranging from 4 to 17. All of the patients had congenital heart disease. Cardiopulmonary bypass time ranged from 52 minutes to 2 hours and 42 minutes. For pump priming, Ringer's lactate without any colloidal solution was used in five patients and Ringer's lactate with a small amount of low molecular weight dextran was used in three patients. The femoral artery occlusion time lasted at least 3 hours. Usually, they were prolonged due to low output syndrome or other complications. Besides complications due to ischemic myopathy and myoglobinuria, renal failure appeared in three patients and two of them required peritoneal dialysis. Severe respiratory failure occurred in two patients and in one of them it was followed by ventricular fibrillation. One of these eight patients died of infection and respiratory failure 3 months after operation.

The authors emphasized the following distinctive features observed in these cases:

1. The femoral artery occlusion time exceeded 3 hours without exception.
2. It occurred in predominantly younger age groups and the majority of them were male.
3. The pump priming fluid for hemodilution contained nothing of colloidal solution.

The authors are not ready to state what the predisposing factors were for this complication. However, after several attempts, the use of hypothermia was used prophylactically, apparently quite successfully in preventing the occurrence of the ischemic myopathy with myoglobinuria. After various attempts for the prevention of this complication, they found the most effective limb protection was a local cooling of the entire cannulated limb. The cooling was about 20° centigrade and was achieved by a special cooling blanket. The experience accumulated with this procedure extended from 1967 to 1974.

Since the last date (July 1974), this group of surgeons performed 444 cases of cardiopulmonary bypass with femoral artery cannulation, but using local cooling applied in all cases. Kugimiya points out, however, that in the recent 100 cases, femoral artery cannulation was used in 27%, while in the remaining 73%, aortic cannulation was the preferred site. The problems contraindicating the aortic site were the small size of the aorta and unacceptable pathological changes of the aortic wall.

The risk factors, as reported by Kugimiya, involved in the cardiac cases with femoral artery cannulation, are: (1) pediatric-adolescent patients; (2) prolonged femoral artery occlusion under low blood pressure (for more than 3 hours); and (3) low colloid osmotic pressure during cardiopulmonary bypass (excessive hemodilution with noncolloidal fluid).

Such complications as reported in this chapter are encountered much more rarely, due to awareness of them and much better handling of the ischemic metabolites.

However, certain reports in the literature dealing with similar technical problems raise serious questions about the validity of the diagnosis and management. Thus, it is known that a number of renal complications occur as a result of these operations. Whether a renal dysfunction following cardiac surgical procedures is due to myoglobinuria in these cases remains a problem open to question in the absence of specific biochemical documentation. One may only speculate on the possible contribution of myoglobinuria to a number of renal complications reported in connection with open-heart surgery. Abel et al.,[1] in reviewing 507 surviving patients from open-heart operations, found that 198 patients or 39% had developed serious renal complications, some with acute tubular necrosis with a mortality rate of 30.3% in this group. Except for BUN and serum creatinine, no other biochemical determinations, especially myoglobin, were mentioned. Awareness of this muscle metabolite which may cause some cases of renal failures in open-heart surgery may help its prevention if treated vigorously in the time before irreversible damage occurs (for details see Chapter 14).

III

Unusual Metabolic Complications

24

Metabolic Complications of Intra-Arterial Use of Streptokinase

Intra-Arterial Use of Streptokinase

Introduction

It is generally accepted that at low doses intra-arterial streptokinase for managing thromboembolic occlusions either of native arteries or grafts is a relatively safe, acceptable method for dealing with recent thrombi. However, some complications may always result from use of thrombolytic agents in certain cases. A review of a few recent typical reports will illustrate the various chemical aspects of this therapy.

Mori et al.[196] reported their experience with selective intra-arterial infusion in 50 arteries in 45 patients. The most common regimen was 5,000 units of SK/hour for 24 to 48 hours with a simultaneous heparin infusion of 250 to 500 units/hour. Significant lysis occurred in 80% of cases. There were minor (30%) and major hemorrhages (8%), the latter requiring blood transfusions. Among other serious complications were 8% of tissue damage consisting of two with limb necrosis and two with compartment syndromes. One of these died of disease progression with leg amputation and acute renal tubular necrosis. These authors concluded that this method of selective low-dose SK infusion provides a moderate gain in benefit-risk ratio over systemic infusion.

Cohen et al.[41] reported the use of intraoperative streptokinase injected directly into the arterial tree following balloon-catheter embolectomy on 13 occasions in 12 patients. The purpose was to remove residual thrombus that could not be mechanically retrieved in patients with imminent limb (10 patients) or kidney (two patients) necrosis. Effective lysis was achieved in 11 of 13 trials (85%). There were five deaths, one related to therapy, and six limbs were salvaged. The average total dose of SK used, 110,000 units, was given in intermittent boluses of 25,000 to 50,000 units. While initially the arterial patency was excellent, the ultimate results, as stated above, were five deaths and seven limbs not salvageable. There is no mention of any metabolic complications related to muscle ischemia, although a number (at least 50%) of limbs were severely affected.

In connection with the use of thrombolytic agents, it is also useful to mention an example of limited experience reported with urokinase. Thus, McNamara and Fischer treated 93 thromboembolic occlusions of peripheral arteries or grafts in 85 patients with high-dose urokinase. Of these, 75 (81%) resulted in clinical improvement. However, they stated that "in an effort to minimize serious complications," they emphasize that only patients with severe ischemia developed compartment syndromes, respiratory distress syndromes, and acute renal tubular necrosis in spite of successful thrombolysis. Other systemic complications were also noted (hyperkalemia, lactic acidosis, congestive heart failure, disseminated intravascular coagulation). While this method is effective, it is not without serious complications.

Lang[160] reported a frequency of complications which is quite unusual. Among others, he presented "an inordinately high rate of renal complications encountered among 35 patients treated for thrombotic or thromboembolic occlusions of the leg by injection of streptokinase into a bypass graft or a native artery."

What follows is a summary by the author. Five patients demonstrated massive myoglobinuria following restoration of flow to ischemic and necrotic tissues; acute tubular necrosis developed in two of them, and one patient died as a result of renal shutdown, electrolyte imbalance, hypofibrinogemia, and mediastinal and retroperitoneal hemorrhage. Massive myoglobinuria was also noted in five out of 13 patients with compartment syndrome but there was no evidence of ischemic necrosis. This complication could be lessened by fasciotomy and resection of the upper third of the fibula. Although myoglobinuria and complications such as acute tubular necrosis are only rarely reported, they are not unexpected following muscular ischemia. Lang concluded that attempts to salvage irreparably damaged tissues by reestablishing circulation appear to carry an unacceptably high risk of renal complications and may even threaten the life of the patient.

Principles

Because of the unusual complications reported in this paper,[160] it is essential that the method used in the delivery of streptokinase into the arterial tree be described in more detail. Low-dose intra-arterial streptokinase therapy was carried out in 86 patients with thrombotic or thromboembolic arterial occlusion. The study group included 71 men and 15 women ranging from 38 to 77 years of age. Streptokinase was injected into the primary artery in 37 patients, a prosthetic aortorenal graft in four, an occluded renal artery (transplanted from a cadaver) in one, a bovine graft in nine, and an occluded prosthetic bypass graft or native artery of the leg in 35 patients. These were selected in compliance with generally accepted criteria, i.e., tolerance of ischemia, no operative procedure within the last 10 days, no history of an ulcer, cerebral infarct, or other potential bleeding site, and no history of prior treatment with streptokinase (and hence a lack of antibodies to it). Despite inclusion of tolerance of ischemia as criterion for selection, streptokinase therapy was instituted in 18 patients who were facing amputation, usually with the hope of limiting the amputation to below the knee.

Technique

A 5F catheter having both end and side holes within the last 5 cm is advanced through the artery and its tip embedded in the clot. Streptokinase is perfused at the rate of 5,000 U/hr, usually delivered by an arterial pump in 20 to 50 ml of carrier solution. Next, 200 to 1,000 U/hr of heparin is added, titrating the solution to maintain partial thromboplastin time (PTT) at 1½ to 2 times normal. When the clot begins to dissolve, the catheter is advanced farther distally and reembedded in the clot, repeating the procedure until flow throughout the occluded segment has been restored. If PTT rises above 3 times normal because of excessive depletion of fibrinogen, cryoprecipitates are administered intravenously until hypofibrinogenemia is corrected to at least 50% of normal levels. Streptokinase is continued until the entire clot is lysed or for at least 72 hours, whichever occurs first. Therapy is terminated if there are no tangible results within 72 hours or if necessitated by complications. Fractional heparinization is continued for 5 days after successful thrombolysis or until surgical intervention, in order to maintain a PTT of 1½ times normal.

Complications

Hemorrhage

Bleeding from the catheter entry site occurred in seven patients (20%). In one patient, this happened after only one day of streptokinase therapy and was coupled with hypofibrinogenemia and a PTT 3 times normal, necessitating discontinuation of streptokinase and institution of intravenous cryoprecipitates. In another patient who was being treated for thromboembolic occlusion of the native femoral artery and resultant ischemic necrosis of the forefoot, streptokinase was perfused for 54 hours and massive mediastinal and retroperitoneal hemorrhage developed 5 days later. He died of renal shutdown, electrolyte imbalance, and massive bleeding.

Distal Emboli

Distal emboli were observed in one patient on the same day that thrombolysis was successfully completed.

Myoglobinuria

Significant myoglobinuria was observed as already mentioned in 10 patients, using agar gel electrophoresis. Among the 17 patients with no evidence of ischemic necrosis or compartment syndrome, three had only trace myoglobinuria, which in one case was present prior to streptokinase therapy.

Out of 13 patients with compartment syndrome but no evidence of ischemic necrosis, massive myoglobinuria developed in five on the same day as thrombolysis. In two of them who had undergone fasciotomy, it cleared several days later; trace myoglobinuria had been present prior to streptokinase therapy in one of them and developed at the time of thrombolysis in the other. Of the other three patients who had had no fasciotomy, one later demonstrated acute tubular necrosis and two continued to have massive myoglobinuria for 5 days despite management with intravenous fluids and furosemide. Of the five patients with both ischemic necrosis and compartment syndrome, two had trace myoglobinuria and three had 1+ myoglobinuria prior to institution of streptokinase therapy.

Comment by Dr. Lang[160]

"While previous articles have noted the frequency of hemorrhagic complications following low-dose intra-arterial streptokinase therapy, there has been little mention of complications arising from renewed perfusion of ischemic muscle. Generally referred to as the 'crush syndrome,' shock, myoglobinuria, oliguria, hyperkalemia, and irregular heartbeat are the characteristic expressions of this condition. While tolerance of ischemia is advocated as a prerequisite for streptokinase therapy, I was tempted to also employ it to improve limb salvage in patients who would otherwise require amputation. My experience, involving 35 patients with thromboembolic occlusion of the leg causing variable ischemic compromise, substantiates the usefulness of streptokinase therapy but also reveals a number of limitations. Following renewed perfusion, the volume of the previously ischemic tissue increases, which can lead to compartment syndrome in the leg in particular. Unless the muscle is properly decompressed by fasciotomy (and fibulectomy if the deep and lateral compartments are affected), perfusion may be compromised further and result in myoglobinuria. These suppositions are supported by the observation that significant myoglobinuria did not occur in the 17 patients who had neither ischemic necrosis nor compartment syndrome, whereas it was present in 10 out of 18 patients with compartment syndrome. The efficacy of fasciotomy is supported by the fact that significant myoglobinuria developed in two out of eight treated with fasciotomy, compared to three out of five who were not. Myoglobinuria was either noted for the first time or intensified after circulation to ischemic tissue had been reestablished. Adverse effects such as acute tubular necrosis became manifest after myoglobinuria intensified. When severe temporary ischemia caused by compartment syndrome resulted in damage to the muscle, fasciotomy and fibulectomy normalized perfusion and myoglobinuria subsided after several days. However, if necrotic tissue was involved, it had to be removed surgically. In fact, reestablishment of perfusion to areas laden with necrotic material caused severe aggravation of myoglobinuria and led to acute tubular necrosis. Salvage of irreparably damaged tissue by means of reestablishing circulation and perhaps converting an 'above the knee' to a 'below the knee' amputation entails an unacceptable risk of ensuing renal complications as well as a possible threat to the life of the patient."

Discussion

The report presented by Lang appears to be unique among the papers which described the use of streptokinase in the management of acute thrombosis either of a native artery or a graft. The description by Lang indicates that he was fully conversant with the problems of acute complications and especially with the effects of myoglobinuria upon the kidney. There is no doubt that the descriptions were entirely consistent with the knowledge of the problem of acute arterial ischemic complications. This is in contrast to several of the papers on streptokinase about lysis of acute occlusion of the arteries, in which there appeared to be failure to note similar complications. On the other hand, Lang's cases may have been just an unusual group of patients, although it seems that Lang's methods and the selection of the patients were completely in keeping with the established procedures.

Other surgeons have reported intraoperative streptokinase as an adjunct to mechanical thrombectomy in the management of acute ischemia. Their results appeared to be effective in clearing the thrombus not amenable to mechanical extraction, thus leading to improved patency and tissue salvage. But as already pointed out in this report, there was no mention of complications similar to those reported by Lang.

In 1983, Bergman et al. described their experience successfully treating chronic external iliac arterial occlusion with local low-dose streptokinase infusion directly into the thrombus. This technique may provide an effective method of treating chronic thromboses and may be applied to patients previously thought unsuitable for fibrinolytic therapy.

The treatment of acute intra-arterial thrombosis with systemic streptokinase may be effective, although one must keep in mind the potential complications of bleeding associated with high-dose intra-arterial or intravenous infusions of streptokinase which make such therapy hazardous or plainly dangerous. This opinion was shared for quite a long time by others. However, more recently, by contrast to the intra-arterial injections, a number of reports indicate that successful systemic streptokinase therapy in both acute and chronic arterial occlusion may be successful and entail fewer hazards.

25

Malignant Hyperpyrexia

Introduction

Malignant hyperpyrexia is a rare condition but one that produces considerable problems for anesthetists. Apparently healthy individuals undergoing routine surgery can develop an alarming and often fatal hyperpyrexia which was described in Australia in the 1960s. Typically, after anesthesia is induced, muscle stiffness is noted in the patient accompanied by a rapid rise in body temperature, increase in plasma potassium and lactate, and subsequent cardiac failure. Myoglobinuria and renal damage are accompanying problems. If these signs are not recognized early during anesthesia and treatment is not begun promptly, the prognosis is poor, death resulting in about 50% of the cases. It is now clearly established that the participating factors are the use of halothane as an anesthetic agent and/or the use of suxamethonium as a muscle relaxant.

Genetic Inheritance

The condition is inherited as an autosomal dominant trait, i.e., it appears in at least three successive generations, is exhibited by about half of the members of an affected family, afflicts both males and females but mostly the former, and is directly transmitted from father to son. In a few cases, malignant hyperpyrexia may be acquired from such nonhereditary muscle diseases as polymyositis or electrolyte abnormalities such as hypomagnesemia or hypercalcemia.

The condition is most common in children, adolescents, and young adults. A certain muscle bulk is necessary before a crisis can be triggered. In old age, declining muscle mass may account for the reduced frequency of episodes. Also, crises seem more apt to occur if the muscle has been recently damaged by vigorous exercise, trauma, or infection.

Although apparently heathy and athletic by nature, susceptible individuals have muscles that when examined on biopsy frequently have a number of abnormal features, most noticeably internal nuclei, small angular fibers, target fibers, and "moth-eaten" fibers. With electron microscopic examination, areas of sarcomere disruption and Z-band streaming can be seen.

The diagnosis of susceptible individuals can be made with reasonable confidence by use of an *in vitro* muscle preparation, which, when compared with normal human muscle, shows a greater propensity to contracture in the presence of caffeine. An alternative diagnostic technique may be to measure the proportion of the active form of phosphorylase in muscle. Willner et al.[297] have shown this to be considerably raised in muscle from susceptible subjects.

Blood Biochemistry Findings

About two-thirds of these individuals, and some of their relatives, exhibit moderate serum elevation of enzymes normally confined to skeletal muscle.

Creatine phosphokinase (CPK) shows the greatest and most consistent rise. This is probably because most of this enzyme is normally located in the skeletal muscle, while large amounts of other enzymes such as SGOT, lactic dehydrogenase (LDH), and aldolase are also found in tissues such as lung, liver, and kidney. Although the rates of elevation of these biochemical factors vary individually or from family to family, in some, however, the elevations are slight and in others are quite high. However, CPK remains the most typical factor for which it is important to screen the individual as a useful diagnostic tool.

Other Diagnostic Findings

Electromyography abnormalities can be detected in many patients, particularly in those who have muscle rigidity. EMG abnormalities, however, while suggestive of this condition, are not diagnostic, since they are also seen in other myopathies.

Muscle biopsy studies present a most accurate method for diagnosing malignant hyperpyrexia according to a number of investigators. The specimen should be obtained from the vastus lateralis or vastus medialis muscles.

Histogram analysis of ATPase stains shows that in some patients the mitochondrial-rich type I fibers have more variability in diameter than do the sarcoplasmic reticulum-rich type II fibers.

The major biochemical defect in the muscle of malignant hyperpyrexia patients appears to be in the control of intracellular calcium and the mechanisms involved in the control of excitation-contraction coupling. Other reported changes already mentioned are found in mitochondria and the sarcoplasmic reticulum which are probably of secondary nature.

Radioactive calcium uptake into isolated sarcoplasmic reticulum (SR) may be measured both in the absence and in the presence of halothane. Without halothane, hyperthermic SR is even more inhibited. On the other hand, halothane moderately accelerates calcium uptake into the normal SR. This latter effect is more pronounced at low doses of halothane (0.5% to 2.0%), than at high concentrations (5.0%). This study supports the view that the calcium-storing membranes of these malignant hyperpyrexia muscle patients are less able to accumulate calcium than are those of normal muscle and that halothane exacerbates this effect.

Calcium is central to the cell's energy-producing processes. The key to elucidating its role in malignant hyperpyrexia has come from understanding its role in normal muscle cells. In the latter, calcium is released from its storage site, the sarcoplasmic reticulum, in response to a signal from a neuron. As calcium concentrations increase, the catalytic enzyme, phosphorylase, goes into action, mediating the breakdown of glycogen into lactic acid, carbon dioxide, and heat. This provides the energy for cellular activities.

When calcium concentrations rise even higher, another enzyme, myosin ATPase, is activated. It acts on the energy-containing molecule, adenosine triphosphate (ATP) formed from creatine phosphate (CP) and adenosine diphosphate (ADP), breaking one phosphate ion from the molecule and releasing heat and free energy. The energy produced from this reaction activates another enzyme, which in turn promotes the cross-bridge linking of the contractile proteins, actin and myosin. When they link together, muscle fibers contract.

The excess of intracellular calcium forces the cell into a state of hypermetabolism. Stores of oxygen, which is necessary for ATP production are used up faster than they can be replenished. Thus, ATP levels begin to fall and the cell's housekeeping functions decline. Cell membranes become depolarized, and ions such as potassium, magnesium, and phosphate leak into the plasma. They are followed by larger molecules, including myoglobin.

The chemical imbalance which results from the various biochemical interactions mentioned initiate the collapse of the coagulation system.

Dantrolene, the specific drug for combatting malignant hyperpyrexia, as will be discussed later, interrupts this catastrophic chain of events by staunching the flow of calcium from the sarcoplasmic reticulum. To be effective, it must be given before all the calcium has escaped, because it does not promote calcium's reentry into the organelle.

Of interest is a veterinarian experience which creates a condition similar to hyperpyrexia seen in patients. This has been described in Pietrain and Landrace pigs. These animals are particularly sensitive to stress and develop muscle rigidity, acidosis, and hyperkalemia and die of heart failure and stressful conditions. This entity is of considerable economic importance because the meat from such animals tends to go into rapid contracture postmortem, extruding water and leaving a pale and unattractive product. Like humans, susceptible pigs are sensitive to halothane and depolarizing muscle relaxants. In pigs, however, stress plays a much greater part in precipitating attacks. Although stress may sensitize susceptible human subjects, it is not the primary precipitating factor. Nonetheless, the muscle abnormalities of pigs and humans appear to be very similar.

Clinical Manifestations

Malignant hyperpyrexia is a rare disease and occurs only once in every 40,000 adult and 15,000 pediatric surgery cases. It has been recognized only since 1960, and was not incorporated in the International Classification of Diseases until 1983. Thus, while many anesthesiology residents can give a textbook recitation of the symptoms of malignant hyperpyrexia, most anesthesiologists don't expect to see them. But they should be looking for the earliest possible sign—an increase in the end-tidal carbon dioxide. Those who lack the equipment to monitor the exhaled gas should be on the alert for unexplained tachycardia, and an increase in core temperature, however subtle. Because temperature usually falls during anesthesia, any reversal can signal the onset of malignant hyperpyrexia. At this kind of a sign, the operation should be discontinued together with the halothane anesthesia, and the rubber tubing on the anesthesia machine should be changed and the patient should be hyperventilated with 100% oxygen. These procedures should be followed by the intravenous administration of 1 to 2 mEq/kg sodium bicarbonate and 2.5 mg/kg dantrolene sodium. Finally, they should use cold solutions in almost any way they can to lower the patient's temperature on the body surface, intravenously, intragastrically, intrarectally, and in the wound itself. They should also begin intravenous insulin and glucose to treat hyperkalemia.

The crisis is not over when the stabilized patient leaves the operating room. In severe cases, malignant hyperpyrexia can flare up again hours later. Thus, the patient's temperature, electrolytes, urine output, and electrocardiograph readings should be monitored in the intensive care unit for at least 24 hours. Oral dantrolene at 4 mg/kg per day is usually effective in averting recurrent episodes. In addition to the above measures, one should make sure that urine myoglobin and renal complications are looked for and treated accordingly.

The management of susceptible patients requires careful monitoring of body temperature and the avoidance of known precipitating agents and stress. If hyperpyrexic attack develops, intravenous dantrolene should be administered and strenuous efforts made to limit the rise in body temperature, plasma lactate, and potassium concentrations.

26

Role of Free-Radicals in Post-Ischemic Skeletal Muscle Reperfusion Injury

Introduction

It is clear from the foregoing chapters that the metabolic syndrome secondary to acute arterial occlusions is primarily related to the ischemic consequences of the skeletal muscles. This syndrome is essentially characterized by biochemical elements emerging from the acute ischemic rhabdomyolysis. They are released from the muscular fibers via their transmembranes. Release of metabolites is due to morphological alterations of the latter that lead first to its increased permeability and subsequently to metabolic changes and tissue necrosis. This, in essence, is the sequence of events of the initial metabolic manifestations.

Recently, in addition to the initial sarcolemmal membrane-dependent biochemical factors, it has been shown that a second phase of metabolic changes takes place. They occur during reperfusion of post-ischemic tissues due to biochemical parameters of oxygen-derived free-radicals, the latter being then incriminated for further inducing damage of the originally ischemic tissues.

While the latter phase is still currently being investigated, it is nevertheless thus far clear that it is a secondary phenomenon derived from the ischemic skeletal muscle.

It appears, therefore, that the overall biochemical events characterizing the metabolic syndrome due to acute arterial occlusions may be classified into two phases:

1. The *initiating ischemia* of the skeletal muscle, or rhabdomyolytic phase, and
2. The *free-radicals-induced ischemia* or the *reperfusion* phase, resulting in additional superimposed necrosis.

Biological Background

In the past few years, a large body of evidence has been accumulated, mostly in connection with ischemically induced myocardium, resulting either by primary occlusion of the coronary arteries or secondarily during coronary bypass surgery. In the latter instance, due to total or global ischemia, which is part of the vascular procedure itself, a different set of biochemical parameters occurs producing additional injury to the original ischemic lesion. This reperfusion syndrome phase appears to be essentially caused by oxygen-derived free-radicals.

It has become increasingly clear that during reflow or reperfusion into a region of a hypoxic or ischemic myocardium or skeletal muscle, one may observe a paradoxical result consisting of marked increase of ischemic damage. This phenomenon led to the evaluation of the mechanism of increasing myocardial cell resistance to the changes that occur during early reoxygenation or reperfusion. It has been shown that oxygen free-radicals exert a cytotoxic effect through lipid peroxidation of cell membranes resulting in subcellular and cellular disruption, all of which are a result of protracted regional or global ischemia of the myocardium. The involvement of cell membranes of the myocardium through the cytotoxic effects appears to be engendered by lipid peroxidation. By analogy, a similar mechanism appears to occur in the skeletal muscle cell membranes. Therapeutically, it has been shown that scavengers in the presence of free-radicals in the ischemic myocardium or, more importantly, at onset of post-ischemic reperfusion, may block the conversion of molecular oxygen to these toxic species and reduce the membrane damage that results from these radicals (Figure 26-1).

Skeletal Muscle Free-Radicals

In contrast to the increasing number of free-radicals studies in relation to coronary occlusion and myocardial ischemia, minor interest was shown relating to the role of oxygen-derived free-radicals in ischemia of skeletal muscle, experimentally or clinically. Unlike the heart and brain, where the results of ischemia are often immediate and catastrophic, the arterial deprivation of skeletal muscle requires a slightly longer period ranging between 1 and 6 or possibly several hours before metabolic changes occur or become apparent. Indeed, with ischemic periods of up to at least 6 hours, these changes become obvious and irreversible. Since the ultimate morphological manifestations observed in the skeletal muscles are somewhat similar to the ischemic changes of the heart, by analogy the latter provides some basis for understanding the mechanisms associated with ischemic injury to skeletal muscle.

A number of experimental studies mentioned earlier (see Chapter 12, *Tourniquet Ischemia: Metabolic Responses*) have shown that blood flow to skeletal muscle obstructed for one-half to several hours may result in edema formation after release of the occlusion. The reflow or reperfusion after occlusion of less than 3 hours leads to a small increase in fluid efflux that results from increased capillary pressure and microvascular surface area. Longer periods of ischemia may lead to a more pronounced edema formation primarily due to changes in vascular permeability. The greater increase in edema is proportional to the damage of the microvascular system as a result of reoxygenation of the ischemic tissues. Several factors have been incriminated in the mechanism of this increased permeability, one of which was histamine. Recently, the role of oxygen-derived free-radicals was added to and superseded that of histamine, both of which are considered the most probable mediators of ischemia by induced increases in permeability.

Such effects have been observed in the myocardium and brain following reconstructive arterial surgery, and by analogy their mechanism may be conceivably found in other similar areas, such as in acute arterial occlusions of the lower extremities.

Thus, recently these were demonstrated in ischemic-reperfusion injury in skeletal muscle carried out by clinical and experimental investigations. Indeed, Korthuis et al.[155] and Harris et al.[123] have shown that prolonged ischemia followed by reperfusion produces morphological alterations in skeletal muscle similar to those seen after reperfusion of ischemic myocardium, intestine, brain, and kidney. Korthuis et al. have shown in skeletal muscle studies that the role of oxygen-derived free-radicals in the genesis of increased vascular permeability could prevent the production of active oxygen species when subjected to pre-treatment with specific oxygen radical scavengers. These investigators have concluded that the results of their study had suggested that oxygen radicals are produced in ischemic skeletal muscle by a mechanism similar to that proposed in studies for small intestine.

According to their method, ATP is converted to adenosine monophosphate (AMP) during ischemia. The elevated AMP is catabolized by hypoxanthine, a substrate for xanthine oxidase. These particular biochemical conversions have been shown earlier in these various other studies with different organisms such as heart, brain, intestine, etc. Thus, xanthine oxidase which normally exists in the cell as NAD^+-reducing dehydrogenase, is formed by the action of a protease in response to the low oxygen tension produced by ischemia. These investigators noted that most of the damage to skeletal muscle occurred not during the ischemic period, but rather after reoxygenation is restored. As to the mechanism, it appears that there is a large amount of evidence which supports that xanthine oxidase is a source of oxygen radicals in ischemic muscle. The conclusions drawn by other investigators seem to propose that oxygen radical generation may constitute an important mechanism of cell damage in post-ischemic muscle. It is of interest to note that ATP levels do not decrease appreciably during the first 2 to 3 hours of ischemia, although longer periods of ischemia result in a substantial reduction of ATP stores. This observation may account for the fact that ischemia of less than 3 hours in duration does not result in an increase of permeability, but longer periods do. This is because no appreciable catabolism of ATP occurs in these first hours, as a result of which hypoxanthine levels would not be expected to increase significantly.

Harris et al.[123] have also shown that the changes in intramuscular metabolites vary with the duration of ischemia. At 2 hours, minimal ultrastructural damage occurred with complete regeneration of intramuscular phosphagens and glycogen on reperfusion with complete normalization of lipid oxidation products. In contrast, one 7-hour ischemic insult resulted in profound injury at the ultrastructural level with inability to restore intramuscular phosphagens and glycogen on reperfusion. Their results pointed out that there was "prolonged glycolytic activity of skeletal muscle during global ischemia which could be documented by increased production of oxygen free-radical-mediated lipid oxidation products in irreversibly injured muscle."

The decline in ATP levels in skeletal muscle appeared considerably slower than in heart muscle, especially during the first 3 hours of ischemia. Harris et al., based on the above, concluded that there exist several important differences between the reponse of skeletal and heart muscle to ischemia. The relative resistance of skeletal muscle to prolonged ischemic stress compared with that of the heart, as already noted by other investigators, may be due to lower energy demand of ischemic skeletal muscle as compared to that of heart ischemic lesions.

Korthuis et al. similarly state that although the results of their study clearly establish a role for oxygen-derived free-radicals in the genesis of ischemia-induced increases in vascular permeability, the mechanism whereby free-radicals increase permeability still remains uncertain. Another important conclusion from this experimental study relates to the ischemia reperfusion-induced damage to the microvascular membrane which may be related to the fact that oxygen radicals promote granulocyte accumulation and adhesion to the endothelium and subsequent activation (Figure 26-1).

It is of interest that these experimental studies have shown that histamine is not involved in the ischemia increase in vascular permeability, but the involvement of oxygen-derived free-radicals in this response of the muscle is clearly established. This is in part

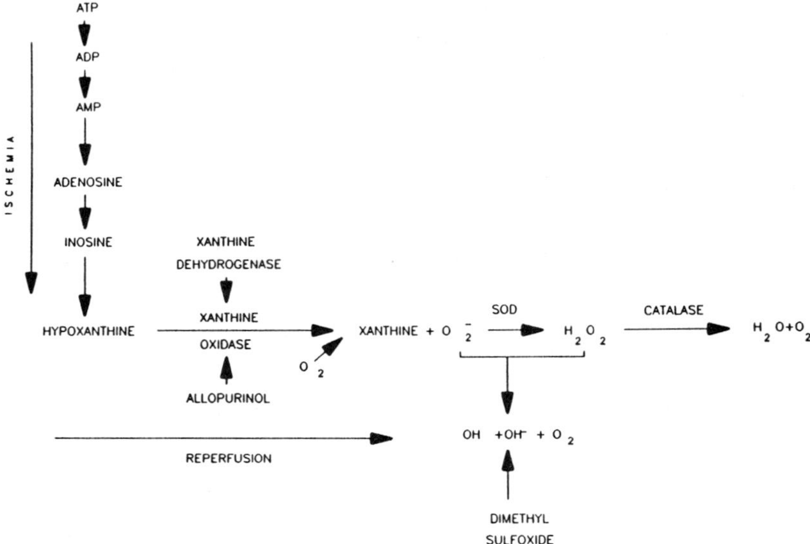

FIGURE 26-1: Biochemical mechanisms of reperfusion of ischemic muscle. This phase of the ischemic skeletal muscle is produced by oxygen radicals as a result of conversion of ATP to ADP followed by adenosine monophosphate (AMP). The elevated AMP is catabolized to hypoxanthine, a substrate for xanthine oxidase. For the production of oxygen radicals, molecular oxygen is required before hypoxanthine and xanthine oxidase can react to form superoxide anion. O_2 represents the hydroxyl radical. Most of the damage to skeletal muscle occurs after reoxygenation is restored, due essentially to *xanthine oxidase* which appears as the source of oxygen radicals in ischemic skeletal muscle. (Figure modified from Korthuis et al.[155])

based not only on the findings of the dynamics of the changes in the skeletal muscle and the vasculature but also by administration of allopurinol, superoxide dismutase, and catalase, all of which reduce ischemic injury to skeletal muscle. This demonstrates the protective effect achieved by pre-treatment with a hydroxyl radical scavenger, a suggestion that this secondary radical is primarily responsible for the injury associated with skeletal muscle ischemia. In addition, as mentioned by other investigators, xanthine oxidase may represent the primary source of oxygen-derived free-radicals in ischemic skeletal muscle.

From a therapeutic aspect, it is extremely important to emphasize that the ischemia followed by reperfusion is significantly reduced by the use of free-radical scavenging agents such as superoxide dismutase, catalase and mannitol. Their use results in significantly better recovery of the left ventricular function following reperfusion. The manner in which oxygen-derived free-radicals may be harmful is related to the possibility that these toxic species are involved in the exacerbation of the ischemic injury that develops upon reflow and reoxygenation as shown in the hearts, brains, kidneys, intestines, and other organs examined. That a similar exacerbation of the injury may occur in the skeletal muscle is very likely, but it has not been extensively used experimentally to substantiate this analogy.

Role of Scavenging Agents

Ischemia induced in skeletal muscle regardless of the cause results in vascular permeability at the microvascular level. The mechanism underlying the increase in permeability is not entirely elucidated. Reperfusion of ischemic skeletal muscle results in a more dramatic increase in microvascular permeability, leading to additional tissue necrosis.

Recent investigation of a few substances, called scavenging agents, have the ability to alter the permeability increase. Of the main agents already noted above, used mostly experimentally, are superoxide dismutase, allopurinol, catalase, and mannitol.*

Morphological alterations in skeletal muscle appear to be similar to those seen after reperfusion of ischemic myocardium, intestine, brain, and kidney. These changes were characterized by endothelial cell swelling, interstitial edema, and subsequent tissue necrosis.

Oxygen-derived free-radicals resulting from increased vascular permeability in ischemic skeletal muscle were prevented by pre-treating them with specific scavenging agents. *Superoxide dismutase*, which is a superoxide anion scavenging enzyme, has the ability to significantly decrease microvascular permeability in-

*Alpha tocopherol has been recently used as a scavenging agent (see Chapter 13), and is being added to this test.

duced by ischemia. Similar action is displayed by *dimethyl sulfoxide*, which is a hydroxyl radical scavenger. In addition, *allopurinol* has been used, which as a competitive inhibitor of xanthine oxidase is as effective as the two previous agents. There is considerable experimental and clinical evidence suggesting that allopurinol provides protection against ischemic reperfusion in many other tissues besides skeletal muscle. Furthermore, the oxygen radicals are produced in ischemic skeletal muscle by a mechanism in which ATP is converted to adenosine monophosphate (AMP) during ischemia. The elevated AMP is catabolized to hypoxanthine, a substrate for xanthine oxidase.

The results of the Korthius experimental investigation clearly indicate that the oxygen-derived free-radicals are involved in this entire process. The use of allopurinol, superoxide dismutase, and catalase prevent ischemic injury to skeletal muscle.

Hyperosmotic mannitol is known to reduce ischemic cell swelling and to minimize myocardial necrosis. This agent has a wider use in cardiac surgery and great potential in vascular surgery. The timing of administration of mannitol is of critical importance. For example, when given following ischemic arrest of the heart and reperfusion, timing of its administration appears critical in order for it to have a beneficial effect on myocardial structure and function.

Clinical evaluation of most of the above agents is still at an experimental and initial stage, especially in arterial diseases. Of these, the physiologic and therapeutic properties of mannitol are more clearly establishd for some time already, preceding the era of free-radicals, in post-ischemic reperfusion lesions.[9] The following shall be confined to mannitol use, primarily in acute arterial occlusions.

Hyperosmotic Mannitol

Heart Ischemia

A number of experimental data indicate that administration of hyperosmotic mannitol in the management of canine heart ischemia has resulted in improvement of function and a lessening of the extent of ischemic injury as assessed by electrocardiographic studies. In addition, there was improved total collateral blood flow and overall metablism of the myocardium. It appeared that mannitol dilated large collateral conductance vessels in addition to improving blood flow to the region of myocardial ischemia.

The mechanism whereby hyperosmotic mannitol acts is by reducing cell swelling in the heart as well as in the kidney. The studies in experimentally induced myocardial ischemia have shown elevation of extracellular osmolality at the same time that there is a lessening of the extent of ischemic injury. Similar experimental data were reported in the management of myocardial injury associated with ischemia and reperfusion. Three scavenging agents such as superoxide dismutase, catalase, and mannitol all resulted in significantly better recovery of left ventricular function following reperfusion.

The critical importance as already mentioned of timing of mannitol administration and preservation of myocardial structure and function indicated that administration immediately prior to aortic cross-clamping or at the onset of reperfusion are essential and could prevent the reperfusion injuries resulting from the free-radicals-induced injuries. Most studies carried out on ischemically induced hearts concluded independently that hypersmolar mannitol is extremely helpful in these reperfusion situations.

Use of Mannitol in Post-Ischemic Revascularization of Extremities

In a recent study, hypertonic mannitol proved to be quite remarkable both experimentally and clinically. Buchbinder et al.,[26] using an experimental set-up of an isolated canine hind limb model, performed revascularization of the limb via an inserted Dacron graft in the aortoiliac area. After reperfusion for 2 hours, the low flow state (50% of control) was associated with thrombosis at the anastomosis of the graft. Use of the hypertonic mannitol reversed the reperfusion syndrome and prevented the graft thrombosis. Histologically, transmission electron micrographs of muscle biopsy specimen taken 60 minutes after reperfusion in untreated dogs showed intracellular edema and mitochondrial swelling and disruption. In contrast, transmission electron micrographs of muscle biopsy specimen taken 60 minutes after reperfusion in mannitol-treated dogs showed absence of changes seen in the previous specimen.

Clinical studies carried out in acute arterial occlusions of the lower extremity in 15 consecutive patients were evaluated and treated with mannitol. Emergency vascular reconstruction was carried out in these 15 patients with the diagnosis of acute arterial occlusion and threatened limb loss. After thromboembolectomy or arterial bypass, and prior to reestablishment of blood flow, all of these patients were given 100 ml of 20% mannitol as an intravenous bolus, followed by an infusion of 10 gm per hour of mannitol. This was continued for 6 to 24 hours. Duration of mannitol treatment was determined by the severity of the preoperative ischemia, level of occlusion, and overall condition of the patients. Fourteen patients had embolism presumed to originate from the heart, with the exception of one patient with thrombosis of the femoral artery associated with secondary polycythemia. All of these patients had concomitant cardiovascular disease: six had old myocardial infarctions, two had congestive heart failure, and nine had atrial fibrillation. Following this treatment, 14 patients had survived during the 30-day postoperative observation period; only one died 3 days after embolectomy. One patient had preoperative myoglobinuria which cleared postoperatively. These patients were not treated with heparin, either preoperatively or postoperatively, but all received a single dose of 3,000 units of heparin during arterial cross-clamping.

Buchbinder[26] pointed out that based on the experimental observations ischemic muscle may not be immediately returned to its normal metabolic state. The continued hypoperfusion of the limb may persist after revascularization which in turn may release a variety of toxins into the systemic circulation. The revascularization syndrome may be due to the flushing out of metabolites such as lactic acid, which can cause an abrupt fall in systemic pH or an increase in potassium level, either of which can result in acute myocardial depression and death. Similar studies have been reported in detail earlier and represent the metabolic syndrome associated with acute arterial occlusions. Anderson et al.[4] studied metabolic changes in blood and changes in adenosine triphosphate, adenosine diphosphate, and creatinine phosphate levels in skeletal muscle of patients undergoing periods of aortic cross-clamping during aortic surgery. These studied have been reported earlier in connection with cross-clamping of the aorta (see Chapter 15, *Temporary Ischemia of the Lower Extremity Secondary to Clamping of Major Arteries*).

The actual mechanism of the metabolites genesis is the oxygen-derived free-radicals that the authors were apparently unaware of at the time of their study.

Subsequent studies of the reperfusion syndrome in acute arterial occlusions of the extremities which has been described in brain, myocardium, and kidney had shown similarities with the present study. The free-radicals were incriminated in all of the complications of the reperfusion syndrome. Regardless of this mechanism, after a period of ischemia with blood flow reestablished, resistance and tissue edema increased and blood flow decreased. These changes have been shown to be prevented by the use of hypertonic mannitol. Morphologically it was found that after reperfusion, vascular endothelium was edematous, with about nearly complete occlusion of the small vessels. Pretreatment with hypertonic mannitol prevents this endothelial swelling. Similarly, in the canine hind limb, preoperative hypertonic mannitol reduced tissue edema, decreased vascular resistance, and increased blood flow. This increased blood flow was associated with absence of thrombosis at anastomotic sites.

The authors noted that when hypertonic mannitol was administered prior to revascularization, the signs and symptoms of reperfusion syndrome were absent. Furthermore, there was an improvement of survival along with a higher rate of limb salvage than in previously reported series. Thus, in a controlled group of 12 patients with acute arterial occlusions studied during the same period, there were four deaths and three limb amputations. Further experience using larger numbers of patients is obviously necessary in support of its effectiveness. The present study on free-radicals and usefulness of scavenging agents has been emphasized above.

The clinical trials in these cases suggest that revascularization of an acutely ischemic limb with hypertonic mannitol would appear to be extremely useful in saving the limb and preventing the complications of reperfusion.

Prospective Views of the Free-Radicals in Management of Vascular Problems

As already mentioned in the beginning of this chapter, the problem of free-radicals and use of their antidotes in the management of vascular diseases is only at its relatively early stages. A great deal of research both in laboratories and in the management of patients is being carried out. The field is in the midst of its expansion and no definitive statements are yet available. Based on current research, however, it is anticipated that in addition to the above-mentioned scavengers, new substances are potentially displaying similar properties.

As an example, in a recent experimental study of the cause and treatment of acute arterial occlusions, alpha-tocopherol has been reported as a scavenger agent. The results appeared encouraging. Alpha-tocopherol is vitamin E and its properties, among others, have been found to exert those of a scavenger of free-radicals.[140a]

Del Maestro,[52] based on a detailed review of an approach to free-radicals in medicine and biology, has provided a list of agents which could be or are being experimentally used as therapeutic drugs. The following is a tentative list of conditions and agents having scavenger properties. It is mentioned here for the sake of completeness, although their usefulness has not been completely tested as yet.

*Therapeutic Considerations**

A. Increased intracellular generation

1. Hydrophobic scavengers
   - Vitamin E (alpha-tocopherol)
   - Barbituric acid derivatives
2. O_2 control
3. Liposomes + SOD

B. Increased extracellular generation

1. Enzymatic scavengers
   - SOD
   - Catalase
   - SOD and catalase
2. Hydrophilic scavengers
   - Ascorbic acid
   - Glutathione-SH
   - L-methionine

*(From Del Maestro published in *Acta Physiol Scand* 1980, (Suppl) 492:153–168.)

C. Increased extracellular and intracellular

1. Enzymatic scavengers
2. Hydrophilic scavengers
3. Hydrophobic scavengers
4. Tissue O_2 decrease
   - Microspheres
5. Liposomes + SOD

D. Decreased scavenger mechanisms

1. Tumor therapy

IV

Management of Rhabdomyolytic Syndromes and Their Metabolic Complications

27

Management of Rhabdomyolytic Syndromes and Their Metabolic Complications

Introduction

The management of the various syndromes of rhabdomyolysis and their metabolic complications varies somewhat with the entity which is dominating the clinical picture. In these acute conditions, it is essential to pay close attention concomitantly to both local and systemic manifestations. *Awareness* of potential complications represents the key to the diagnosis, prevention, and their immediate and specific treatment. Besides a number of specific situations, a set of general principles are applicable to all the entities: (1) acute arterial occlusions with myonephropathic metabolic syndrome; (2) traumatic lesions of the crush syndrome; (3) vascular trauma, and (4) nontraumatic rhabdomyolysis with renal complications.

Acute Arterial Occlusions with Myonephropathic-Metabolic Syndrome

In the presence of this syndrome, two major signs must be first ascertained: (1) the presence of a dark red urine containing myoglobin as detected by the tests previously described, and (2) rigidity of the calf muscles including edema of the extremity due to severe muscle ischemia.

After evaluation of the patient's overall vascular condition and its exact location (aortoiliac or femoral popliteal), the patient may be prepared for angiography for identification of the lesions before the surgical procedure is undertaken without too much delay. First, the essential biochemical parameters from the systemic, and from the involved limb, are to be ascertained, such as the pH, myoglobin, CPK, pCO_2, PO_2, blood volume, etc. Arterial and venous lines should be established without delay.

Fluid replacement and restoration of electrolyte balance is a first step for appropriate treatment of blood loss, using fluids and electrolytes as immediate management. In the vast majority of these individuals with acute arterial occlusions and metabolic complications, the initial chemical markers are still minor evidence of what is going on in the kidney as well as in the skeletal muscle compartments. There is a slight elevation only of serum creatine or transient diminution of the urinary output. However, restoration of their intravascular volume is absolutely essential.

Whether the color of the urine is dark red and myoglobin is detectable or not, sodium bicarbonate must be used to correct a possible or definite presence of acidosis. Usually, 1.5 to 2 mEq/kg of body weight should be given over a 20 to 60 minute period depending on the cardiac status of the patient. Glucose and insulin may be started intravenously, in some of these cases, using 50 gm hypertonic glucose (20–50% solution) associated with 15 units of insulin (i.e., 3 to 4 gm of glucose require one unit of insulin).

If there is evidence of rigidity of the skeletal muscle in the calf or higher up, fasciotomy is mandatory, even before arterial repair. The fasciotomy of the leg may involve one or three compartments, or all four, depending on the extent of the edema of the muscles and the viability of the tissue observed. Biopsies of the muscle should be obtained routinely.

Operative Procedure

Following these measures, thromboembolectomy or any other reconstructive arterial procedure, as the case may be, should be undertaken at that point. (See Chapter 26 for a discussion on the use of mannitol.)

Post-Revascularization Stage

After the early reestablishment of blood flow of the acutely ischemic extremity has been completed, prevention of muscle damage by use of mannitol and alkalinization of the patient should be continued during and after the operation until the blood pH, especially in the involved limb, has been restored to a normal level. This treatment is all the more essential if myoglobin is present or suspected, since it precipitates readily in the renal tubules in the acid milieu. Concurrently, reestablishment of electrolyte balance, especially including reducing serum potassium to normal levels, is essential. Use of insulin combined with intravenous glucose may be sometimes indicated. In the presence of severe renal dysfunction, hemodialysis should be started rather than peritoneal dialysis until renal function can be restored. This may sometimes take several days to several weeks.

Amputation, which is obviously necessary in the presence of frank gangrene, is sometimes indicated even in the absence of frank necrosis as a prophylactic measure to eliminate the source of metabolites from the ischemic skeletal muscles, more particularly if severe and extensive rhabdomyolysis is present.

During *fasciotomy*, the nonviable skeletal muscle, especially in the delayed procedures, should be excised and only the viable tissues attached to the limb should be left. Occasionally, one may excise a large mass of muscle down to the interosseous membrane. Healing by secondary intervention may be achieved, thus salvaging the limb.

Traumatic Muscular Lesions (Crush Syndrome)

As in the acute arterial occlusions, administration of fluid and alkali is mandatory. Patients with severe muscle damage who are delayed in arriving at the emergency room of the hospital may suffer from a lack of fluids and may be hypotensive. As a result of the metabolic acidosis, they should be given, immediately upon arrival, sodium bicarbonate or other mild alkali or THAM until the pH of the urine is no longer in the acidotic range. The alkalinization of the patient should be continued over the next 2 or 3 days in order to prevent any possible damage to the kidneys. In addition to sodium bicarbonate, isotonic sodium lactate should be given intravenously at the same time, either before or during the surgical procedure that may be needed in these cases. In order to be effective, alkalinization should be early and thorough, and should be monitored for the reaction of the urine.

Most of these patients with traumatic shock or crush syndrome, in addition to having lost blood due to damage to the blood vessels, may be leaking plasma into the injured area, sometimes without outward signs if the trunk is affected. "Oligemic shock," although the blood pressure remains normal for a time because of vasoconstriction, should not mislead the physician examining the patient. Prompt treatment of these patients is indicated as if they were in shock, although some of the symptoms are not yet available. Serum and plasma should be given before the blood pressure falls in the stage of hemoconcentration.

The injured limb should be kept cool either with ice bags or other means available, such as a cooling blanket, in the emergency room or on the operating table. The damaged muscle or skin which appear to be irreversibly necrotic should be excised. Fasciotomies, as in the previous group of patients, should be considered in the presence of an enlarged extremity with edema and bulging muscles.

Vascular reconstruction in such cases may be necessary, if in addition to the crushed muscles there is also evidence of contused or occluded major arteries. *Amputation* of the leg may be necessary if it is severely damaged, appearing not only useless but mostly dangerous to the patient due to the invasion of the circulation by metabolites from the necrotic muscle.

The surgical problems associated with crush syndrome consist primarily of immediate fasciotomy, debridement of necrotic muscles, which must be removed completely, leaving only the neuromuscular bundles which appear to be within normal limits of viability.

Renal Problems. The most serious of the major complications threatening the life of the patient are renal problems. Although all patients with this condition receive from the time of arrival to the emergency set-up 4,500 to 10,000 ml of crystalloid solution intravenously during the first 24 hours, it is also necessary to provide these patients with furosemide and mannitol. The use of mannitol is doubly essential for combatting the superoxide radicals in its indication of the reperfusion phase of the extremity should revascularization be carried out (see below for details). In the presence of anuria because of the hypercatabolic state, hemodialysis may have to be carried out daily for 6 to 8 hours. Improvement of renal function may take, in some severe cases, between 5 and 30 days after appearance of renal failure. Nonoliguric acute renal failure may be achieved provided early massive fluid therapy is used.

In addition to the renal problems, the patients with crush syndrome are potential candidates of *local infection* and *systemic septicemia*. Most of these patients present pseudomonas as cultured in their blood, as well as *E. coli*. In addition to the excision of the necrotic nonviable tissues, appropriate antibiotics should be given systemically in order to overcome, if possible, the septic shock which is present due to pseudomonas.

Respiratory failure may occur in some of these patients as a result of microemboli from the involved extremity or as a result of the systemic infection noted in these patients.

Vascular Trauma

Vascular trauma *per se* is usually only part of a wider picture of multiple severe injuries. The relative incidence of post-traumatic necrosis associated with myoglobinuria and secondary renal shutdown is difficult to estimate in these cases.

In such instances, as in the crush syndrome, resuscitation of the patient and control of breathing with control of open wounds are the immediate preoccupation of the trauma surgeon. Vascular damage usually takes second place which may account also for the common late revascularization in the presence of critical ischemia. It is in these latter cases that myonecrosis, myoglobinuria, and renal problems appear to take precedence over other critical aspects of the total trauma picture. Keen awareness of potential metabolic complications arising from ischemic muscles is probably the greatest prerequisite for diagnosis and immediate treatment.

In brief, the awareness of the metabolic complications either in acute arterial occlusions or in the crush syndrome or in post-traumatic arterial lesions, is essential to replace first the volume of blood before treating the other components of the metabolic syndrome. Hyperkalemia and myoglobinuria are, of course, the two major dangers both to life and limb of the patient.

Specific Factors

Management of these patients, in general, is of an emergency nature, involving limb- or life-threatening conditions. Their management upon arrival at the hospital, after vital signs assessment, should be handled in a similar fashion for acute vascular and muscular lesions.

Myoglobinuria. Within a few hours of the onset of these conditions, whether it is an acute occlusion, or crush syndrome, the urinary output is usually decreased and the urine displays a dark cherry red or burgundy color, due to myoglobin.

In the presence of or if myoglobinuria is anticipated, alkalinization should be continued throughout the first 2 days until the blood pH, especially from the blood of the involved limb, has been restored to a normal level.

Hyperkalemia. In severe cases of myonecrosis, increased serum potassium is noted after revascularization. It usually represents a poor prognostic factor translating in advance the degree of muscle cytolysis. Its sudden release after removal of a tourniquet or arterial clamp may lead to cardiac arrest. Should hyperkalemia and BUN fail to yield to appropriate fluid and electrolyte replacement, hemodialysis must be considered.

Rhabdomyolysis. The degree of ischemic damage to the skeletal muscle is of central significance, since it determines the viability of the limb and to a great extent the severity of the metabolic syndrome.

Focal lesions can be excised as already mentioned and an attempt can still be made to salvage the limb. Wide debridement is often necessary, unless amputation is unavoidable.

Acute Renal Failure. This has been discussed above, and need not be repeated here.

Mannitol

Hypertonic mannitol, advocated in the 1960s by Barry[9] and others, for its use in the prevention of renal shutdown during aortic surgery, is again being strongly recommended in vascular reconstructive surgery, this time for additional biological reasons. Experimental and clinical data suggest that its administration may play the role of a scavening agent of oxygen-derived free-radicals. The current clinical data indicate that mannitol, like superoxide dismutase, catalase, and allopurinol, can significantly reduce the extent of lesions during reperfusion of ischemic tissues. The mechanism of action of mannitol and the other allied substances is not entirely clear. The clinical results of their use in myocardial, brain, and intestinal ischemic injuries have been most encouraging. Similarly, administration of mannitol in cases of skeletal muscle ischemia, especially in the prevention of the revascularization syndrome after acute arterial ischemia, seems to respond to the same mechanism of action. Hypertonic mannitol administered prior to revascularization may prevent the signs and symptoms of reperfusion syndrome. The survival rate and limb salvage rate may improve significantly.

Hypertonic mannitol (20%) should first be given as an intravenous bolus of 100 cc to be followed by an infusion of 10 gm/hr, the latter schedule to be continued for 6 to 24 hours. The duration of this treatment is determined by the severity of the ischemia and the overall condition of the patient. Its administration, to be thoroughly effective, should start before any reconstructive procedure is initiated.

Nontraumatic and Nonocclusive Arterial Rhabdomyolysis with Acute Renal Failure

Such entities are observed in a wide number of medical subspecialties in which neither trauma nor acute arterial occlusions are at the etiologic basis of their occurrence. These cases are of widely different natures including myopathies, bacterial or viral infections, burns, epilepsy, toxic materials, prolonged coma, etc. (see Chapter 21). Their clinical pictures are due to a number of metabolic complications found in all cases except in some which display only specific entities. As a rule, the following therapeutic guidelines are applicable in these cases depending on the nature of the complications: (1) acute renal shutdown should be started without delay on hemodialysis; (2) antibiotic therapy as needed; (3) in inflammatory myopathies, steroid therapy should be started as soon as the biochemical and biopsy findings confirm the nature of the rhabdomyolysis; (4) in cases of comatose patients, due to drug abuse or toxic factors, relief of pressure due to body weight or extraneous objects should be achieved immediately to prevent necrosis of the involved compressed parts, especially of the extremities.

Because of the wide variety of causative factors, the patient's clinical condition should be carefully identified in terms of the main complications: (1) myoglobinuria, including myoglobinemia; (2) renal function (oliguria, anuria); (3) hypo- or hypercalcemia; (4) muscle biopsy; (5) status of arterial circulation of the extremities.

In brief, due to the above multiple causative factors, the management may require a thorough understanding of the biochemical alterations, muscular and renal lesions, and the application of appropriate therapy for their complex picture, as outlined in the preceding three major groups of entities.

Role of Scavenging Agents

As previously stated (Chapter 26), ischemia induced in skeletal muscle, regardless of the cause, results in increased vascular permeability at the microvascular level. Its mechanism is not entirely elucidated. However, reperfusion of skeletal muscle results in a more dramatic increase in microvascular permeability, leading to additional tissue necrosis. The so-called scavenging agents have the ability to alter beneficially the permeability increase.

Oxygen-derived free-radicals resulting in ischemic skeletal muscle can be prevented by pre-treating with the specific scavenging agents. Superoxide dismutase, a superoxide anion scavenging enzyme, has the ability to significantly decrease microvascular permeability induced by ischemia. Similar action is displayed by dimethyl sulfoxide, a hydroxyl radical scavenger. In addition, allopurinol, a competitive inhibitor of xanthine oxidase, is as effective as the two previous agents. There is considerable experimental and clinical evidence suggesting that allopurinol provides protection against ischemia reperfusion in many other tissues besides skeletal muscle. Furthermore, the oxygen radicals are produced in ischemic skeletal muscle by a mechanism in which ATP is converted to adenosine monophosphate (AMP) during ischemia. The elevated AMP is catabolized to hypoxanthine, a substrate for xanthine oxidase.

With the exception of superoxide dismutase (SOD), the most recent of these agents, the others are well-known chemicals and are considered to be effective scavenging agents. SOD provides significant protection following resumption of blood flow after total blockage of vessels. Development of this enzyme is the subject of intense research of several technology companies, which are studying its possible use in the treatment of a variety of medical problems.

Among the latter, the post-ischemic phase of acute arterial occlusions is a most illustrative example. Usefulness of this enzyme is obvious. It is at the present time at an experimental stage primarily in post-ischemic myocardial damage.

Studies that have shown that oxygen-derived free-radicals have a direct toxic effect on myocardial structure, and function seems to be benefitted by the use of SOD. Likewise, free-radical scavengers can, therefore, reduce myocardial infarct size in some but not in all models. The role of the white blood cell in mediating reperfusion injury and the role of free-radicals in mediating the phenomenon of prolonged post-ischemic myocardial dysfunction and the role of free-radicals in cardiac surgery may prove to be of great significance in the near future.

28

Summation: An Epilogue

A short summation, in contrast to a summary of a mere recapitulation of the data, may provide a more selective view of the entire subject. A summation's scope may confine itself to a few concluding remarks and briefly point out primarily some of the highlights of the main facets of this monograph. Furthermore, an attempt will also be made to indicate the major trends of the evolving concepts of the interrelationships between acute arterial ischemia and its effects on the skeletal muscle.

Based on the components of the metabolic complications in acute arterial occlusions, a new biological vision emerged concerning the role of the ischemic striated muscle. As a result, the latter assumes usually the central source of the factors causing the metabolic syndrome, and finally, as a corollary, it dominates the outcome of the severe acute arterial occlusions.

For a comprehensive understanding of the above-mentioned role played by the skeletal muscle, it was important to delve into its biological responses to acute ischemia, both from morphological and biochemical points of view.

To illustrate the significance of the physical muscular mass in relation to the entire body, it should be pointed out that the muscles, as an anatomic entity, constitute about 42% of the body weight. Furthermore, the muscular mass of the lower extremity offers the relatively larger percentage, representing 76% of its volume. The muscular arteries, especially the intramuscular components, play a significant role down to their minute divisions into capillaries. It is at this latter level that when obstructions occur the ischemic changes become irreversible in spite of the fact that the extramuscular arteries may still remain patent to some degree.

Biochemically, it should be stressed that the skeletal muscle is a tissue which incorporates a multitude of biochemical substances in its structural complex. Being highly vulnerable to anoxia of whatever cause, the muscle may respond by releasing into the circulation some or most of these biochemical elements which may be highly harmful or even fatal to the patient. These elements are precisely responsible for the substrate of the metabolic repercussions of the acute ischemic muscle entities.

Knowledge of the morphology and biochemistry of the skeletal fiber is basic for further comprehension of the pathophysiology and clinical findings which are at the core of this clinicopathological syndrome.

As an illustration, one morphological element that plays a cardinal role in the interchanges of the biochemical components is the sarcolemma or membrane of the muscle fiber. It is a multicomponent structure covering the entire surface of the fiber and is divided into an innermost component, an inner basal lamina and an external reticular lamina.

The metabolic complications resulting from ischemic skeletal muscle are due to the derangement of transport processes across the membranes. The latter plays a fundamental role in the biochemical functions of the various components. Changes in permeability of membranes under traumatic or simply ischemic conditions may induce severe biochemical alterations in the internal space of the sarcolemmal reticulum and outside of it.

The physiological integrity of the membrane, which includes neural components, can be affected by decreased ATP. Since the latter is markedly reduced in ischemic muscle, it follows that abnormal membrane permeability in the presence of reduced ATP represents the underlying mechanism of the biochemical changes. In spite of these facts, little is still known about the exact mechanism of the interchange between biochemical substances from the muscle fiber into the interstitial space or from the latter into the retromembrane structures. The muscle may act under aerobic and anaerobic conditions to a certain extent, so as to provide its many varied functions.

Of the biochemical substances, myoglobin has been singled out in the early studies as a main marker of the biochemical derangement representing the pathophysiology of the skeletal muscle. It took several decades for its chemical study, but clinically it became known only since 1942. Myoglobin, when associated with metabolic acidosis, may precipitate in the renal tubules, and thus represents a major danger to the kidney function, which if unrecognized or not treated vigorously, may lead to renal shutdown and even death of the patient.

Of the many other substances, creatine phosphokinase (CPK) is an important index of muscle ischemia or necrosis, depending on its serum level and duration.

The ultimate dysfunction of the biochemical elements taking place in the skeletal muscle fiber result in rhabdomyolysis. The degree and extent of the latter range from diffuse cell injury to variable necrosis, to frank massive gangrene. The degree of rhabdomyolysis is usually assessed, among other factors, by the level of CPK.

The three major etiologic types of rhabdomyolysis are due to: (1) acute arterial occlusions; (2) traumatic lesions directly applied to the muscular tissue; and (3) nontraumatic lesions, including a wide spectrum of entities in which diffuse muscle cell injuries dominate but in which occasionally extensive muscular necrosis may also occur.

The most sigificant biological alterations associated with the rhabdomyolytic processes are the following:

1. Metabolic acidosis (increased lactates and pyruvates).
2. Enzymatic changes: CPK, LDH, SGOT. Of these, as mentioned earlier, CPK is the most characteristic index of muscle damage, a severity ranging from transient cellular ischemia to extensive necrosis.
3. Oxidative phosphorylations: ATP → ADP → AMP, the central role of ATP in the muscle metabolism was pointed out earlier.
4. Electrolyte changes (Na, K), PO_2, pCO_2.

While all these biological alterations associated with rhabdomyolysis play significant roles, the major one that stands out among them is metabolic acidosis. It plays a decisive role in the metabolic syndrome and has to be treated immediately, as soon as the diagnosis of the metabolic syndrome is made. The treatment consists of buffer solutions to block the acidotic manifestations of these agents by the use of either bicarbonates or THAM (see the discussion later in this chapter on experimental evidence of the role of buffer substances used in suppressing the metabolic complications by reducing other metabolites which are released by the ischemic or necrotic skeletal muscle).

The clinical entities that constitute the major scope of this monograph deal essentially with acute ischemic changes under a variety of conditions. The prototype of these clinical entities may be considered to be represented by the acute arterial embolism. Actually, this entity had been at the origin of this entire work when the metabolic syndrome was uncovered as shown in the original publication. The clinical manifestations of an acute arterial embolism are classified into three phases: (1) ischemia or devascularization; (2) revascularization; and (3) reperfusion of ischemic tissues.

As stated in the introduction, only highlights and major significant facets will be presented in this summation. Therefore, one will have to consider the important and striking manifestations that occur either at the onset or later in the development of the clinical syndrome. Among the more striking and characteristic initial features of the ischemic phase is the rigidity of the extremity or rigor mortis. Muscular contracture and stiffness of the joints are very pronounced, to the point that passive or active motion is completely abolished due to the "frozen" aspect of the joints. The pain is extreme and prevents any motion of any part of the involved extremity. The rigidity of the limb can then be considered as an "alarm signal" of acute muscular ischemia and most probably is associated with myoglobinuria. This sign of rigidity or contracture of the muscles should evoke immediately the presence of an incipient metabolic syndrome and all measures should be taken to overcome the metabolic factors enumerated above.

The major factors that will determine the clinical course and prognosis of such a severe ischemia depend on several features, of which the most important are: (1) the number, extent, and level of arterial occlusions; (2) the duration of the occlusions; (3) the extent of involvement of intramuscular arterioles and venules; (4) the awareness and early recognition of this syndrome; and (5) the immediate aggressive treatment of the ischemia and its early metabolic manifestations.

While revascularization of the extremity is an important and urgent maneuver, one must keep in mind that the initiating ischemia of the skeletal muscle results in rhabdomyolysis, but the reperfusion phase is further complicated by free-radicals-induced ischemia leading to additional superimposed necrosis. Antioxidants or antidotes to this phase of the skeletal muscle reperfusion injury are available and will be mentioned in the discussion on management.

Pathogenesis has been alluded to earlier and the role of the membrane of the muscular fiber has been discussed and emphasized. One more mention may be of value in stating that the morphological alterations are not only the result of the ischemic changes *per se*, but that the chemical changes occur at the cellular level where CPK, myoglobin, potassium, etc., are released into the blood and lymph streams, all of which contribute to the complexity of the metabolic syndrome. The basic morphological derangement resides in the membrane of the muscle fibers due to decreased ATP as a result of ischemia of the membrane.

The preceding highlights referred essentially to arterial embolism. One should remember that this entity was taken as a prototype of acute arterial occlusions in which rhabdomyolysis and severe metabolic complications are illustrated by the hallmark of the cardinal events in the acute arterial entities described in this monograph. It is clear that not all clinical entities in this section are characterized by the identical manifestations described in Chapter 14, *Arterial Embolism,* although the basic rhabdomyolytic and metabolic complications are to be found in every one of the entities described.

It may be repetitious to attempt to point out highlights from the other clinical entities which as mentioned may be identical or similar to the ones encountered in arterial embolism. One may only mention, for instance, that acute thrombosis of abdominal aortic aneurysms may have a severe prognosis if unrecognized immediately after onset, which may result in bilateral lower extremity gangrene, renal shutdown, and a high mortality rate. Similarly, acute abdominal aortic occlusions in nonaneurysmal cases may offer a less severe prognosis, with a decreased mortality, as compared to the aneurysmal variety.

Myoglobinuria, being one of the highlights of the metabolic syndrome, may be found in a variety of conditions and may be the cause of acute renal failure due to blockage of the renal tubules by this pigment, myoglobin. A great variety of conditions may be associated with this complication secondary to myoglobinuria. Its early detection and treatment is essential to prevent renal shutdown and other associated facets that accompany myoglobinuria. One important point to emphasize is that when myoglobin is released through the membrane, there are other substances that are also released, such as CPK, LDH, SGOT, etc., and may produce a variety of other complications besides myoglobinuria.

Nontraumatic and nonocclusive arterial rhabdomyolysis is differentiated from the acute arterial occlusions and the crush syndrome as far as its etiologies are concerned, but the major hallmark distinguishing this entity from the others is acute renal failure which always accompanies the various metabolic alterations. Therefore, in the absence of the usual etiologic factors, namely acute arterial occlusion or direct muscular injury, it should be pointed out that a great variety of toxins, either exogenous or endogenous, are the usual factors responsible for inducing damage to the muscle and producing a similar rhabdomyolytic syndrome as seen in the classic occlusive arterial and muscular trauma syndromes.

Myocardial infarction was included among the clinical entities for a simple reason—that the metabolic changes which occur in the infarction of the cardiac muscle may exhibit a certain number of biochemical findings similar to those in skeletal muscle ischemia. The presence of these metabolic factors seen in myocardial ischemia may serve only as an adjuvant in the diagnosis, in which other specific criteria are available for determining the diagnosis of myocardial infarction. Nevertheless, this was included in this group of clinical entities to show the universality of response of the skeletal muscle and that of the cardiac muscle to ischemia. Their similarities are quite striking and provide a common ground for the pathogenesis of the biochemical responses of this tissue.

While enumerating briefly the common denominators of

some of these clinical entities, the divergence between them due to some specific differences of the pathological and clinical manifestations have also been pointed out.

Before reviewing briefly the highlights of management, it is important to mention the role of free-radicals in post-ischemic skeletal muscle reperfusion injury, as already mentioned earlier. This is a novel aspect in the physiopathology and management of arterial occlusions of the extremities. It is based on the experimental studies and clinical findings in the management of cardiac ischemia. By analogy, the ischemia of the skeletal muscle has proven to show some similarities from a physiopathological point of view and has provided an open field for research in the management of the acute ischemia of the extremities with the antioxidants and the use of scavengers in the presence of free-radicals in the skeletal muscle ischemia. Indeed, recent investigations of a few substances, called scavenging agents, have the ability to alter the capillary permeability increase due to the superoxide free-radicals. The main agents used already, mostly experimentally and some clinically, are superoxide dismutase, allopurinol, catalase, and mannitol. Recently, alpha-tocopherol has been added as a scavenging agent in experimental studies of this syndrome. Clinically, hyperosmotic mannitol is the most appropriate and most available scavenging agent at the present time.

Management of the rhabdomyolytic syndromes and their metabolic complications may vary somewhat with the entity that dominates the clinical picture. However, in these acute conditions, it is essential to pay close attention concomitantly to both local and systemic manifestations. The key to successful management and suppression of the metabolic factors is based on awareness of potential complications and prevention, together with immediate and specific blockage of the metabolites. Since metabolic acidosis is one of the major factors leading to severe complications, it is essential to use appropriate and immediate buffers to block and suppress this condition. It consists of the use of bicarbonate in appropriate amounts in order to reverse the acidotic pH level and reduce it to a normal one above 7.2. Metabolic acidosis, a constant biological disturbance in these cases, is related to the toxemia emerging from the rhabomyolysis. Once the rhabdomyolytic tissue is excised or blocked by medical means, metabolic acidosis may be easily controlled. Among the chemical substances able to block and reverse these metabolic complications is THAM, as shown by several investigators in the past few years. It is used either intravenously or by reperfusion of the limb before releasing the arterial clamp, so that the "wash out" of the limb involved in the source of the metabolites is more or less purified of these noxious metabolites.

Whether the experimental data are applicable to a great extent at the clinical level remains to be proven. Likewise, whether the scavenging agents would provide a lot of therapeutic help in blocking the superoxide free-radicals by using scavengers remains a problem for the future. The premises upon which some of these investigations are based are concerned with the cause of the rhabdomyolysis by focusing on the lipid peroxidation by the active free-radicals of superoxide nature. Their effectiveness as a prophylaxis before release of the clamp or at the time when the metabolic complications are still at the early phase, is an open question left for future evaluation of these new agents. In any event, this problem of *myonephropathic-metabolic syndrome* has been recognized by a number of centers worldwide and it is hoped as a result of recent progress that these complications may be blocked before they appear or initiate harm locally or systemically as demonstrated throughout this monograph.

Bibliography

1. Abel RM, Wick J, Beck CH Jr: Renal dysfunction following open heart operations. *Arch Surg* 108:175, 1974.
2. Adams CA Jr, Elliott TA: Urinary myoglobin in myocardial infarction. Letter to *JAMA* 211:1013–1014, 1970.
3. Alemany J: Metodos, resultados y complicaciones en las desobliteraciones tardias de las occlusiones arteriales agudas perifericas. *Angiologia* 21-81, 1969.

3a. Alpert J, Goldenkranz RJ, Brief DK, et al: Limb ischemia during intra-aortic balloon pumping: Indication for femoro-femoral crossover graft. *Ann Thorac Cardiovasc Surg* 79:729, 1980.

4. Anderson J, Eklof B, Neglen P, Thomson D: Metabolic changes in blood and skeletal muscle in reconstructive aortic surgery. *Ann Surg* 283–293, 1979.
5. Arcangeli P, Digiesi V, Massala B: Metabolism of skeletal muscle following incomplete ischemia. *Angiology* 24:114, 1973.
6. Arruda JH, Kurtzman NA: Heroin addiction and renal disease. *Contrib Nephrol* 7:69–78, 1977.
7. Aub JC, Wu H: Studies in experimental traumatic shock. III. Chemical changes in the blood. *Am J Physiol* 54:416, 1920.
8. Baker WH, Munns Jr: Aneurysmectomy in the aged. *Arch Surg* 110:531, 1975.

9. Barry KG, Cohen A: Mannitolization. I. Prevention and therapy of oliguria associated with cross-clamping of the abdominal aorta. *Surgery* 50:335–337, 1961.
10. Baue AE, McClerkin WW: A study of shock: Acidosis and the declamping phenomenon. *Ann Surg* 161:40, 1965.
11. Bell JW: Acute thrombosis of the subrenal abdominal aorta. *Arch Surg* 95:681–684, 1967.
12. Benichoux R: Metabolic acidosis following regional circulatory arrest: treatment by THAM, hyperventilation and hyperbaric oxygen. *J Cardiovasc Surg* 14:573, 1973.
13. Berman LB: When the urine is red. *JAMA* 237:2752–2754, 1977.
14. Biglioli P, Santa A, Ferrozi G: Renal function after revascularization. *J Cardiovasc Surg* 14:578, 1973.
15. Biörk G: On myoglobin and its occurrence in man. *Acta Med Scand* 226(Suppl):1–216, 1949.
16. Bizet LMO, Lopez FF, Villalobos MC, Roque CT: Clampeo aortico infrarenal: Cambios metabolicos y su repercusion sobre la funcion renal. *Angiologia* 34:21–20, 1982.
17. Blaisdell FW: Traumatic shock: the search for a toxic factor. *Am Coll Surg Bull* 68:2–10, 1983.
18. Blaisdell GS, Steele M, Allen RE: Management of acute lower extremity arterial ischemia due to embolism and thrombosis. *Surgery* 84:822, 1978.
19. Bogaerts Y, Lameire N, Ringoir S: The compartmental syndrome: A serious complication of acute rhabdomyolysis. *Clin Nephrol* 17:206–211, 1982.
20. Bole PV, Purdy RI, Munda RT: Civilian arterial injuries. *Ann Surg* 183:13–23, 1976.
20a. Bowman W: On the minute structure and movements of voluntary muscle. *Philos Trans Royal Soc London* 130:457–501, 1840. (In *Skeletal Muscle*, Chapter 2, Peachey LD, et al., p 24.)
21. Bradley EL: The anterior tibial compartment syndrome. *Surg Gynecol Obstet* 136:289–297, 1973.
22. Breger PR, Guenel J, Lebeaupin R, Lemeillet Y: Une complication rare de la chirugie reparatrice des plaies arterielles graves: Le syndrome de Bywaters. *Mem Acad de Chir* 83:886–889, 1957.
23. Bridges KG, Donnelly JC Jr: Acute occlusion of an abdominal aortic aneurysm complicated by bilateral lower extrem-

ity venous thrombosis: A case report. *Cardiovasc Dis Bull Texas Heart Inst* 8:93–107, 1981.

24. Brodkin HM: Myoglobinuria following epsilon-aminocaproic acid (EACA) therapy: Case report. *J Neurosurg* 53:690–692, 1980.
25. Bruner JM: Time, pressure and temperature factors in the safe use of the tourniquet. *The Hand* 3:39, 1970.
26. Buchbinder D, Karmody AM, Leather RP, Shah DM: Hypertonic mannitol, its use in the prevention of revascularization syndrome after acute arterial ischemia. *Arch Surg* 116:414–421, 1981.
27. Bulkley GB, Morris JB: Role of oxygen-derived free radicals as mediators of post-ischemic injury: A clinically oriented overview. In *Superoxide and Superoxide Dismutase in Chemistry, Biology and Medicine*, Rotilio G (Ed.), Elsevier Science Publishers B.V., Amsterdam, 1986, pp 565–570.
28. Burton KP, McCord JM, Ghai G: Myocardial alterations due to free radical generation. *Am J Physiol* 246:H776–783, 1984.
29. Burton W, Holderness MC, John HT: Circulatory and acid-base changes during operations for abdominal aortic aneurysms. *Lancet* 2:782, 1964.
30. Busuttil RW, Keehn G, Milliken J, Paredero VM, Baker JD, Machleder HI, Moore WS, Baker WF: Aortic saddle embolus: A twenty-year experience. *Ann Surg* 197:698–706, 1983.
31. Bywaters EGL: Ischemic muscle necrosis, crushing injury, traumatic edema, the crush syndrome, traumatic anuria, compression syndrome: A type of injury seen in air raid casualties following burial beneath debris. *JAMA* 124:1103–1109, 1944.
32. Campbell GS: Physiological and technical factors in the surgical treatment of abdominal aortic aneurysms. *Surgery* 62:789–792, 1967.
33. Cannon WB: *Traumatic Shock*. Appleton, New York, pp 142–159, 1923.
34. Campion DS, Arias JM, Carter NW: Rhabdomyolysis and myoglobinuria: Association with hypokalemia of renal tubular acidosis. *JAMA* 220:967–969, 1972.
35. Camus J, Pagniez P: Hemoglobinurie musculaire. *Compte Rend Acad Sci* 135:1010, 1902.
36. Carlström B: Uber die Atiologie und Pathogenese der

Kreuzlahme des Pferdes. *Skand Arch Physiol* 61:161, 1931.
37. Cassar JP: Contribution a l'etude des troubles metaboliques lies a l'ischemie aigue des membres: Leurs variations au cours des gestes therapeutiques. Thesis, Universite Scientifique et Medicale de Grenoble, 1974.
38. Chawla SK, Najafi H, et al: Acute renal failure complicating ruptured abdminal aortic aneurysm. *Arch Surg* 110:521, 1976.
39. Chiu D, Wang HH, Blumenthal MR: Creatine phosphokinase release as a measure of tourniquet effect on skeletal muscle. *Arch Surg* 111:71–74, 1976.
40. Chugh KS, Nath IVS, Ubroi HS, Singhal PC, Pareek SK, Sarkar AK: Acute renal failure due to nontraumatic rhabdomyolysis. *Postgrad Med J* 55:386–392, 1979.
41. Cohen LH, Kaplan M, Bernhard VM: Intraoperative streptokinase. *Arch Surg* 121:708–175, 1986.
42. von Colmers: *Arch Klin Chir* 90:701, 1909.
43. Corcoran AC, Page IH: Renal damage from ferroheme pigments myoglobin, hemoglobin and hematin. *Texas Rep Biol Med* 3:528, 1945.
44. Cormier JM, Devin R: Traitement des obliterations arterielles aigues des membres: Consequences generales de l'ischeimie aigue. 7th Congres Francais de Chirurgie, 1969.
45. Cotton RT, Bedford DR: Symmetric peripheral gangrene complicating acute myocardial infarction. *Am J Med* 20:301–307, 1956.
46. Criado FJ: Acute thrombosis of abdominal aortic aneurysm. *Texas Heart Inst* 9:367, 1982.
47. Cullen MJ, Appleyard ST, Bindoff L: Morphologic Aspects of Muscle Breakdown and Lysosomal Activation. *Ann NY Acad Sci* 371:440–463, 1979.
47a. Coffler et al: Quoted by Grossman et al: Nontraumatic rhabdomyolysis and acute renal failure. *N Engl J Med* 291:807, 1974, ref 94.
47b. Cooley DA, Reul GJ, Wukash DC: Ischemic contracture of the heart: "Stone heart." *Am J Cardiol* 29:575-577, 1972.
48. D'Agostino RS, Arnett EN: Acute myoglobinuria and heroin snorting. *JAMA* 241:277, 1979.
49. Dahlback L: Effects of tourniquet ischemia on striated muscle fibers and motor end-plates. *Scand J Plast Reconstr Surg* 7(Suppl):7–91, 1970.

50. Dahlback LO, Rais O: Morphologic changes in striated muscle following ischemia: immediate postischemic phase. *Acta Chir Scand* 131:430–440, 1966.
51. Danto LA, Fry WJ, Kraft RO: Acute aortic thrombosis. *Arch Surg* 104:569–572, 1972.
52. Del Maestro RF: An approach to free radicals in medicine and biology. *Acta Physiol Scand* 492(Suppl):744–748, 1980.
53. Del Maestro RF, Bjork J, Arfors KE: Increase in microvascular permeability induced by enzymatically generated free radicals. *Microvasc Res* 22:239–254, 1981.
54. De Meis L: Mechanism of ATP synthesis by sarcoplasmic reticulum ATPase. *Ann NY Acad Sci* 402:535–548, 1982.
55. Demopoulos HB, Flamm FS, Pictronigro DD, Seligman ML: The free radical pathology and the microcirculation in the major control nervous system disorders. *Acta Physiol Scand* 492(Suppl):91–120, 1980.
56. DeWall RA, Vasko KA, Stanley EL, Kezdi P: Responses of the ischemic myocardium to allopurinol. *Am Heart J* 82:362–370, 1971.
57. Dixon SH Jr, Fuchs JCA, Ebert PA: Changes in serum creatine phosphokinase activity following thoracic, cardiac, and abdominal operations. *Arch Surg* 103:66–68, 1971.
58. Doolan PD, Wiggins RA, Thiel GB, Lee J, Martinez E: Acute renal insufficiency following aortic surgery: A discussion of the pathogenesis and a consideration of gangrene of an extremity as a complication. *Am J Med* 28:895–904, 1960.
59. Drabkin DL: Crystallographic and optical properties of human hemoglobin. *Am J Med Sci* 209:268, 1945.
60. Drexel H, Dienstl F: Myoglobinemia and reperfusion in myocardial infarction. *N Engl J Med* 309:1457, 1983.
61. Dunant J, Nosbaum J, Waibel P: Metabolic changes during induced ischemia of the leg. *J Cardiovasc Surg* 14:586, 1973.
62. Duncan GW, Blalock A: The uniform production of experimental shock by crush injury: Possible relationship to clinical crush syndrome. *Ann Surg* 115:684–697, 1942.

62a. Deterling RA, Vargas LL, McAllister FF: Follow-up studies of patients with embolic occlusion of the aortic bifurcation. *Ann Surg* 155:383–391, 1962.

63. de Duve C: A spectrophotometric method for the simultaneous determination of myoglobin and hemoglobin in

extracts of human muscle. *Acta Chem Scand* 2:264–289, 1948.

64. Edwards RHT, Jones DA: Malignant hyperpyrexia. In *Skeletal Muscle,* Peachey LD, Adrian RH, Geiger SR (Eds.), American Physiological Society, Bethesda, Maryland, 1983, Chapt. 20:657–659.
65. Edwards RHT, Jones DA: Nuclear Magnetic Resonance. In *Skeletal Muscle,* Peachey LD, Adrian RH, Geiger Sr (Eds), American Physiological Society, Bethesda, Maryland, 1983, Chapt. 20:637.

65a. Edwards RHT, Wiles CM, Gohil K, Krywawych S, Jones DA: Energy metabolism in human myopathy. In *Disorders of the Motor Unit,* D. Schottland (Ed.), John Wiley, Boston, MA, 1981, pp 715–728.

65b. Edwards RHT, Wilkie DR, Dawson MJ, Gordon RE, Shaw D: Clinical use of nuclear magnetic resonance in the investigation of myopathy. *Lancet* 2:725–731, 1982.

66. Eiken O, Nabseth DC, Mayer RF, Deterline RA Jr: Limb replantation II: The pathophysiological effects. *Arch Surg* 88:54–56, 1964.
67. Eisenberg BR: Quantitative Ultrastructure of Mammalian Skeletal Muscle. In *Skeletal Muscle,* Peachey LD, Adrian RH, Geiger SR (Eds.), American Physiological Society, Bethesda, Maryland, 1983, Chapt. 3:73–112.
68. Eklof B, Neglen P, Thomson D: Temporary incomplete ischemia of the legs induced by aortic clamping in man. *Ann Surg* Jan: 89–98, 1981.
69. Elek SD, Anderson HF: Paroxysmal paralytic myoglobinuria. *Br Med J* 533:536, 1953.
70. Elliott JP, Hageman JH, Szilagyi DE, Ramakrishnan V, Bravo JJ, Smith RF: Arterial embolization: Problems of source, multiplicity, recurrence and delayed treatments. *Surgery* 88:833–845, 1980.
71. Enger EA, Jennische E, Medegard A, Haljamae H: Cellular restitution after 3 h of complete tourniquet ischemia. *Eur Surg Res* 10:230–239, 1978.
72. Engler HS, Ellison LT, Moretz WH, Simpson JG, Gleaton HE, Freeman RA: Shock following release of aortic cross-clamping. *Arch Surg* 86:791–797, 1963.
73. Esato K, Nakano H, Ohara M, Nomura S, Mohri H:

Methods of suppression of myonephropathic metabolic syndrome. *J Cardiovasc Surg* 26:473–478, 1985.

74. Falk K, Rayyes AN, David DS: Myoglobinuria with reversible acute renal failure. *NY State J Med* 73:537, 1973.
75. Famos M, Radu EW, Harder F: Rhabdomyolysis and the compartment syndrome in heroin addiction. *Helv Chir Acta* 50:745–747, 1984.
76. Fishback DK, Fishback HR: Studies of experimental muscle degeneration. *Am J Path* 12:193–217, 1932.
77. Fisher RD, Fogarty TJ, Morrow AG: Clinical and biochemical observations of the effect of transient femoral artery occlusion in man. *Surgery* 68:323–328, 1970.

77a. Fiske CH, Subbarow. The isolation and junction of phosphocreatine. *Science* 67:169–170, 1928.

78. Flatt AE: Tourniquet time in hand surgery. *Arch Surg* 104:190–192, 1972.
79. Fleischman AH: Ischemic necrosis of tibialis anticus muscle with renal syndrome. *Bull Hosp Joint Dis* 22:146, 1961.
80. Fletcher WM, Hopkins FG: The respiratory process in muscle and the nature of muscular motion. *Proc Royal Soc London Ser B* 89:444–467, 1917.
81. Fontaine R, de Sousa-Pereira A: Obliterations et resections veineuses experimentales; contribution á l'etude de la circulation collaterale veineuse. *Rev Chir* (Paris) 75:161, 1937.
82. Frankenthal L: *Virchows Arch Pathol Anat Physiol* 222:332, 1916.
83. Francisco J Jr, Miranda F Jr, Barros N Jr, Delmonte CA, Burihan E: The Haimovici-LeGrain-Cormier syndrome in arterial embolectomy: The myonephropathic-metabolic syndrome. Personal communication, to be published.
84. Fry WJ, Keitzer WF, Kraft RO: Prevention of hypotension due to aortic release. *Surg Gynecol Obstet* 116:301, 1963.
85. Gardner TJ, Stewart JR, Casale AS, Downey JM, Chambers DE: Reduction of myocardial ischemic injury with oxygen-derived free radical scavengers. *Surgery* 94:423–427, 1983.
86. Gautier R, Bonneton G, Guidicelli H, Cordonnier D, Guignier M, Debru J: Traumatismes arteriels femoro-poplites avec ecrasement de membre: Etude critique de l'operabilite. *Chirurgie* 98:479–485, 1972.

87. Gilmour JR: Myoglobinuria and the crush syndrome. *Lancet* 1:524, 1941.
88. Glenn AM: Temporary vascular occlusion ending fatally in uremia. *Br Med J* 2:875, 1941.
89. Goodwin JN, Berne TV: Symmetrical peripheral gangrene. *Arch Surg* 108:780–784, 1974.
90. Green HN: Shock producing factor(s) from striated muscle isolation and biological properties. *Lancet* 24:147, 1943.
91. Green RM, deWeese JA, Rob CG: Arterial embolectomy before and after the Fogarty catheter. *Surgery* 77:24, 1975.
92. Grey DP, Shemin R, Couch N: Acute infrarenal aortic thrombosis during aortoiliac reconstruction. *Texas Heart Inst* 9:101–103, 1982.
93. Griffiths DL: Volkmann's ischaemic contracture. *Br J Surg* 28:239–260, 1940–1941.
94. Grossman RA, Hamilton RW, Morse BM: Nontraumatic rhabdomyolysis and acute renal failure. *N Engl J Med* 291:807, 1974.
95. Günther H: Uber den Muskeliarbstoff. *Virchows Arch* 230:146, 1921.
96. Günther H: Kasuistische Mitteilung uber Myositis myoglobinurica. *Virchows Arch Pathol Anat Physiol* 251:141, 1924.
97. Gutierrez-Carreño R, Sanchez Fabela C: Sindrome miopatico metabolico renal post revascularizacion de los miembros inferiores. *Rev Mex Angiologia* 4:5–8, 1977.
98. Haimovici H: Arterial embolism with acute massive ischemic myopathy and myoglobinuria: Evaluation of a hitherto unreported syndrome with report of two cases. *Surgery* 47:739, 1960.
99. Haimovici H: Arterial circulation of the extremities. In *Structure and Function of the Circulation*, Vol I, Plenum Press, New York, 1980, p 425.
100. Haimovici H: Arterial embolism of the lower extremity. In *Vascular Emergencies*, Haimovici H (Ed.), Appleton-Century-Crofts, New York, 1982, pp 163–180.
101. Haimovici H: Acute atherosclerotic thrombosis. In *Vascular Emergencies*, Haimovici H (Ed.), Appleton-Century-Crofts, New York, 1982, pp 213–223.
102. Haimovici H: Arterial embolism, myoglobinuria and renal tubular necrosis, *Arch Surg* 100:639–645, 1970.
103. Haimovici H: *Ischemic Forms of Venous Thrombosis: Phleg-*

masia Cerulea Dolens, Venous Gangrene. Charles C. Thomas, Springfield, Illinois, 1971.

104. Haimovici H: Late arterial embolectomy. *Surgery* 46:775, 1959.
105. Haimovici H: Metabolic complications of acute arterial occlusions. *J Cardiovasc Surg* 20:349–357, 1979.
106. Haimovici H: Metabolic syndrome secondary to acute arterial lesions. In *Vascular Emergencies,* Haimovici H, Appleton-Century-Crofts, New York, 1982, pp 267–289.
107. Haimovici H: Myopathic-nephrotic-metabolic syndrome associated with massive acute arterial occlusion (Editorial), *Arch Surg* 106:628–629, 1973.
108. Haimovici H: Myopathic-nephrotic-metabolic syndrome associated with massive acute arterial occlusions. *J Cardiovasc Surg* 14:589–593, 1973.
109. Haimovici H: Muscular, renal and metabolic complications of acute arterial occlusions: Myonephropathic-metabolic syndrome. *Surgery* 85:461–468, 1979.
110. Haimovici H: Rhabdomyolysis secondary to sudden arterial occlusions: A key to renal metabolic complications. *Contemp Surgery* 17:33–44, 1980.
111. Haimovici H, Maier N, Spiegler E: Effects of infrarenal aortic clamping on renal function: An experimental study in the dog. *J Cardiovasc Surg* 2:206–213, 1961.
112. Haimovici H, Moss CM, Veith FJ: Arterial embolectomy revisited. *Surgery* 78:409–410, 1975.
113. Haimovici H: *Myonephropathic-Metabolic Syndrome.* Key address to the XVII Japanese Cardiovascular Surgery Congress, Tokyo, May 1–2, 1987.
114. Haljamae H, Enger E: Human skeletal muscle energy metabolism during and after complete tourniquet ischemia. *Ann Surg* 182:9–14, 1975.
115. Haljamae H, Jennische E, Medegard A: Transmembrane potential measurements as an indicator of heterogeneous distribution of nutritive blood flow in skeletal muscle during shock. *Acta Physiol Scand* 101:458–464, 1977.
116. Hamilton RW: Acute tubular necrosis caused by exercised induced myoglobinuria. *Ann Intern Med* 77:77–82, 1972.
117. Hardy JD, Timmis HH: Abdominal aortic aneurysms: Special problems. *Ann Surg* 173:945, 1971.
118. Hargens AR, Schmidt DA, Evans KL, Gonsalves MR,

Cologne JB, Garfin SR, Mubarak SJ, Hagan PL, Akeson WH: Quantitation of skeletal-muscle necrosis in a model compartment syndrome. *J Bone Joint Surg* 63-A:631–636, 1981.

119. Harken AH: Lactic acidosis. *Surg Gynecol Obstet* 142:593–606, 1976.
120. Harman JW: A histological study of skeletal muscle in acute ischemia. *Am J Pathol* 23:551–565, 1947.
121. Harman JW: The significance of local vascular phenomena in production of ischemic necrosis in skeletal muscle. *Am J Pathol* 24:625–641, 1948.
122. Harman JW, Gwinn RP: The recovery of skeletal muscle fibers from acute ischemia as determined by histologic and chemical methods. *Am J Pathol* 25:741, 1949.
123. Harris K, Walker PM, Mickle DAG, Harding R, Gatley R, Wilson GJ, Kuzon B, McKee N, Romaschin AD: Metabolic response of skeletal muscle to ischemia. *Am J Physiol* 250:H213–H219, 1986.
124. Helzlsouer KJ, Hayden FG, Rosol AD: Severe metabolic complications in a cross-country runner with sickle cell trait. *JAMA* 249:777–779, 1983.
125. Herman BE, Wallace HW, Gadboys HL: Anterior crural syndrome as a complication of cardiopulmonary bypass. *Thorac Cardiovasc Surg* 52:755, 1966.
126. Herrero Mateo LM, Ros Die E, Sanchez Fernandez Bravo J: Modifications del pH muscular y otros parametros medidores de la hipoxia tisular en el ejercicio intenso y prolongado. *Angiologia* 29:118, 1977.
127. Hibrawl H, Blaker RG: Improved estimation of urinary myoglobin by counter-immunoelectrophoresis, as compared with the double-immunodiffusion technique. *Clin Chem* 21:765–768, 1975.
128. Hill R: Oxygen dissociation curves of muscle haemoglobin. *Proc Royal Soc* B120:472, 1936.
129. Horsley BL, Nelson RM: Metabolic acidosis in the ischemic limb during open heart surgery. *Ann Thorac Surg* 4:474, 1967.
130. Horton VH, Bernatz PE, Fairbairn JF II: Acute arterial occlusion. In *Peripheral Vascular Diseases*, Fairbairn JF II, Juergens JL, Spittell JA Jr (Eds.), Saunders, Philadelphia, Pennsylvania, 1972, p 259.

131. Huckabee WE: Relationship of pyruvate and lactate during anaerobic metabolism, III. *J Clin Invest* 37:264–271, 1958.
132. Hughes JR: Ischemic necrosis of anterior tibial muscle due to fatigue. *J Bone Joint Surg* 30B:581, 1948.
133. Humphries AW, DeWolfe VG, Young JR: Evaluation of the natural history and the results of treatment in occlusive arteriosclerosis involving the lower extremities in 1850 patients. In *Fundamentals of Vascular Grafting*, Wesolowski SA, Dennis C (Eds.), McGraw-Hill, New York, 1963, p 423.
134. Husfeldt E, Bjering T: Renal lesion from traumatic shock. *Acta Med Scand* 91:279, 1937.
135. Inesi G, Watanabe T, Coan C, Murphy A: The mechanism of sarcoplasmic reticulum ATPase. *Ann NY Acad Sci* 402:515–534, 1982.
136. Jacobs, AL: *Arterial Embolism in the Limbs*. Livingston, Edinburgh, 1959, p 60.
137. Janetta PJ, Roberts B: Sudden complete thrombosis of an aneurysm of the abdominal aorta. *N Engl J Med* 264:434–436, 1961.
138. Jennische E, Enger E, Medegard A, Appelgren L, Haljamae H: Correlation between tissue pH, cellular transmembrane potentials, and cellular energy metabolism during shock and during ischemia. *Circ Shock* 5:251–260, 1978.
139. Jepson P: Ischemic contracture: Experimental study. *Ann Surg* 84:785–795, 1926.
140. Johnson JM, Gaspar MR, Movius HJ, Rosenthal JJ: Sudden complete thrombosis of aortic and iliac aneurysms. *Arch Surg* 108:792–794, 1974.

140a. Ikezawa T: Personal communication.

141. Johnstone JH, Lawson LJ, Mucklow RG: Metabolic changes after aortoiliac occlusion. *Br Med J* 2:974, 1965.
142. Jolly SR, Kane WJ, Baillie MB, Abrams GD, Lucchesi BR: Canine myocardial reperfusion injury: Its reduction by the combined administration of superoxide dismutase and catalase. *Circ Res* 54:277–285, 1984.
143. Justis DL, Law EJ, MacMillan BG: Tibial compartment syndrome in burn patients: A report of four cases. *Arch Surg* 3:1004–1008, 1976.
144. Kagen LJ: Immunologic detection of myoglobinuria after cardiac surgery. *Ann Intern Med* 67:1183, 1967.

144a. Kagen LJ, Gurevick R: Localization of myoglobin in human skeletal muscle using fluorescent antibody technique. *J Histochem Cytochem* 15:436–441, 1967.

144b. Kagen LJ: Immunofluorescent demonstration of myoglobin in the kidney: Case report and review of 43 cases of myoglobinemia and myoglobinuria identified immunologically. *Am J Med* 48:649, 1970.

145. Kagen LJ: *Myoglobin: Biochemical, Physiological, and Clinical Aspects*. Columbia Univ Press, New York, 1973, 1–451.

146. Kagen J: Myoglobinemia in inflammatory myopathies. *JAMA* 237:1448–1452, 1977.

147. Kaiser HF, Spaar U, Sold G, et al: Radioimmunoassay for diagnostic significance in myocardial infarction. *Klin Wochenschr* 57:225–235, 1979.

148. Keaveny TV, O'Boyle A, Fitzgerald PA: Effect of surgical procedure on muscle ATP. *J Cardiovasc Surg* 14:601, 1973.

149. Kievit EL, Boontje AH: Myoglobinuria in arterial circulatory disorders of the legs. *Ned Tijdschr Geneeskd* 124(23):910–913, 1980.

150. Klinkerfuss G, Bleisch V, Dioso MM, Perkoff PT: A spectrum of myopathy associated with alcoholism II: Light and electron microscopic observations. *Ann Intern Med* 67:493–510, 1967.

151. Knochel JP: Exertional rhabdomyolysis. *N Engl J Med* 287:927–929, 1972.

152. Knochel JP, Schlein EM: On the mechanism of rhabdomyolysis in potassium depletion. *J Clin Invest* 51:1750–1758, 1972.

153. Koffler A, Friedler RM, Massry SG: Acute renal failure due to nontraumatic rhabdomyolysis. *Ann Intern Med* 85:23, 1976.

154. Kornmesser TW, Trippel OH, Haid SP: Acute occlusion of the abdominal aorta. In *Surgery of the Aorta and Its Body Branches*, Bergan JJ, Yao JST (Eds.), Grune & Stratton, New York, 1979.

155. Korthuis RJ, Granger DN, Townsley MI, Taylor AE: The role of oxygen-derived free radicals in ischemia-induced increased in canine skeletal muscle vascular permeability. *Circ Res* 57:599–609, 1985.

156. Kreitzer SM, Ehrenpreis M, Migue E: Acute myoglobinuric renal failure in polymyositis. *NY State J Med* 78:295, 1978.

157. Krise LP, Milne FJ, Margolius KA, Bayliss CB: Rhabdomy-

olysis and renal failure–unusual complications of drug abuse: A case report. *S Afr Med J* 64:253–254, 1983.

158. Kuffler SW: The relation of electrical potential changes to contracture of skeletal muscle. *J Neurophysiol* 9:367-377, 1946.
159. Kugimiya T, Shirabe J, Kusaba E, Hadama T, Kaku K: Myonephropathic-metabolic syndrome as a complication of cardiopulmonary bypass. *Jap J Surg* 13(5):431–437, 1983.
160. Lang EK: Streptokinase therapy: Complications of intra-arterial use. *Radiology* 154:75–77, 1985.
161. LaPorta MA, Linde HW, Bruce DL, Fitzsimons EJ: Elevation of creatine phosphokinase in young men after recreational exercise. *JAMA* 239:2685–2686, 1978.
162. Larsson J, Hultman E: The effect of long-term arterial occlusion on energy metabolism of the human quadriceps muscle. *Scand J Clin Lab Invest* 39:257–264, 1979.
163. Lazar HL, Buckberg GD, Manganaro AJ, Becker H, Maloney JV Jr: Reversal of ischemic damage with amino acid substrate enhancement during reperfusion. *Surgery* 88:702–709, 1980.
164. van Leeuwenhoek A: Quoted by Peachey et al: Structure and function of membrane systems of skeletal muscle cells. In *Skeletal Muscle*, p 27, ref. 214.

164a. Lefemine AA, Kosowsky B, et al: Results and complications of intraaortic balloon pumping in surgical and medical patients. *Am J Cardiol* 40:416–420, 1977.

165. Legros-Clark WE, Blomfield LB: The efficiency of intramuscular anastomoses with observations on the regeneration of devascularized muscle. *J Anat* 79:15–32, 1945.
166. Leser E: *Saml Klin Vortr* 3:2087, 1884. Quoted in Brooks B: Pathologic changes in muscle as a result of disturbances of circulation. *Arch Surg* 5:188, 1922.
167. Letac R, Letac S, Chassaigne JP: Syndrome de Bywaters apparu á la suite d'une plaie de l'artere femorale commune sans traumatisme musculaire. *Ann Chir Thorac Car* 2:469, 1963.
168. Lie JT, Sun SC: Ultrastructure of ischemic contracture of the left ventricle ("stone heart"). *Mayo Clinic Proc* 51:785–793, 1976.
169. Lim RC, Bergentz SE, Lewis DH: Metabolic and tissue

blood flow changes resulting from aortic cross-clamping. *Surgery* 65:304–310, 1969.

170. Little JM, Ferguson DA: The incidence of hypothenar hammer syndrome. *Arch Surg* 105:684, 1972.
171. Littooy FN, Baker WH: Acute aortic occlusion: A multifaceted catastrophe. *J Vasc Surg* 4:211–216, 1986.
171a. Lwebuga-Mukasa JS, Libby P, Bloor CM, Maroko PR: The evaluation of serum myoglobin following experimental coronary occlusion. (Abstr) *Circulation* 48(Suppl IV):IV-129, 1973.
172. Luft FC, Hamburger RJ, Dyer JK, Szwed JJ, Kleit SA: Acute renal failure following operation for aortic aneurysm. *Surg Gynecol Obstet* 141:374–378, 1975.
173. Luginbuhl WH: Immunologic investigation of preparations of human myoglobin. *Am J Clin Pathol* 38:487, 1962.
174. Lytton B, Blandy JP: Anterior tibial syndrome after embolectomy. *Br J Surg* 48:346, 1960–1961.
174a. Malan E, Tattoni G: Physio- and anatomopathology of acute ischemia of the extremities. *J Cardiovasc Surg* 4:212, 1963.
175. Malan E, Haimovici H: Round table on acute ischemia of the limbs and revascularization syndrome: XXI Congress of the European Society of Cardiovascular Surgery. *J Cardiovasc Surg* 14:573, 1973.
176. Mansberger AR Jr, Cox EF, Flotte CT, Buxton RW: "Washout" acidosis following resection of aortic aneurysms: Clinical metabolic study of reactive hyperemia and effect of dextran on excess lactate and pH. *Ann Surg* 163(5):778–786, 1966.
177. Markowitz H, Wobig GH: Quantitative method for estimating myoglobin in urine. *Clin Chem* 23:1689–1693, 1977.
178. Martonosi AN, Beeler TJ: Mechanism of CA^{2+} transport by sarcoplasmic reticulum. In *Skeletal Muscle*, Peachey LD, Adrian RH, Geiger SR (Eds.), Bethesda, Maryland, American Physiological Society, 1983, p 417.
179. Matolo NM, Cheung L, Albo D, Lazarus HM: Acute occlusion of the infrarenal aorta. *Am J Surg* 126:788, 1973.
180. McClelland JC: Anuria: Report of three types of cases. *Canad MAJ* 45:332, 1941.
181. McCombs R, Roberts B: Acute renal failure following resec-

tion of abdominal aortic aneurysm. *Surg Gynecol Obstet* 148:175–178, 1979.

182. McCord JM: Oxygen-derived free radicals in postischemic tissue injury. *N Engl J Med* 312:159–163, 1985.
183. Mehl RR, Paul HA, Beattie EJ Jr: Successful treatment of shock after experimental replantation of extremities severed for long periods. *Lancet* 1:1419, 1964.
184. Meyer-Betz F: Beobachtungen an einem eigenartigen mit Muskellahmungen vergunden Fall von Hamoglobinurie. *Deut Arch Klin Med* 101:85, 1911.
185. Meyerhoff O, Schulz W: Uber die Energieverhaltnisse bei der enzymatischen Milchsaurebildung und der Synthese der Phosphagene. *Biochem Z* 281:292,305, 1935.
186. Michaelson M, Taitelman U, Bursztein S: Management of crush syndrome. *Resuscitation* 12:141–146, 1984.
187. Miller HH, Welch CS: Quantitative studies on the time factor in arterial injuries. *Ann Surg* 130:428–438, 1949.
188. Miller SH, Price G, Buck D, Neeley J, Kennedy TJ, Graham WP III, Davis TS: Effects of tourniquet ischemia and postischemic edema on muscle metabolism. *J Hand Surg* 4:457–555, 1979.
189. Millikan GA: Experiments on muscle haemoglobin in vivo, the instantaneous measurement of muscle metabolism. *Proc Royal Soc London* B123:218, 1937.
190. Millikan GA: Muscle hemoglobin. *Physiol Rev* 19:503, 1939.
191. Minami S: Uber Nierenveranderungen nach Verchuttung. *Arch Pathol Anat Physiol* (Virch) 245:247, 1923.
192. Moloney WC, Stovall SL, Spring DH Jr: Renal damage due to ischemic muscle necrosis. *JAMA* 131:1419, 1946.
193. Montagnani CA, Simeone FA: Observations on the liberation and elimination of myohemoglobin and of hemoglobin after release of muscle ischemia. *Surgery* 34:169, 1953.
194. Moon BC, Girotti MJ, Dawson R, Wren SF: PMN superoxide radical production following a metabolic-endocrine simulation of trauma. *Ann Surg* 203:246–249, 1986.
195. Moore DH, Ruska H, Copenhaven WM: Electron microscopic and histochemical observations of muscle degeneration after tourniquet. *J Biophys Biochem Cytol* 2:755–764, 1956.
196. Mori KW, Bookstein KJ, Heeney DJ, Bardin JA, Donnelly KJ, Rhodes GA, Dilley RB, Warmath MA, Bernstein EF:

Selective streptokinase infusion: Clinical and laboratory correlates. *Radiology* 148:677–682, 1983.

197. Morton JH, Southgate WA, DeWeese JA: Arterial injuries of the extremities. *Surg Gynecol Obstet* 123:611, 1966.
198. Mullick S: The tourniquet in operations upon the extremities. *Surg Gynecol Obstet* 146:821, 1978.
199. Nadel SM, Jackson JW, Ploth DW: Hypokalemic rhabdomyolysis and acute renal failure: Occurrence following total parenteral nutrition. *JAMA* 241:2294–2296, 1979.
200. Natali J, Lacombe M, Bruchou P, Vinardi G: Les traumatismes arteriels vus tardivement conduite a tenir en leur presence. *Presse Med* 39:2273–2278, 1964.
201. Neglen P, Eklof B, Thomson D: Prevention of deleterious effects on central hemodynamics and skeletal muscle metabolism of extracorporeal shunting during reconstruction of abdominal aortic aneurysms. Paper presented at XIV World Congress, International Cardiovascular Society, San Francisco, 1979.
202. Nevins MA, Saran M, Bright M, Lyon LJ: Pitfalls in interpreting serum creatine phosphokinase activity. *JAMA* 224:1382–1387, 1973.
203. Nichikai M, Homma M: Circulating autoantibody against human myoglobin in polymyositis. *JAMA* 237:1842–1844, 1977.
204. Nolan B, McQuillan WM: A study of acute traumatic limb ischaemia. *Br J Surg* 52:559, 1965.
205. O'Connor JV, Iyer SK: Myoglobinuria associated with parainfluenza type 2 infection. *NYS J Med* Sept:1469–1470, 1982.
206. O'Donnell TF Jr, Clowes GHA Jr, Browese HL, Ryan NT, Blackburn GL: A metabolic approach to the evaluation of peripheral vascular disease. *Surg Gynecol Obstet* 144:51–57, 1977.
207. Olerud JE et al: Incidence of acute exertional rhabdomyolysis. *Arch Intern Med* 136:692–697, 1976.
208. Ong L, Reiser P, Coromilas J, Scherr L, Morrison J: Left ventricular function and rapid release of creatine kinase MB in acute myocardial infarction: Evidence for spontaneous reperfusion. *N Engl J Med* 309:106, 1983.
209. Ong L, Reiser P, Coromilas J, Scherr, Morrison J: Reply to Drs. Drexel and Dienstl. *N Engl J Med* 309:1458, 1983.

210. Otani H, Engelman RM, Rousou JA, Breyer RH, Lemeshow S, Das DK: Cardiac performance during reperfusion improved by pretreatment with oxygen free-radical scavengers. *J Thorac Cardiovasc Surg* 91:190–195, 1986.
211. Parks DA, Buckley GB, Granger DN: Role of oxygen free radicals in shock ischemia and organ preservation. *Surgery* 94:428–432, 1983.
212. Parks DA, Granger DN: Ischemia-induced vascular changes: Role of xanthine oxidase and hydroxyl radicals. *Am J Physiol* 245:G285–G289, 1983.
213. Pasque MK, Wechsler AS: Metabolic intervention to affect myocardial recovery following ischemia. *Ann Surg* 200:1–12, 1984.
214. Peachey LD, Adrian RH, Geiger SR: *Skeletal Muscle*. Bethesda, Maryland, American Physiological Society, pp 1–688, 1983.
215. Peachey LD, Armstrong CF: Structure and function of membrane systems of skeletal muscle cells. In *Skeletal Muscle*, Peachey LD, Adrian RH, Geiger SR (Eds), Bethesda, Maryland, American Physiological Society, 1983, pp 23–71.
216. Penneys R, Wilkinson JH: Elevation of serum creatine kinase following amputation of the leg. *Surgery* 67:302–305, 1970.
216. Perdue GD: Thrombosis of aneurysms of the abdominal aorta. *J Med Assoc Ga* 52:201–202, 1963.
217. Perkoff GT, Hardy P, Velez-Garcia E: Reversible acute muscular syndrome in chronic alcoholism. *N Engl J Med* 274:1277, 1966.
218. Pernow B, Saltin B, Wahren J: Leg blood flow and muscle metabolism in occlusive arterial disease of the leg before and after reconstructive surgery. *Clin Sci Med* 49:165, 1975.
219. Perry MO: The hemodynamics of temporary abdominal aortic occlusion. *Ann Surg* 168:193–200, 1968.
220. Perry MO: Vascular trauma. *Bull NY Acad Med* 61:638–649, 1985.
221. Perutz MF, Kendrew JC, Watson HC: Structure and function of hemoglobin. II. Some relations between polypeptide chain configuration and amino acid sequence. *J Mol Biol* 13:669, 1965.
222. Pietri P, Alagni G, Domeniconi R: Isquemias agudas de las arterias perifericas. *Angiologia* 29:161, 1975.

223. Pirovino M, Neff MS, Sharon E: Myoglobinuria and acute renal failure with acute polymyositis. *NY State J Med* 79:764, 1979.
224. Planell ES: Emergency thrombectomy in the treatment of acute arterial thrombosis. J Cardiovasc Surg (Special issue) XI World Congress, International Cardiovascular Society, Barcelona, Spain, 1973.
225. Polson AG: Quoted by G Biörk: Researches on the diffusion constants of the proteins. Thesis 1937, p 146, ref 15.
226. Potter DJ, Hopkins JG: Reversible paraplegia and acute renal failure due to occlusive disease of the abdominal aorta. *Ann Intern Med* 69:777–780, 1968.
227. Powell WJ, DiBona DR, Flores J, Leaf A: The protective effect of hyperosmotic mannitol in myocardial ischemia and necrosis. *Circulation* 54:603, 1976.
228. Powers CA: The ischemic paralysis and contracture of Volkmann. *JAMA* 48:759, 1907.
229. Powers SR, Boba A, Stein A: The mechanism and prevention of distal tubular necrosis following aneurysmectomy. *Surgery* 142:146, 1957.
230. Provan JL, Fraenkel GJ, Austen WG: Metabolic and hemodynamic changes after temporary aortic occlusion in dogs. *Surg Gynecol Obstet* 544–550, 1966.
231. Quenu: Quoted by Cannon in *Traumatic Shock. Revue de Chirur* 56:204, 1918, ref 33.
232. Qvarfordt P, Christenson JT, Eklof B, Ohlin P: Intramuscular pressure after revascularization of the popliteal artery in severe ischemia. *Br J Surg* 70:539–541, 1983.
233. Ray GB, Paff GH: A spectrophotometric study of muscle hemoglobin. *Am J Physiol* 94:521, 1930.
234. Reichlin M, Visco JP, Klock FJ: Radioimmunoassay for human myoglobin: Initial experience in patients with coronary heart disease. *Circulation* 57:52–56, 1978.
235. Rheingold OJ, Greenwald RA, Hayes PJ, Tedesco FJ; Myoglobinuria and renal failure associated with typhoid fever. *JAMA* 238:341, 1977.
236. Reznik M: Aspect ultrastructural de la degenerescence due muscle strie ischemie. *Ann Anat Pathol* 12:209, 1967.
237. Rich NM, Spencer FC: *Vascular Trauma,* Philadelphia, WB Saunders, 1978, pp 1–610.
238. Richter RW, Challenor YB, Pearson J, Kagen LJ, Hamilton

LL, Ramsey WH: Acute myoglobinuria associated with heroin addiction. *JAMA* 216:1172–1176, 1971.

239. Robbs JV, Baker LW: Late revascularization of the lower limb following acute arterial occlusion. *Br J Surg* 66:129, 1979.
240. Rizza RA, Scolnick S, Conley CL: Myoglobinuria following aminocaproic acid administration. *JAMA* 236:1845–1846, 1976.
241. Rossi-Fanelli A: Crystalline human myoglobin: Some physico-chemical properties and chemical composition. *Science* 108:15–16, 1948.
242. Robbs JV, Baker LW: Major arterial trauma: Review of experience with 267 injuries. *Br J Surg* 65:532–538, 1978.
243. Rowland LP, Fahn S, Hirschberg E, Harter DH: Myoglobinuria. *Arch Neurol* 10:537, 1964.
244. Rowland LP: Myoglobinuria 1984. *Can J Neurol Sci* 11:1–13, 1984.
245. Roy RS, McCord JM: Superoxide and Ischemia: Conversion of xanthine dehydrogenase to xanthine oxidase. In *Oxy Radicals and Their Scavenger Systems* Vol II, Greenwald RA, Cohen G (Eds.), New York, Elsevier/North Holland Biomedical Press, 1983, pp 143–153.
246. Russell SM, Bleiweiss S, Brownlow K: Ischemic rhabdomyolysis and creatine phosphokinase isoenzymes. *JAMA* 225:632, 1976.
247. Ryback JJ, Thomford NR: Acute occlusion of the infrarenal aorta from blunt trauma. *Am Surg* 35:444–447, 1969.

247a. Sachs G, Chang HH, Rabson E, et al: *J Biol Chem* 251:7690–7698, 1976. Quoted by Pederson PL, in *Ann NY Acad Sci* 402:1–20, 1982.

248. Saha SP, Nunn DB: Sudden thrombotic occlusion of abdominal aortic aneurysm: A report of two patients. *Am Surg* 40:246, 1974.
249. Saltin B, Gollnick P: Metabolic Capacity. In *Skeletal Muscle*, Peachey LD, Adrian RH, Geiger SR (Eds.), Bethesda, Maryland, American Physiological Society, 1983, pp 19:589–601.
250. Saltin B, Gollnick P: Muscle Fiber Composition in Human Skeletal Muscle. In *Skeletal Muscle*, Peachey LD, Adrian RH, Geiger SR (Eds.), American Physiological Society, Bethesda, Maryland, 1983, pp 571–573.
251. Sanderson RA, Foley RK, McIvor GWD, Kirkaldy-Willis

WH: Histological response on skeletal muscle to ischemia. *Clin Orthoped* 113:27–35, 1975.
252. Sapir DG, Dandy WE Jr, Whelton A, Cooke CR: Acute renal failure following ruptured abdominal aneurysms: An improved clinical prognosis. *Crit Care Med* 7:59–62, 1979.
253. Saranchak HJ, Bernstein SH: A new diagnostic test for acute myocardial infarction: The detection of myoglobinuria by radioimmunodiffusion assay. *JAMA* 228:1251–1255, 1974.
254. Sarrazin R: Metabolic troubles in limb ischemia and their variations during surgical therapy. *J Cardiovasc Surg* 14:627, 1973.
255. Saunders H, Lawrence J, Maciver DA, Nemethy N: The concept of the Macromesh and Micromesh as Illustrated by the Blood Supply of Muscles in Man. In *Peripheral Circulation*, Grune & Stratton, New York, 1957, pp 113–145.
256. Sautot J, Traeger J: Anurie apres thrombo-endartereictomie de l'aorte abdominale: Epuration renale: Guerison: Resultat eliogne (Quatre ans). *Mem Acad Chir* 88:577–585, 1962.
257. Savelyev VS, Zatevakhin II, Stepanow NV: Artery embolism of the upper limb. *Surgery* 81:367, 1977.
258. Schaff HV, Flaherty JT, Bulkley BH, Goldman RA, Gott VL: Hyperosmolar reperfusion following ischemic cardiac arrest: Critical importance of timing of mannitol administration on myocardial structure and function. *Surgery* 89:141–150, 1981.
259. Scully RE, Hughes CW: The pathology of ischemia of skeletal muscle in man: A description of early changes in muscles of the extremities following damage to major peripheral arteries on the battlefield. *Am J Pathol* 32:805–829, 1956.
260. Scully RE, Shannon JM, Dickersin GR: Factors involved in recovery from experimental skeletal muscle ischemia produced in dogs, I: Histologic and histochemical pattern of ischemic muscle. *Am J Pathol* 39:721, 1961.
261. Sederholm M, Sylvan C: Relation between ST and QRS vector changes and myoglobin release in acute myocardial infarction. *Cardiovasc Res* 17:589–594, 1983.
262. Seddon H: Volkmann's ischemia. *Br Med J* 1:1587–1592, 1964.

263. Seidenberg B, Stern J, Hurwitt ES: Thrombotic occlusion of abdominal aortic aneurysm following distal embolization. *Circulation* 25:995–996, 1962.
264. Siegel AJ, Silverman LM, Evans WJ: Elevated skeletal muscle creatine kinase MB isoenzyme levels in marathon runners. *JAMA* 250:2835–2837, 1983.
265. Sjostrom M, Neglen P, Friden J, Eklof B: Human skeletal muscle metabolism and morphology after temporary incomplete ischaemia. *Eur J Clin Invest* 12:69–79, 1982.
266. Smith et al: Quoted by Nadel: Incidence of acute exertional rhabdomyolysis. *Arch Int Med* 136:692–697, 1976, ref 207.
267. Synder DD, Campbell GS: Humoral effects of experimental crush syndrome. *Surgery* 47:2, 1960.
268. Solonen KA, Hjelt L: Morphological changes in striated muscle during ischemia. *Acta Orthop Scand* 39:13, 1968.
269. Sorlie D, Huseby NE, Kluge T: Ischemia during arterial reconstructive surgery: Biochemical changes as reflected in popliteal vein samples. *Scand J Thor Cardiovasc Surg* 11:151–158, 1977.
270. Soule TI, Cunningham GR: Herbicola lathyri septicemia, myoglobinuria and acute renal failure. *JAMA* 223:1265–1266, 1973.
271. Stallone RJ, Blaisdell FW, Cafferata HT: Analysis of morbidity and mortality from arterial embolectomy. *Surgery* 1:207, 1969.
272. Stenger RJ, Spiro D, Scully RE: Ultrastructural and physiologic alterations in ischemic skeletal muscle. *Am J Pathol* 40:19, 1962.
273. Stenstrom JD, Ford HS, MacKay MI: Ruptured abdominal aortic aneurysms: A 10-year study. *Am Surg* 38:608, 1972.
274. Stewart JR, Crute SL, Loughlin V, Hess ML, Greenfield LJ: Prevention of free radical-induced myocardial reperfusion injury with allopurinol. *J Thorac Cardiovasc Surg* 90:68–72, 1985.
275. Stewart JSS, Mostert JW, Hilton DD, McGrath D: Bicarbonate therapy during embolectomy: Prevention of acidosis shock and acidosis arrest. *Lancet* 25:1320–1323, 1965.
275a. Shumacker H: Surgical treatment of aortic aneurysms. *Postgrad Med* 25:535–548, 1959.
275b. Strock PE, Majno G: Microvascular changes in acute ischemic rat muscle. *Surg Gynecol Obstet* 129:1213–1224, 1969.

276. Stipa S, Cavallaro A, Privitera L: Treatment of shock following prolonged ischemia of the limbs. *J Cardiovasc Surg* 8:529, 1967.
277. Stock W, Bohn HJ, Isselhard W: Metabolic changes in rat skeletal muscle after acute arterial occlusion. *Vasc Surg* 5:249–255, 1971.
278. Stokes JM, McAfee CA: Increasing limb survival in vascular injury with fracture. *J Trauma* 5:162, 1965.
279. Strandness DE Jr, Parrish DG, Bell JW: Mechanism of declamping shock in operations on the abdominal aorta. *Surgery* 50:488–492, 1961.
280. Subram AN, Duncan JM: Acute limb ischemia from sudden thrombosis of an abdominal aortic aneurysm: A case report. *Texas Heart Inst J* 9:97–99, 1982.
281. Swartz WM, Cha CJM, Clowes GHA Jr, Randall HT: The effect of prolonged ischemia on high energy phosphate metabolism in skeletal muscle. *Surg Gynecol Obstet* 147:872–876, 1978.
281a. Sylven C: Release of myoglobin and creatine-kinase into serum following acute myocardial infarction. *Eur J Cardiol* 9:483–491, 1979.
282. Taheri Sa, Heffner R, Williams J, Lazar L, Elias S: Muscle changes in venous insufficiency. *Arch Surg* 119:929–931, 1984.
283. Theorell H, de Duve C: Crystalline human myoglobin from heart muscle and urine. *Arch Biochem* 12:113, 1947.
284. Thompson WW, Campbell GS: Studies on myoglobin and hemoglobin in experimental crush syndrome in dogs. *Ann Surg* 149:235–242, 1959.
285. Trazzi R, Pannacciuli E, Blasi G: Experimental metabolic modifications in acute ischemia. *J Cardiovasc Surg* 14:635, 1973.
286. Tuller MA: Acute myoglobinuria with or without drug usage. *JAMA* 217:1868, 1971.
287. Veress B, Kerenyi T, Huttner I, Jellinek H: The phases of muscle necrosis. *J Pathol Bact* 92:511-517, 1966.
287a. Volkmann RV: Die ischaemischen Muskellähmungen und Kontraktwen. *Zentralbl Chir* 8:801, 1881.
288. Vortel V, Bryzek V: Myoglobinuric nephrosis after embolectomy in the common iliac artery. *Sb Ved Pr Lek Fak Univ Karlovy* 6:291, 1963.
289. Walker PM, Lindsay TF, Labbe R, Mickle DA, Romaschin

AD: Salvage of skeletal muscle with free radical scavengers. *J Vasc Surg* 5:68–72, 1987.

290. Weeks SR: The crush syndrome. *Surg Gynecol Obstet* 127:369–374, 1968.
291. Wei EP, Christman CW, Kontos HA, Povlishock JT: Effects of oxygen radicals on cerebral arterioles. *Am J Physiol* 248:H157–H162, 1985.
292. Welborn MB, Sawyers JL: Acute abdominal aortic occlusion due to nonpenetrating trauma. *Am J Surg* 118:112-116, 1969.
293. Whelton A: Post-traumatic acute renal failure. *Bull NY Acad Med* 55(2):151–162, 1979.
294. Whipple GH: The hemoglobin of striated muscle. II. Variations due to anemia and paralysis. *Am J Physiol* 76:608, 1926.
295. Whipple GH: The hemoglobin of striated muscle. I. Variations due to age and exercise. *Am J Physiol* 76:693, 1926.
296. Willerson J, Powell WJ Jr, Guney TE: Improvement in myocardial function and coronary blood flow in ischemic myocardium after mannitol. *J Clin Invest* 51:2989–2998, 1972.
297. Willner JH, Wood DS, Cerri C, Britt B: Increased myophosphorylase in malignant hyperthermia. *N Engl J Med* 303:138–140, 1980.
298. Willhoite DR, Moll JH: Early recognition and treatment of impending Volkmann's ischemia in the lower extremity. *Arch Surg* 100:11–16, 1970.
299. Winninger A: Biopathological disturbances in the revascularization stage of ischemic limbs. *J Cardiovasc Surg* 14:640–648, 1973.
300. Winninger A: Consequences generales de la revascularisation apres ischemie aigue des membres. Thesis, Marseilles Medical School, 1969.
301. Wrogemann K, Pena SDJ: *Lancet* 1:672–674, 1976. Quoted by Cullen MJ, ref. 47.
302. Zamecnick RC, Aub JC, Brues AM: The toxic factors in experimental shock, V: Chemical and enzymatic properties of muscle exudate. *J Clin Invest* 24:859, 1945.
303. Zuber WF, Gaspar MR, Rothchild PD: Anterior spinal artery syndrome: A complication of abdominal aortic surgery. *Ann Surg* 172:909–915, 1970.

Index